Interpreting Professional Self-Regulation

Regulation of professions is coming under increasing scrutiny. There has been serious questioning of medical performance recently and doubt about how far it is in the public interest that professions regulate themselves. Government is introducing new forms of inspection and monitoring, and client groups are increasingly calling for greater protection for vulnerable service users and for participation in decisions about standards of education, practice and conduct in the health field.

This book provides a history of the UKCC – the body that maintains a register of nurses, midwives and health visitors – from its inception under legislation in 1979 to the present day. It covers the decade of battle before the legislation, and tells the story of major reform of pre-registration education and pioneering work to set standards for demonstrating competence to stay on the register. It also analyses the disciplinary work of the UKCC in removing people from and restoring them to the register.

Interpreting Professional Self-Regulation provides a deeper understanding of what regulators do than has been available previously. It lays bare the tensions between different groups within the professions and notes how the powers of National Boards and Central Council have come into question. It shows just how much behind-the-scenes negotiation there has been in contexts where the public debate in parliament has been minimal and calls for much wider debate on professional accountability.

This is an important text for all those who teach on professional and policy issues in nursing, giving them a factual background that has never been brought together before, enabling them to bring discussion of post-registration education, discipline and other professional matters more firmly into the curriculum.

Celia Davies is Professor of Health Care, School of Health and Social Welfare, The Open University. **Abigail Beach** is Research Fellow, School of Health and Social Welfare, The Open University.

Interpreting Professional Self-Regulation

A history of the United Kingdom
Central Council for Nursing, Midwifery
and Health Visiting

Celia Davies and Abigail Beach

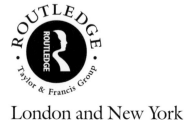

London and New York

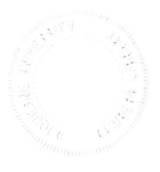

First published 2000
by Routledge
11 New Fetter Lane, London EC4P 4EE

Simultaneously published in the USA and Canada
by Routledge
29 West 35th Street, New York, NY 10001

Routledge is an imprint of the Taylor & Francis Group

Typeset in Galliard by
BOOK NOW Ltd
Printed and bound in Great Britain by
TJ International Ltd, Padstow, Cornwall

British Library Cataloguing in Publication Data
A catalogue record for this book is available
from the British Library

Library of Congress Cataloging in Publication Data
Davies, Celia, 1945–
    Interpreting professional self-regulation : a history of the United Kingdom Central
Council for Nursing, Midwifery and Health Visiting / Celia Davies and Abigail Beach.
        p.   cm.
    Includes bibliographical references and index.
    1. United Kingdom Central Council for Nursing, Midwifery, and Health
Visiting—History. 2. Nurses—Licenses—Great Britain. 3. Nursing—Law and
legislation—Great Britain. 4. Nursing—Standards—Great Britain. 5.
Midwives—Licenses—Great Britain. 6. Midwives—Legal status, laws, etc.—Great Britain.
7. Midwifery—Standards—Great Britain. I. Beach, Abigail. II. Title.
    RT11 .D38 2000
    610.73'02'1841—dc21
                                                                            00-027211

ISBN 0 415 23033 0

Contents

Figures

Foreword

The 1979 Nurses, Midwives and Health Visitors Act heralded far-reaching changes in the regulation of these three professions. The new Act brought together nine bodies previously responsible, in whole or in part, for separate regulation of the three professions within the United Kingdom. The United Kingdom Central Council for Nursing, Midwifery and Health Visiting and four National Boards established by the new Act created, by far, the largest regulatory body for any health care profession.

Following implementation of the new legislation, the profundity, frequency and pace of change in health care management and provision was unparalleled in the history of health care. The extent of critical focus on professional regulation by consumers, government, the three professions and the national and professional press also could not have been expected. The 'shadow' and subsequent consecutive three Councils spanning an eighteen-year period – the period of this historical review – had different challenges to anticipate and respond to. These included, by the time of the Third Council, implementing significant changes arising from the 1992 amending Nurses, Midwives and Health Visitors Act and contributing to the Government's second quinquennial review of non-departmental public bodies in 1997.

In 1996, the Council commissioned a history of its achievements and a review of its activities in setting standards for education and conduct, the results of which are recorded in these pages. Given the size of the three professions which the UKCC regulates and therefore the mammoth volume of activity within the organisation, together with the major projects undertaken throughout the eighteen-year period, the authors Celia Davies and Abigail Beach were presented with a diverse and complex task. The result of their work is a detailed, factual analysis and record of events, captured in a way that reveals the different and significant contributions which the 'shadow' and three Councils have made to professional self-regulation. In doing this they have highlighted in a constructive manner the strengths and weaknesses, 'warts and all', and have given due and fair consideration to the tensions that surfaced from time to time, particularly between nurses and midwives. But the text is much more than a factual record. It is balanced by critical scrutiny and reflection on events of professional self-regulation. The authors pose significant challenges at a time when fundamental questions are being raised about the future form of regulation of all health care professions and the relationship between self-regulation and the aspirations of government. Whatever structure emerges from the current debate must be informed by our history and influenced by both the professions and consumers.

The UKCC has enabled the growth of an ethical base for the professions through the Code of Conduct and the development of practice via the enabling *Scope of Professional Practice*. Openness to outside consumer involvement has shaped both policy creation and the key Council activity of professional conduct. There is much to celebrate in these achievements, not least that they have been brought about through a democratic process by the professions of nursing, midwifery and health visiting. The challenge for those who follow is that they learn from our mistakes and build upon our successes – remembering always that this endeavour must be firmly and clearly rooted in the public interest.

Mary Uprichard DBE RSCN RGN RM MTD
President of the UKCC, 1993–8

Alison Norman CBE HonDSc RGN RM RHV
President of the UKCC, 1998–

Acknowledgements

We have amassed a large number of debts of gratitude in the course of producing this book. Members of a Project Advisory Group set up by the UKCC commented diligently on numerous drafts and entered willingly into debates and discussions with us. We would like to thank Mary Uprichard, Sue Norman, George Castledine, Eva Jacobs, Pam Walter, as well as the two external academics, Judith Allsop and Frank Honigsbaum. The staff of the UKCC were unfailingly helpful as we tried to find our way about their organisation. We would particularly like to thank Tariq Burney, Viren Hindocha, Paul Hutchinson, Eva King, John Knape, Mandie Lavin, Stuart Skyte, Lesley South, Richard Stanwell, Sarah Waller and Sonja Wolfskehl, as well as a number of administrative and secretarial staff whose knowledge of working systems was invaluable. Several people interrupted busy retirements to talk to us in the early stages, patiently suffering our repeated contacts with them as the work progressed. We are grateful to Anne Bent, Reg Pyne, Maude Storey, Maggy Wallace, Jane Winship and Heather Williams, and we would particularly like to thank Reg and Heather for taking on the further and onerous task of reading the final draft. We would also like to thank the following people for giving up their time to be interviewed: Margaret Auld, Christine Chapman, Audrey Emerton, Tariq Hussain, Margaret Green, David Ravey, Audrey Males, John Rogers, Tony Smith, and Joan Wheeler. Many of these people attended a day seminar in June 1999 which the UKCC kindly agreed to organise. Both the seminar and the interviews were helpful in testing out emerging interpretations and giving new leads. Last, but not least, we would like to thank Jane Lewis. A full member of the team for the first 18 months, commitments made it impossible for her to continue. We have probably not situated the study enough in the contemporary health and social policy context, which she understands so well. Such failures of imagination, together with such inaccuracies and errors as might have crept in, are the responsibility of the authors alone.

Abbreviations

BMA	British Medical Association
CCNS	Committee for Clinical Nursing Studies
CEPP	Community Education and Practice Project
CETHV	Council for Education and Training of Health Visitors
CFP	Common Foundation Programme
CMB	Central Midwives Board
CSC	Care Sector Consortium
COHSE	Confederation of Health Service Employers
CPSM	Council for Professions Supplementary to Medicine
DipHE	Higher Education Diploma
DHSS	Department of Health and Social Services
DNJC	District Nursing Joint Committee
EC	European Community
EEA	European Economic Area
ENB	English National Board for Nursing, Midwifery and Health Visiting
EN	Enrolled Nurse
EPAC	Educational Policy Advisory Committee
EU	European Union
GDC	General Dental Council
GMC	General Medical Council
GNC	General Nursing Council
HVA	Health Visitors' Association
HVJC	Health Visiting Joint Committee
JBCNS	Joint Board for Clinical Nursing Studies
LAG	Legislative Advisory Group
LSA	Local Supervising Authority
NALGO	National and Local Government Officers Association
NBNI	National Board for Nursing, Midwifery and Health Visiting for Northern Ireland
NBS	National Board for Nursing, Midwifery and Health Visiting for Scotland
NCC	National Consumer Council

NCHCNC	Nursing and Community Health Care Nursing Committee
NHS	National Health Service
NICNM	Northern Ireland Council for Nurses and Midwives
NUPE	National Union of Public Employees
PADNT	Panel of Assessors for District Nurse Training
PCC	Professional Conduct Committee
PPC	Preliminary Proceedings Committee
PREP	Post-Registration Education and Practice
PREPP	Post-Registration Education and Practice Project
PSR	Professional Self-Regulation
RCGP	Royal College of General Practitioners
RCM	Royal College of Midwives
RCN	Royal College of Nursing
RMN	Registered Mental Nurse
RNMH	Registered Nurse Mental Handicap
RNMS	Registered Nurse Mental Subnormality
SCM	State Certified Midwife
SEN	State Enrolled Nurse
SHHD	Scottish Home and Health Department
SPRINT	Single Professional Register and Index of Training
SRN	State Registered Nurse
TUC	Trades Union Congress
UKCC	United Kingdom Central Council for Nursing, Midwifery and Health Visiting
WNB	Welsh National Board for Nursing, Midwifery and Health Visiting
YTS	Youth Training Scheme

Introduction

The statutory self-regulation of professions is a shadowy subject. The work that is done by bodies granted a legal entitlement to maintain a register of qualified professionals, to determine entry to it and removal from it, is not well understood. Practitioners and public alike tend to confuse the roles of regulatory bodies with those of professional associations. It is only perhaps those with direct experience of working within the regulatory structures, who could begin to hazard a guess about how many registering bodies there are, what exact powers they have, what the rationale for those powers is and how they carry out their responsibilities.

Gaining legal recognition for the establishment of a register of qualified practitioners, deciding on appropriate initial education and restricting practice to those whose competence is recognised through registration lies at the heart of what is known as professional self-regulation (PSR). PSR has been a particularly significant feature of the health field. The forerunner to today's General Medical Council (GMC) dates back over 130 years; the Central Midwives Board (CMB) opened its doors almost a century ago in 1902. Nurses, dentists, opticians, a growing group of what have been known as professions supplementary to medicine, as well as more recently chiropractors and osteopaths, have been granted the right to maintain a register and to enjoy the protection of status that goes with it. The professions themselves have fought hard for this form of regulation. They prize the status and recognition that it gives and they are careful to remind themselves of the privilege that it implies – the trust accorded to them to maintain the register in the interests not just of the profession but of the public as a whole. The underlying rationale for PSR has always been the protection of the public – the giving of an assurance that those who are registered are competent in and committed to their practice. In an inquiry into the regulation of the medical profession in the mid-1970s, it was suggested that PSR can be seen as a contract between the public and the profession with advantages on both sides. It is a contract 'by which the public go to the profession for medical treatment because the profession has made sure it will provide satisfactory treatment'.[1] It was self-evident to that committee that the profession should keep the register because it was only members of the profession who had the knowledge and experience to decide on the competence of their peers.

Much, however, has changed. The regulatory bodies have faced public questioning not only of the decisions they have made on matters such as educational requirements for entry, but also of the rulings they have made on removing names from and restoring them to the register. It is this latter activity in particular that has begun to bring self-regulation into doubt. If the rationale for the regulation of professions is the protection of the public, should professions themselves play so strong a part? Can they be trusted always to work in the public interest? These questions have grown in importance since the 1980s and have erupted particularly strongly onto the public agenda at the end of the 1990s. A detailed study of the working of PSR in what is by far the largest of the regulatory bodies is thus particularly timely.

The significance of the UKCC

Created under legislation in 1979, The United Kingdom Central Council for Nursing, Midwifery and Health Visiting (UKCC) may seem too youthful an institution to attract a full-length history of its own. Three features, however, mark it out as particularly interesting. First, there is the timing of its creation. Its birth coincided with the start of a long period of Conservative government and an altogether more insistent questioning of the costs, quality and organisation of welfare services. Public-sector professionals came under scrutiny as never before. The managerial and market mechanisms that were brought into state-run services, including the NHS, marked a clear break with the public trust in and deference to professions that had been a feature of the post-war period. Attention, however, focused on the workplace. Conservative governments of the time were reluctant to question the conditions for registration or to bring a debate about the relevance of PSR to the present day into the public arena. This did not mean that self-regulation was given free rein. Government restrained the ambitions of the UKCC, especially over educational reform that would affect expenditure and flexibility in the NHS. The regulatory bodies, however, contrary to popular belief, have never had the powers to control numbers of entrants to the profession or to shape the skill mix in the delivery of care. The extent to which the nursing and midwifery professions can in practice regulate themselves has always been curtailed by the state, and this history provides detailed documentation of this.

The second feature that makes the UKCC of particular interest is its scale and its scope. The 1979 Act created a Central Council and four National Boards to cover what had previously been separately regulated professions of nursing and midwifery in the various parts of the UK. It also brought under its umbrella bodies that had been set up to control the education and training of health visitors, district nurses and areas of specialist clinical practice. Once the records of these bodies had been amalgamated and updated, it was clear that over half a million practitioners fell within its remit. Alongside the preparation of policies and guidance on standards of education, conduct and practice, lies the lesser-known routine of the UKCC – adding new names to the register, managing periodic re-registration, handling removals, restorations and confirmations of registration for employers, as well as dealing with day-to-day enquiries. Every working day, staff make around 2000 changes to the register, take around 5000 phone calls and receive what can amount to an almost unbelievable 14,000 items of post.

The third particular feature of the UKCC has been the ambition of its activities in rethinking regulation and adapting it to changing circumstances and expectations. Both the nurses and the midwives who held office in the early years were keen to see changes to the frameworks of regulatory rules. Nurses in particular wanted to move away from the old regulatory equation of close control of a curriculum and precise specification of tasks and to create a more confident professionalism. They also wanted to see a register that testified to the continuing competence of a registrant, not simply to the fact of qualifying in a particular year. Nurses and midwives wanted to use the professional conduct machinery not to punish a practitioner but to ensure that standards were upheld. The inclusion for the first time of the word 'improve' on the face of the Act gave greater scope to make a reality of this. The story of how far, by the late 1990s, these goals were being achieved, and also of how the UKCC was bringing a consumer voice into more and more of its activities, is a particularly significant one in the present context of regulatory change.

But is it a matter of too little and too late? In 1996, as we embarked on this work, a history of the UKCC looked to be a quiet backwater project, of interest only to the nursing world and perhaps, even then, only to a small minority within that world. In 1999, as we brought the study to publication, PSR was an issue with a much higher public profile. Questions have begun to proliferate. What does the public want of a professional – and how can a standard of performance be assured? What sanctions should there be, not only against those who commit acts of gross misconduct but also against those whose performance is persistently poor? As cases of poorly performing doctors hit the headlines and as the news about restoration to the nursing register of those of who had committed the most serious of crimes emerged, so this kind of questioning has become more persistent. Is it a matter of updating and streamlining, or do the institutions of PSR need total reorganisation? A history cannot provide a definitive answer to such questions but it can help to generate a more informed debate.

The development of the study

The UKCC took a decision in April 1996 to commission this history. The plan was to produce a work of record and a critical reflection covering the first ten years. As researchers, we argued that it was important to go further back. This was not simply to pick up this history at the point where a previous work of record for the GNC for England and Wales had stopped.[2] It was also vital in our view to explore the period prior to the creation of the Council, to examine the government's review of nursing in the early 1970s, the lobbying which followed and the legacies this left. We also wanted to ensure there was scope for the work to be critical rather than celebratory. We wanted to deal with the controversies that emerged, the relations, sometimes very uneasy, with the four National Boards, and to reflect on what so many called 'tribalism' in the nursing professions. These points were accepted and the project formally began in September with a timetable of three years.

At the end of the first year, we came to the Council with a proposal that would substantially alter the scope of the study and have important consequences for its methods. By now, we had begun to understand the importance of legislative amendments in 1992 and to realise how the pattern of the development of Council would not be reflected unless we came much more up to date. Instead of finishing after the first two five-year terms of Council, we proposed to include the third term due to finish in March 1998. It was a courageous decision for the UKCC to agree to this. Council had been enmeshed in unprecedented levels of controversy about its professional conduct work and was still coming to terms with a fundamental reorganisation of its daily working that had followed adverse publicity. It was also a daunting prospect for the researchers – we would not enjoy the distance that time allows to reflect on events, we would have to find ways of keeping up to date with a fast-moving and controversial present. None of us knew at the time that it would be impossible to leave matters in March 1998. In outline at least, it has become important to tell the story of the following year – the one in which it became clear that the Labour Government's commitment to modernising professional self-regulation was to transform both the UKCC and the National Boards.

Our methods and ways of working for what has become a work of contemporary history reflect this trajectory. Archival sources have been used for the period before the formation of the UKCC. We were fortunate in gaining early access to the extensive DHSS archive on the Briggs Committee on Nursing and the lead-up to the 1979 Act. Council papers and committee papers have been available to us for the period from the setting up of the shadow body to the present day. The working files of the organisation were open, subject to constraints about personal data and confidential cases coming to the Health Committee. The UKCC's press cuttings and the professional press were also valuable resources. It proved a challenging business sometimes just to track publications and decisions – let alone to generate some perspective on events and bring them to life.

The history of the project and its ways of working have lent both strengths and weaknesses to the ensuing work. We have aimed to produce a work of detailed record, locating key decisions and arguments and indicating where in the voluminous records of Council, the discussions will be found. For some this will be too detailed an account although we have struggled to cut chapters to a readable length and keep referencing manageable. Working so closely with Council sources, we are conscious that we have not been able to trace National Board perspectives on issues as far as we would have liked. We have not considered in a systematic way the view from the professional associations, the trade unions or ordinary practitioners. Oral testimony through interviews was the major casualty of extending the project. We particularly regret the lost opportunity for systematic interviewing of Council members. Whatever judgement one comes to about the merits and demerits of PSR, the personal cost of this kind of service to professions deserves to be much more fully appreciated. The biggest challenge, however, has been that of going beyond the narrative, finding frameworks, making interpretations. It has struck us repeatedly in the course of this study, how little academic work there is that engages with the business of PSR in a direct way.

The book is in three parts. Part I gives an account of the circumstances of the creation of the UKCC and National Boards and the hopes and fears of the different groups that were brought together under the new regulatory structure (Chapter 1). It stresses the skeleton nature of the legislation, emphasising the range of work that had to be completed before the Council proper began (Chapter 2). Chapter 3 gives an overview of developments across the three Councils that are the main subject matter of the book, introducing the main directions of change that have been identified. Part II then covers three key areas of the work of the Council in more depth. Reform of initial programmes of education was the first major task of the new Council. Chapter 4 shows how, as this story ends, the issue was in process of being considered once again. Chapter 5 turns to the question of removal from the register, and the challenges that were faced. Maintenance of standards for those in practice proved to be a confused and confusing issue for the profession. Chapter 6 charts the steps that were taken and the many dimensions which were intertwined.

Part III asks about the 'how?' rather than the 'what?' of PSR. Chapter 7 considers how the many different groups worked together under a single regulatory umbrella, and includes an assessment of the different traditions in nursing and midwifery and the problems of similarity and difference that have dogged their relationship. It also draws attention to the way a reorganisation in 1995 started to offer a new way to listen to minority voices and involve them. Chapter 8 considers the question of lay participation in the work of the Council and the involvement of the 'ordinary' professional. This is a topic that is likely to gain greater prominence in the immediate future as questions are asked about the stakeholders in regulation and how in future they are to work together. The concluding chapters give the reader a brief chronology of events since the end of the Third Council and offer a series of reflections and assessments that are a product of a close encounter with this example of PSR. At a time when PSR has come so recently onto the public agenda, we can only hope to signal lines of questioning and draw attention to some of the complexities. These are issues, however, not just for nursing and midwifery but for all of the professions in health and social care and perhaps for the very notion of profession and professional identity itself.

Notes

1   Report of the Committee of Inquiry into the Regulation of the Medical Profession (Merrison Report), London, HMSO, Cmnd 6018, para 4.
2   Bendall, E. and E. Raybould, *History of the General Nursing Council for England and Wales, 1919–1969*, London, H. K. Lewis and Co., 1969.

Part I

The importance of context

1 'All is not well with nursing'

The Briggs Committee and a new statutory framework[1]

There is a paradox at the heart of the history of the United Kingdom Central Council for Nursing, Midwifery and Health Visiting (UKCC). The origins of the regulatory structure set out in the Nurses, Midwives and Health Visitors Act of 1979 are firmly associated with the Report of the Briggs Committee on Nursing published in 1972, and yet Briggs barely discussed the matter of professional regulation at all.[2]

Set against the background of intense industrial unrest among nurses and other public-sector staff, uncertainty over the consequences of the planned reorganisation of the NHS and growing government pressure for cost containment in the delivery of health care, the Briggs Committee focused its deliberations on the nature and purpose of nurse training, and the management of limited nursing and midwifery resources. Reform of the 'organisational framework', as Briggs termed the existing statutory and training bodies, was discussed only at the end of the document, and in less than ten of the report's 220 pages.[3] This chapter will explore the importance of the Briggs Report, the turmoil that followed and the lobbying that created the UKCC and the four National Boards. The period was one of intense professional disunity, the resulting legislation shot through with compromise. It was a difficult legacy on which to build a completely new structure of professional self-regulation.

The Committee and its context

The establishment of the Briggs Committee in April 1970 came at the end of a decade of disquiet within nursing. The profession's concerns were varied, and included the structure of the nursing service, its status within the NHS and arrangements for, and the standard of, nurse training. In 1964 an increasingly vocal Royal College of Nursing (RCN) published two reports outlining arguments for change.[4] The first, *Administering the Hospital Nursing Service*, argued for a better career structure for senior nurses and greater recognition of the role of nurse administrators: a position that was broadly endorsed by the government following the report of its own Committee on Senior Nursing Staff Structure (Salmon Committee) in 1966.[5] The second RCN report, *A Reform of Nursing Education*, received a much less positive response. Known to the profession as 'Platt' after the chairman of the College's committee of inquiry, the document was an uncompromising statement of the need for radical change, calling for full 'student' status for trainee nurses, higher educational qualifications for entrants, a lower age of entry and fewer, more independent, schools of nursing.[6] To the profession's leadership at the RCN, Platt was an attempt to free nurse education from the worst elements of its historic compromise with the nursing service. Ministers, however, saw an inflexible approach to nurse training that would sit uneasily with plans for health service reorganisation, and a woeful neglect of the cost and manpower implications of such major change.[7] The Platt recommendations were not pursued.[8]

Pressure for a comprehensive review of nurse education, however, refused to go away. Indeed, by the end of the decade the issue had become subsumed within a much wider demand for improved pay and conditions.[9] Ten years of public-sector pay restraint had taken its toll. In 1969, the RCN launched its 'Raise the Roof' campaign, demanding a salary increase amounting to around 28 per cent. For a Labour government committed to the modernisation of major British institutions by discussion and consensual change, this was a major source of embarrassment. Direct industrial action by nurses, together with the 'quieter protest' of high rates of wastage and turnover, now forced the government's hand.[10] In the summer of 1969, the DHSS acceded to the RCN's wish for an independent review of nurse education.[11] The initial plan was for a 'modest exercise' with deliberations confined to basic nurse training in England, Wales and Scotland (not Northern Ireland), and excluding post-registration training, midwifery, health visiting, district nursing and the national statutory arrange-ments.[12] By the end of the year, however, Richard Crossman, the Secretary of State for Social Services, and Prime Minister Harold Wilson had decided that only 'a completely new study of nursing', embracing such issues as 'the nurse's place in society, her status, training, pay and working conditions' would suffice.[13]

On 2 March 1970 Crossman announced the establishment of the Committee on Nursing to the House of Commons. Professor Asa Briggs, Vice-Chancellor of the University of Sussex, was appointed as chairman.[14] It was to be a small committee, with nurses and midwives constituting around half of its membership. The rest were to be drawn from the fields of medicine, health service administra-tion and further and secondary education.[15] While the health departments expected that those appointed would cover a broad range of experience and expertise, members were selected for the individual contribution they could make, rather than as representatives of particular interests.[16] Nevertheless, following a number of representations, the Department did accept the late inclusion of a registered mental nurse, believing that the absence of a member from this distinct and politically sensitive specialty would cause problems if, and when, the com-mittee made recommendations affecting this sector. Similarly, the Department was concerned that all levels of nursing experience were seen to be included. The resignation from the committee of ward sister Susan Cooper in October 1970, for instance, re-opened the issue of the 'balance'. 'Junior nursing staff from the provinces', it was argued, were a significant section of the profession and such a 'gap' could seriously hinder the effectiveness of the committee.[17] The question of membership was to remain a sensitive issue during the lifetime of the committee and beyond. Midwives were uncomfortable with the inclusion of only one practising midwife. The committee, though, was perhaps most vulnerable in the area of primary care. Throughout the period of its deliberations, groups of health visitors and district nurses expressed concern that their work was not being discussed with sufficient specialist expertise.[18] This was to have an enduring impact, creating a wariness long after the publication of the report.

The Briggs Committee began work in April, just days before the 1970 General Election, which returned the Conservatives to power under Edward Heath. Its remit was broad but deliberately focused to reflect key elements of government health policy, particularly the commitment to integrate hospital and local authority health services under a single administrative structure, and to effect this change within existing staffing constraints.[19] The terms of reference were: 'to review the role of the nurse and the midwife in the hospital and the community and the education and training required for that role, so that the best use is made of available manpower to meet present needs and the needs of an integrated health service'.[20] The Committee immediately adopted a 'big picture' approach, seeking opinions on the role of the nurse, the nature of her duties and her relationship to others engaged in the delivery of health care. It was also agreed that evidence should be collected from as wide a range of interested bodies as possible.[21] The signals within the terms of reference, though, were unmistakable. The requirement to work within existing resource levels meant that the Committee's principal focus would be issues of demand rather than supply, and the needs of the service rather than those of the profession.

An important starting point was the high levels of wastage and turnover within nursing. While total nursing and midwifery numbers had risen during the 1960s, the general impression was of a looming crisis. Doubts were reaching the Committee about the 'adequacy and suitability' of current arrangements for nurse and midwife education for a fast-developing health service.[22] One of the most pressing questions identified by the Briggs committee, therefore, was how to develop programmes of education and training that would equip nurses for their varied and changing responsibilities.[23] So, while the Briggs Committee did not explicitly address the activities of the bodies responsible for standards of nurse, midwife and health visitor training in England, Wales and Scotland, its attention was immediately drawn to what could be seen as the failings of the existing statutory arrangements, namely the inflexible system of training and registration that had developed under its auspices.

Three problems, in particular, were identified. First, it was clear that educational resources were inefficiently deployed. In the early 1970s, training for nurses and midwives in Great Britain was taking place 'in a wide range of places, in contrasting conditions and with different teaching strengths, educational methods and social amenities'. By the time the Briggs Committee reported, for instance, there were 665 schools approved for training by the General Nursing Council (GNC) for England and Wales, and sixty-two in Scotland. In addition to these were the 'various centres for the education of midwives, district nurses and health visitors, as well as the numerous places in which different kinds of post-basic courses' were held. Given the marked shortage of tutors and clinical teachers, manpower as well as equipment was particularly 'thinly spread'.[24]

Second, and even more concerning, was the in-built inflexibility of the existing training regime. Nursing's long history of early specialisation, whereby trainees were prepared to care for particular groups of patients – such as children or mentally handicapped people in hospitals – appeared to be grossly out of step with the demands of a reorganised and administratively integrated NHS.[25] If nursing care was to be planned across the current dividing lines of hospital and community, and delivered with as much continuity as possible, then education and training needed to produce 'all-rounders': nurses with a good enough basic education to enable them to function satisfactorily within the nursing team at basic level and to progress from basic to specialist nursing skills with further education.[26]

Third, the Briggs Committee was unconvinced of the value of maintaining two discrete 'portals' of entry to nursing: 'registration', following a three-year training programme; and 'enrolment' following a shorter (usually two-year) and less theoretical course of preparation.[27] Since first accepting the concept of a second level of nurse during the war, the profession's leadership had insisted that a 'sharp distinction' exist between registered and enrolled nurses (though in practice, the level of work assigned to enrolled nurses was often very similar to that assigned to registered nurses in the staff nurse grade). In 1962, for instance, the GNC regained the right to impose minimum educational requirements for those seeking entry to courses leading to registration. Entry to courses leading to enrolment were not to be restricted in this way. The RCN was particularly keen to see an increase in the educational standard of entrants but also campaigned for the development of clearer distinctions between those trained for state registration and those prepared for entry to the roll. The members of the Briggs Committee, however, were convinced that a more flexible approach to training was essential. Given the increasing emphasis on teamwork within nursing and the enormous range of duties expected of the professional nurse, the committee felt that programmes of nurse education should cover 'a range of standards catering for different types of entrant motivated towards and capable of performing different nursing activities'.[28] Moreover, recent experience had demonstrated the growing importance of the State Enrolled Nurse (SEN) grade: between 1962 and 1970 the proportion of trainees who were 'pupils' (i.e. trainees for the roll) rather than 'students' (trainees for the register) had increased from 13 per cent to 42 per cent. Future programmes of nurse training would have to reflect the significance of this source of recruits.[29]

The Committee rejected the RCN's desire to increase the formal qualifications required of recruits, arguing for more attention to be given to the identification of 'motivation' as distinct from 'academic ability'.[30] Educational developments outside the fields of nursing and midwifery were cited in support of this shift. For instance, the 'comprehensive' model of learning, with goals reached through different tracks and at a varied pace, strongly influenced both the substance and the rhetoric of the committee's recommendations.[31] The Briggs Report, there-fore, recommended the introduction of an eighteen-month general basic nurse training, accessible through a number of different modes of entry, and leading to a single statutory qualification – the 'Certificate in Nursing Practice'. Those with the ability and desire to train further would undertake a further eighteen months of training leading to full registration, with some taking additional courses lead-ing to the award of higher certificates in certain specialties.[32] It was a model that both reflected contemporary educational developments and, more importantly, endorsed the need for flexibility to meet health service demands.

Issues for health visiting and district nursing

The Conservative government's continued efforts to integrate the administration of NHS hospital services and the community health services previously provided by local authorities, also shaped the deliberations of the Briggs Committee. Particular attention was given to future educational and clinical arrangements for community-based nurses. Once again, this was a potentially controversial area. The Briggs Report itself acknowledged that 'strong and divergent views' had been expressed in oral and written evidence on the subject.[33]

Within the community nursing sector there were fears that 'integration' of nursing services, when finally translated into practice, would entrench the domi-nation of the hospital. Yet there were also tensions between different types of community practitioner. Health visitors, in particular, were anxious for their future, seeing the distinctive nature of their work under threat from district nurses and midwives eager to assimilate the preventive and curative aspects of community-based care, and from social workers whose role with families affected by health-related problems and with elderly people had been strengthened in England and Wales by the recommendations of the 1968 Seebohm Report and the Local Authority Social Services Act which followed it in 1970.[34] The 1968 National Board for Prices and Incomes Report No. 60 into nursing pay and recruitment, indeed, had stated that 'if the social work content of the health visitor's role grew, consideration should be given to the creation of a "medico-social worker" to take it over'.[35] The Briggs Report was to add fuel to such concerns. Given the on-going manpower constraints, the Committee felt obliged to discuss whether the existing distinction between health visitors and district nurses should continue or be replaced by a single category of 'community nurse', with social workers taking over certain aspects of the health visitors' duties.[36] After hearing the evidence of interested and allied bodies, and on the basis of their assessment of developing needs in the community, members endorsed the continuation of two categories of community nurse, but also recommended a clarification of the role of the health visitor (to be renamed 'family health sister') and its re-orientation towards nursing and the family health team.[37] This was reflected in the Committee's decision to recommend the abolition of the statutory training body for health visiting, the Council for Education and Training of Health Visitors (CETHV) and the transferral of statutory control to a proposed

Nursing and Midwifery Council. This was seen by a large section of the health visiting profession as an unequivocal rejection of their distinctive identity. It was a highly controversial decision, and one that was to have a considerable impact on nursing politics for some years to come.

Issues for midwifery

The Committee's discussion of the future of midwifery raised similar issues of professional identity. In this case, however, sensitivities were compounded by distinct national differences between the English and Welsh, and the Scottish midwifery bodies. This fusion of concerns for professional and national identities was to become an important element in the debates on the implementation of the Briggs Committee's recommendations.

At an early meeting, the Committee held an unstructured discussion of midwifery covering such issues as the impact of increased integration of hospital and community midwifery services, career structure, supply and demand issues, syllabuses for basic and post-basic education, the trend towards closer links with basic nurse training and the crucial question of the future of midwifery as a separate profession. Affirmation was given to the distinctiveness of midwifery. The midwife's prominent role as an educator of student doctors as well as midwives was stressed, as was the legacy of her independent practice.[38] The enduring impact of midwifery's separate historical development was acknowledged much more readily than that of the health visitor.[39] However, the Committee did not accept the arguments of the statutory and professional bodies for midwifery in favour of the continued separation of statutory regulation: the advantages of combination were deemed to far outweigh the disadvantages. In part this stemmed from the Committee's decision that, as already occurred in Scotland, all entrants to midwifery training should be qualified nurses.[40] The amalgamation of statutory responsibilities for the basic and post-basic training of nurses and midwives, it was suggested, would deepen communication between the different branches of the nursing and midwifery professions which had not always been consistent or totally effective. Amalgamation was also advocated on the grounds that it would create 'a more powerful nursing body to negotiate nursing and midwifery policy at the highest level', not only in Britain but, given the Heath government's desire for Britain's entry into the European Economic Community, also in Europe. To safeguard the special interests of midwives,[41] however, it was 'considered essential' that a 'strong standing midwifery committee' be established within the new framework. The Briggs Committee was acutely aware that, given the considerable opposition of sections of the profession, amalgamation was going to be a controversial decision and one that would need to be explained in detail.[42] The implications of amalgamation, indeed, continued to be discussed throughout 1971. A paper produced towards the end of the year by Margaret Auld, the only practising midwife member of the Committee, and two of the nursing members, Sheila Collins and Winifred Frost, suggested that the Committee might wish to reconsider its decision. The resulting discussion, however, confirmed the commitment to unification. The 'concept of comprehensiveness', it was agreed, was too important to be 'eroded by splitting off midwives'.[43]

At the twentieth meeting of the committee in June 1972, therefore, it was finally agreed that midwifery would be represented by a separate committee within a unified central council. This committee would advise the council on all matters relating to midwifery education, and exercise direct control of midwifery practice. This role, moreover, was to be conferred by statute and not simply delegated at the council's discretion.[44]

Discussion of the future of midwifery also revealed the presence of a strong, if sometimes ill-defined, sense of the national differences between Scottish midwives and those from England and Wales. Pressure for continued national autonomy grew in strength and clarity during the implementation phase, and will be discussed in more detail below; yet it is worth noting that the Briggs Committee was not unaware of this potential obstacle to the implementation of its recommendations. The written evidence of the Central Midwives Board (CMB) (England and Wales) conflicted with that of the CMB for Scotland on a number of fundamental points and, in December 1970, the committee had decided that oral evidence, to identify the extent of the discrepancy was necessary and urgently required.[45] The Scottish Board was asked, for instance, about its relationship with other statutory bodies and whether any changes were desirable. The response was emphatic: no changes involving an amalgamation between Scottish and other United Kingdom bodies were favoured. The obstetric services, it argued, 'were further advanced in Scotland than in England partly because the smaller population and fewer training schools made changes, such as the introduction of integrated [nurse and midwife] training easier'.[46] These gains might be lost with amalgamation. Adequate mechanisms for contact with the bodies representing midwifery in England and Wales, and also with the Northern Ireland Council for Nurses and Midwives, it asserted, already existed and relations between them were 'cordial'. It was hoped, however, that 'liaison' with the Scottish GNC would be increased. The GNC for Scotland also stated that it was 'not in favour of assimilating conditions in England and Scotland', basing its argument on the difference between English and Scottish laws.[47]

The Committee's discussions on future arrangements for the training and deployment of nurses, health visitors and midwives were clearly pointing towards a unitary statutory framework of some kind. However, when considering the draft report in April 1972, the chairman found that while there was plenty of material on the role and function of the nurse and midwife, there was plainly 'insufficient on statutory frameworks'. Agreement still had to be reached on the relationship between the various components of the proposed new bodies – which were to include a 'central council' for nursing (including health visiting) and midwifery covering the three countries of Great Britain, 'education boards' for each of the countries and a central midwifery committee with statutory responsibility for standards of midwifery practice. Even the nomenclature was yet to be agreed. Most importantly, final agreement still had to be obtained on whether the committee's 'radical proposals for one body covering not only all the present training bodies, but the three countries of Great Britain, were correct in essence and practical in application'.[48] The arguments for and against were recounted, but the weight of opinion remained for unification. Summarising the Committee's arrival at this decision, the Report stated that while consultation between the existing statutory and training bodies in Great Britain appeared to have improved over recent years, this could not be regarded as a 'good substitute for common participation' in a unified statutory framework, particularly at a time when all parts of Great Britain were experiencing 'the same trends towards integration of the National Health Service (community and hospital)'. Moreover, the Committee's conception of a 'unified and continuous educational process, carefully thought out and planned, with the different parts relating to each other', led it 'naturally [to] an administrative structure which avoids both fragmentation and over-lapping'. If education in nursing and midwifery were to become 'more systematic [and] given a far greater degree of independence from the service sector', its best hope, the Committee argued, lay in a 'central organisation' with 'real powers', and 'which could speak for the profession as a whole'.[49]

Briggs unveiled

The Briggs Report was submitted to the government in the autumn of 1972. The text comprised about 220 pages (with a further 100 pages of appendices) and contained over seventy recommendations. The main proposals were to lower the age of entry into nursing from eighteen to seventeen by 1975; to make entry requirements dependent on a flexible system designed to test motivation and aptitude rather than on formal education requirements; to restructure training, introducing an eighteen-month general training leading to a first statutory qualification (Certificate in Nursing Practice) and a further (optional) eighteen-month course leading to registration; to replace the four specialised parts of the existing nursing register (general, children, mental health, mental handicap) by a single undifferentiated register; to introduce improvements in the career structure in order to achieve a clearer identification of nurses and midwives with advanced clinical qualifications; to discontinue the statutory certification of health visitors, thereby eliminating the need for the CETHV; to set up Colleges of Nursing and Midwifery throughout the country, financed separately from the health service through Area Committees for Nursing and Midwifery; and to replace the separate statutory regulatory bodies by a single Central Nursing and Midwifery Council for Great Britain, with a statutory standing Midwifery Committee, supported by three Nursing and Midwifery Education Boards for England, Wales and Scotland. A scholarly, yet accessible document, the Briggs Report was broadly welcomed by nurses who felt that, at last, their profession had received the in-depth analysis it so badly needed. Much that Briggs said, especially its sensitive appreciation of the distinctive caring role of the nurse and the need to improve the career structure of clinical nurses, was greatly appreciated. Yet, as the Committee's deliberations had already shown, the Briggs Report was not free from controversy. Expressions of unease were already beginning to emanate from health visitors and midwives, and from Scotland.

In conducting its review of nursing and midwifery, the Briggs Committee clearly had a number of differing interests, both within and outside the professions, to satisfy. Its attempt to steer a path through this complex area led to a recommendation for a new regulatory structure for the previously discrete professions of nursing, midwifery and health visiting. Yet nothing had been said in any overt way of the notion of professional self-regulation, or the rights and responsibilities of bodies statutorily charged with maintaining a register of those fit to practise. The establishment of a unified regulatory structure was, in essence, a means to an end – and that end had far more to do with an overhaul of nurse education and with the management of scarce nursing and midwifery resources than anything else. In other words, the Briggs Report was about the proper deployment of nurses and midwives first and professional education second (although Briggs sought firmly to link these), with professional self-regulation only indirectly on the agenda.

Reactions and responses, *c.* 1972–9

The Conservative government's response to the Briggs Report was mixed. While the health departments were broadly supportive of its recommendations and eager to press ahead with their own assessments of the main areas of reform, Treasury ministers and officials were worried about the cost of implementation. Concerned that swift publication of the Briggs Report 'might arouse hopes and encourage pressures for increased expenditure', which, given the 'bleak' outlook were unlikely to be achievable, the Treasury urged tactical delay. It felt that the situation might be 'less embarrassing' for the government if publication came after the grim outlook for public expenditure had become generally known through the publication of the White Paper on Public Expenditure due in November or December 1972.[50] However, the DHSS got its way and the Report was presented to Parliament in October 1972. Three months later the Secretary of State, Sir Keith Joseph, 'initiated the first in a protracted series of consultation exercises' on the Report's recommendations and established an inter-departmental steering group, with representatives from the DHSS, the Scottish Home and Health Department (SHHD), the Welsh Office and an observer from Northern Ireland, to prepare a departmental policy on implementation.[51] Government activity, however, continued to be affected by growing uncertainties about costs and resources. Preparations for a government announcement on the Briggs recommendations continued within the DHSS during 1973, but timetables repeatedly slipped. Keith Joseph's parliamentary statement was deferred first until January 1974, and then to February. By this stage, though, the Heath administration was in serious trouble with the further devaluation of sterling, the economic impact of the Middle East war and mounting problems of industrial unrest. A General Election was called, and on 28 February a minority Labour government was returned to office.[52]

Having set up the Briggs enquiry in 1970, Prime Minister Harold Wilson was under pressure to make known his government's response. Moreover, with industrial action spreading to the NHS the need for swift action was apparent.[53] When it became clear that selective increases in nurses' pay, directed primarily at nurse tutors and ward sisters, were to be announced by the Secretary of State for Employment in May 1974, it became imperative that the government issue a simultaneous statement on its reaction to the Briggs Report 'since the grounds for this award' related directly to its recommendations for increased numbers of teaching staff. On 6 May 1974, therefore, Barbara Castle, the new Secretary of State for Social Services announced the government's acceptance of the main recommendations of the Committee on Nursing.[54]

How did the professions react to the Briggs Report and to the government's belated response? Initial reactions were on the whole favourable. Most expressed relief that a major review had finally been undertaken. The tone of Briggs was greatly welcomed, given the way the Report highlighted 'the unique caring role of nurses and midwives', and insisted that the nurse was not one of the doctor's means of treating people, but was rather the person who cares and co-ordinates care.[55] Briggs's almost passionate defence of nursing, and the space devoted to the need for educational reform, certainly raised expectations. However, as different groups within the profession absorbed Briggs 'in the round', reservations began to be expressed. Both the GNC for England and Wales and the RCN welcomed the recommendation for a single statutory body and the general tenor of the educational reforms. The RCN, however, was concerned about the possible dilution of nursing standards. Having fought hard to achieve a minimum entry requirement in 1962, the Briggs recommendations made it possible that nursing would be the only profession that did not insist on minimum educational entry requirements. The main tensions, however, arose from the professional divisions within nursing, midwifery and health visiting, and from different national identities.

The most challenging criticism came from health visitor organisations. The Health Visitors' Association (HVA), for example, submitted its comments on the report in January 1973. At their heart lay the charge that the nature of health visiting had been misunderstood. This lack of comprehension, it asserted, was reflected in the 'extraordinary and entirely unexplained decision' to recommend a change in title from health visitor to 'family health sister'. Not only did this disregard the recent move to admit men into the occupation, but it ignored the 'considerable success' of health visitors in winning 'public recognition for, and understanding of' their work.[56]

Midwives were also suspicious fearing, like health visitors, the wider implications of the loss of their own statutory body. Scottish midwives were particularly anxious, and asked for an 'assurance' that 'a degree of autonomy' would be given to the National Education Board for Scotland to enable it to plan and execute midwifery policy in the light of Scottish conditions.[57]

Along with the issue of professional identity, indeed, questions of national identity and autonomy pervaded the post-Briggs debate, fuelled and complicated by the contemporary political debate on devolution.[58] Opposition from Scotland to the formation of a powerful central regulatory body was especially strong, and influenced the implementation debate considerably.

Two years, and a change of government on from the publication of the Briggs Report, therefore, the situation was becoming increasingly tense and confused. The concerns of the different professional groups were becoming clearer, and a delicate situation with Scotland was emerging. On top of this, government needed to decide whether Northern Ireland should be included.[59]

Debates about devolution

Control of nursing and midwifery education in Northern Ireland was governed by the 1970 Nurses and Midwives Act (N.I.) which, in many ways, had 'anticipated Briggs in miniature by establishing the Council for Nurses and Midwives as the body responsible for all these matters in Northern Ireland'.[60] Before proceeding with plans for legislation, a decision needed to be reached as to whether this newly created body was to remain, or be incorporated within a new UK-wide framework. While strong advantages for integration were perceived by officials at the DHSS in both England and Northern Ireland, their main reservation was the attitude of the Scots, who were, 'playing noticeably cool on Briggs'. If the Scottish nursing and midwifery bodies decided to oppose a single body for Great Britain, choosing instead 'to integrate separately within Scotland', then the existing situation within Northern Ireland would 'at once become less anomalous' and preferable to a 'link with England alone'.[61] While the Minister of State decided to 'leave the door open for a decision on entry in the light of further local consultations', official attention focused jointly on the reaction of Scottish nursing bodies and on the developing political situation.[62]

During 1974, consultations between the government and the main nursing and midwifery organisations, launched under the previous government, came to focus on the constitution of the new statutory bodies and on the relationship between the Central Council and the national education boards, matters 'on which Briggs had given very little guidance'.[63] In announcing its proposals, the government stated that its 'guiding principle' had been 'that only those issues on which it is important that there should be a uniform decision for the whole of Great Britain should come within the competence of the Central Council and that otherwise there should be maximum decentralisation to the boards'. Yet it quickly became clear that significant differences of opinion were developing between the Scottish bodies and those representing nurses and midwives in England and Wales.[64] One of the main areas of contention was the division of responsibility for professional discipline. In July 1974 a sub-group on disciplinary procedures met at the DHSS, with representatives from the health departments, the GNC for England and Wales, the GNC for Scotland, and the two central midwives boards. Scottish representatives were strongly of the opinion that the investigation of cases of misconduct should be placed at the national level. While powers to suspend, revoke or restore the licence to practise, and to establish an appeals procedure would rest with the Central Council, the investigation of cases should be conducted through a disciplinary committee of the national board.[65] Significant national differences in disciplinary and health service procedures in England and

Wales and in Scotland and, more fundamentally, in the legal systems of the countries, were given as the main reasons. The GNC for England and Wales, however, did not agree with this proposal, believing it to be contrary to the recommendations, and the spirit, of the Briggs Committee. The function of the national education boards, they insisted, should be purely educational.[66]

A parallel argument, centring on the rising political interest in devolution, occurred between officials from the SHHD and those from the DHSS during the later months of 1974 and early 1975. As Ian Sharp of the SHHD noted in a letter to his counterpart at the DHSS,

> . . . we have become increasingly involved in recent months in discussions about devolution to a Scottish Assembly and its implications for the various services, including the health service . . . In this climate the proposal of Briggs that the present statutory bodies should be replaced by a strong Central Council for Great Britain responsible for the maintenance of professional standards, the control of professional discipline, the determination of broad principles of educational policy and the maintenance of registers seems increasingly unlikely to be acceptable to Scottish opinion . . .[67]

Sharp noted that if Briggs legislation came before the House about the same time as legislation on Scottish devolution, 'it would be well-nigh impossible for Scottish ministers to defend' the handing over 'to a Great Britain body functions over which Scotland has exercised its own statutory control for so long'.[68] Given this wider context, consideration needed to be given to an alternative approach – that is, shifting 'the balance of power by giving the main powers to the three national education boards and restricting the powers of the Central Council to the minimum necessary to secure effective co-ordination'. This would mean placing both responsibility for 'professional discipline', and the 'control of midwifery practice' with the national boards.[69] DHSS officials, however, argued that if 'the essence of the Briggs structure' was to be preserved, 'the Council must be an effective body and not just a piece of co-ordinating machinery'. Briggs had envisaged it as 'a standard-setting body, which would establish common professional standards throughout Great Britain'. For this to be realised, 'irreducible minimum functions', in their view, had to include registration, ensuring common disciplinary standards and the establishment of the boundaries of midwifery practice.[70]

The situation in Wales was rather different. Unlike Scotland, Wales did not have its own statutory bodies and therefore did not 'stand to lose anything if the existing proposals for a large measure of centralisation' were pursued. Indeed, it could be argued, 'that the establishment of a national education board in the Principality' was 'itself a nod in the direction of devolution'. Nevertheless, consistency with Scotland was deemed politically prudent.[71] At the end of 1974 and beginning of 1975, therefore, the question of the distribution of functions between a central council and the national boards had, to a large extent, become a political one, with Whitehall waiting for a response from Ministers.[72] Early in the new year, Ministers surprised SHHD officials by reaffirming 'their earlier decision to proceed along the lines recommended by Briggs', accepting the need for 'an effective body capable of speaking for the nursing profession as a whole and safe-guarding professional standards on a Great Britain' or rather, since the Minister for Northern Ireland had agreed to inclusion, a United Kingdom basis.[73] Never-theless, the 'devolutionary theme' continued to be taken seriously: the Bill, it was suggested, needed 'to be seen to provide for the maximum degree of devolution to the National Boards, compatible with the principles enunciated in Briggs'.[74]

Disagreement over the distribution of functions between a central council and the national education boards also made it difficult for representatives from the nursing bodies to come to any firm conclusions on the composition of the new bodies since, it was argued, function would affect the form. The GNC for England and Wales, in line with their view that the national boards should have an educational (plus an associated budgetary) function only, argued that elections should be held for the central council. If, as Briggs had recommended, this was to be the body responsible for professional standards and discipline, then it was right that the profession had a say in its composition.[75] Scottish and Welsh opinion, on the other hand, favoured election to the national boards.

Continuing professional concern

The prolonged discussion of these and associated issues contributed to the delay in the timetabling of the Briggs legislation. While Scottish, Welsh and Northern Irish officials discussed the implications of devolution, and while the Treasury wrestled, in the midst of a deepening economic crisis, with DHSS submissions on the expenditure implications of the Briggs proposals, nurses, midwives and health visitors grew weary of ministerial platitudes and anxious that long-hoped-for reforms would fail to reach the statute book. In a strongly worded memorandum, the Chief Nursing Officer, Phyllis Friend, stated her 'gloom' at receiving the news that the Briggs proposals had not been placed on the reserve list for parliamentary time in the 1975/6 session. The profession was 'already of the opinion that the Briggs Report has been quietly shelved and that there [was] no real intention to implement its recommendations'. This disaffected attitude, she continued, was compounded by 'other "evidence" of a lack of sympathy with the profession', such as the disappointing Halsbury pay recommendations for nurse teachers and the absence of a review of salaries for top posts which had been promised for April 1975.[76] Without a 'definite assurance that the Government still supported Briggs, intend to implement it and back it with money in the foreseeable future', Phyllis Friend argued, nursing morale was bound to 'go from bad to worse, and what could be a constructive and vital element in the NHS at this time could become the opposite'.[77] The 'wait for Briggs', moreover, was seriously affecting the work of the existing statutory bodies, 'causing a stagnation' in their current work, and inhibiting 'preparatory work for the future'.[78] When the Briggs legislation failed to reach the reserve list for the 1976/77 session, the new Secretary of State, David Ennals, agreed to the establishment of a co-ordinating committee to aid the preparation of legislation. With representatives from the statutory bodies, professional organisations and trade unions, the co-ordinating committee was intended 'to act as a shadow advisory organisation or non-statutory council, preparing the way for the statutory bodies to be established when the opportunity was presented'.[79] By 1977, however, the very concept of an integrated education and training for nurses had become extremely fragile. Instead of moving closer together, there was a real danger that the various nursing and midwifery bodies would pull further apart.[80]

The issue of the separate professional identities of health visitors and midwives, which had arisen during the period of the committee and following the publication of its report, remained prominent and, indeed, gained a further dimension as other specialist groups, primarily district nurses and mental health and handicap nurses, grew more vocal. This was to remain a live issue right up to the end of the legislative process, with key amendments sought from the Lords, as well as during the Commons committee stage.

Given the outspoken reaction of health visitor organisations, early attention was given to the health visitors' concerns. Indeed, before the government had expressed its intention to legislate along the lines of the Briggs Report, agreement had already been reached that the term 'health visiting' would be included in the title of the new statutory bodies and that a standing committee for health visiting would be established within the Central Council. The case for this revision, it was argued, rested on the fact that health visitors already had their own statutory body: 'to propose its disappearance without replacement would undermine the moral [sic] of both health visitors in general and of the existing statutory body on whom we are dependent for keeping progress going for the next three years at least.' Also, it was accepted that 'health visitors are sufficiently distinctive in their role for the new statutory bodies to need some form of committee to look after them – making this statutory will do much to avoid a row.'[81] The new Minister of State for Health, Dr David Owen, anticipated a similar reaction from the district nurses, but officials felt that this was unlikely to be strongly expressed and, given their lack of a statutory body at present, the case for a statutory committee would be decidedly weaker than those of midwives and health visitors.[82] Pressure for special committees, nevertheless, did surface and gained in strength once the detail of the promised legislation began to emerge. In November 1977, for example, following a mass demonstration by district nurses, a working party of the Briggs Co-ordinating Committee began to receive evidence from district nurses, (and also from mental health and handicap nurses and occupational health nurses), arguing the case for separate committees.[83] In the meantime, the two general nursing councils began to harden their attitudes, feeling that the whole philosophy of a united profession was about to be eroded by concessions to specialist interests.[84]

From Bill to Act

The Nurses, Midwives and Health Visitors Bill was finally introduced into the House of Commons in November 1978, a full six years after the publication of the

Briggs Report. Considerable differences of opinion within the professions in the four countries of the UK, the political prominence of devolution and the need for consistency with the principles embodied in the Scotland and Wales devolution Bills, the hesitancy of the Treasury (which resurfaced during 1977 after the initial estimates of the cost of educational reform had been revised) and a congested parliamentary timetable had all contributed to the delay. Lobbying by the various professional groups continued right until the last phase of the legislative process. The midwives, arguably, were the most successful, gaining increased authority for the Central Council's Standing Midwifery Committee.[85] The health visitors' demands met stronger resistance, with DHSS ministers anxious that further substantial concessions would not only cause difficulties with nursing groups but act as a precedent for similar treatment for district nurses and mental nurses. Certainly, when the Bill failed to include the specific mention that district nurses were demanding, pressure was put on the House of Lords, which finally accepted the inclusion of an enabling clause for a joint committee for district nurses. As David Rye, director of professional activities at the RCN recalled, 'the Bill started life as non-controversial politically, but professionally it was a different matter'.[86] Far more controversial than had been envisaged, the Nurses, Midwives and Health Visitors' Act finally received Royal Assent on 4 April 1979. 'Crossman's initiative for a review of nursing education thus took more than a decade to yield its first significant fruits.'[87]

Conclusion

The 1970s had been a challenging decade for nurses, health visitors and midwives. New opportunities were clearly emerging – the prospect of a unified and stronger nursing voice, a better balance between hospital and community, to name but two. But in seeking to take them, the professions were forced to consider their histories as well as their futures, and many felt that they could be losing more than they were about to gain. The familiar health service constraints – of costs and workforce planning – appeared to remain firm. Moreover, difficult as its passage had been, the 1979 legislation tackled only one part of the Briggs recommen-dations: the controversial education reforms – which for many professionals were the heart of the matter – were not addressed. In Parliament, this 'limited' interpretation of Briggs was defended as a demonstration of the government's faith in professional self-regulation: it would be for the professions themselves to decide at a later date on the details of their future education and training.[88] The reality, of course, was more complicated. At the very least, it reflected government wariness of the costs of a more comprehensive reform of nursing and midwifery. The Briggs Report had spoken of the need for the recruitment of 14,500 additional nurses over a period of seven years if its proposals for educational reform were to be meaningful. In 1979 it still remained to be seen whether this extra investment would be forthcoming.

   The difficulty that was experienced in getting any part of Briggs onto the statute book revealed a number of tensions that were to continue to be important in the new regulatory structure. The rivalries between the different groupings within nursing, especially between nurses, midwives and health visitors, but also between nurse managers, clinicians and educators, and between different grades of nurse, were laid open. If Margaret Stacey's comment (in the course of her account of the GMC) that 'a united profession is needed for self-regulation to work' is correct, then this foretold difficulty for the new UKCC.[89] Nor did the legislation, any more than the Briggs Report, give a clear steer as to what the nature of the regulatory powers of the UKCC would entail. The new statutory bodies were conceived by governments operating without a definite majority in an atmosphere of economic uncertainty, and in the context of the drive towards devolution. As we shall see in the next chapter, the Central Council and National Boards, established in shadow form in November 1980, had much to do to establish viable internal structures, develop effective relationships between the five bodies and between the several professional groups, and to begin to articulate a clear and authoritative voice for professional standards.

Notes (see Appendix 5)

1 RCN, *Annual Report for 1971*, London, HMSO, 1971, para. 7.
2 *Report of the Committee on Nursing* (Briggs Report), Cmnd 5115, London, HMSO, 1972.
3 The existing statutory bodies were the General Nursing Councils (GNC) for England and Wales and for Scotland, the Central Midwives Boards (CMB) for England and Wales and for Scotland, and the Council for the Education and Training of Health Visitors (CETHV). This latter body did not have a disciplinary role. There were also three non-statutory training bodies, the Panel of Assessors for District Nurse Training (PADNT); the Joint Board of Clinical Nursing Studies (JBCNS) and the Committee for Clinical Nursing Studies (Scotland) (CCNS). The regulatory body in Northern Ireland was the Northern Ireland Council for Nurses and Midwives (NICNM) but the situation in this part of the UK was not included within the remit of the Briggs Report.
4 Dingwall, R., A. M. Rafferty and C. Webster, *An Introduction to the Social History of Nursing*, London, Routledge, 1988, p. 113.
5 RCN, *Administering the Hospital Nursing Service*, London, RCN, 1964; Ministry of Health and Scottish Home and Health Department, *Report of the Committee on Senior Nursing Staff Structure* (Salmon Report), London, HMSO, 1966. Salmon accepted the need to integrate hospital-based nurses into the NHS management structure and proposed a new structure of nursing grades based on three tiers of management responsibility. A parallel review for local authority nursing services was established at the end of 1968 under the chairmanship of E. L. Mayston. See C. Webster, *The Health Services since the War. Vol. 2. Government and Health Care. The National Health Service 1958–1979,* London, HMSO, 1996, pp. 249–53.
6 RCN, *A Reform of Nursing Education* (Platt Report), London, RCN, 1964. See also Webster, *The Health Services*, pp. 249–59.
7 Throughout this book we have followed terminologies in use in documents and reports and at the UKCC at the time. When making an overall assessment we have reverted to more modern conventions, thus shifting, for example, from 'manpower' to non-sexist terminology.
8 Records from the DHSS show that the government's view of the nursing profession during the middle and later 1960s was a distinctly unflattering one. It doubted whether the profession, in the form of either the RCN or the GNC, had the inclination

or the capabilities to appreciate the manpower and cost implications of widespread reform of nurse education. See Public Record Office, London, Kew, MH165/152, 25 October 1968, memo by D. Somerville on the establishment of a committee on nurse training; PRO, MH165/146, 20 October 1968, meeting on proposed departmental inquiry into nurse training; 4 August 1969, weekly policy meeting on nurse training.

9 Partial support for the RCN's case for educational reform was contained within the report of the National Board for Prices and Incomes, *Pay of Nurses and Midwives in the National Health Service*, Report no. 60, Cmnd 3585, London, HMSO, 1968. The DHSS responded by setting up a Departmental Committee on Nurse Tutors (chaired by the Chief Nursing Officer, Dame Kathleen Raven). This fell into abeyance shortly after producing a report on potential improvements in nurse training in early 1970. Webster, *The Health Services*, pp. 254–5, pp. 260–1.

10 Dingwall *et al.*, *An Introduction to the Social History of Nursing*, p. 113, p. 205. See also Webster, *The Health Services*, pp. 253–9, and Webster, C., *The National Health Service: A Political History*, Oxford, Oxford University Press, 1998, pp. 70–3.

11 PRO, MH165/146, Nurse training: future development.

12 Webster, *The Health Services*, p. 262.

13 PRO, MH165/146, policy meeting on nurse training, 24 October 1969. See also Crossman, R. H. S., *The Crossman Diaries: Vol. III*, London, Hamish Hamilton/ Jonathan Cape, 1977, p. 759 and Webster, *The Health Services*, p. 263.

14 The announcement of the Committee's establishment came in a statement outlining the agreement achieved on nurses' pay. Briggs's acceptance of the chairmanship had been conditional on a satisfactory settlement of the nurses' pay claims. *Parliamentary Debates* [Commons], 797, 2 March 1970, cols 36–43; PRO, MH165/146. See also Webster, *The Health Services*, p. 259.

15 For a full list of the eighteen members see the *Report of the Committee on Nursing*, iii. Elisabeth Singleton of the DHSS Nursing Division was appointed Secretary. It is notable that no links were being drawn with the contemporary expansion of higher education.

16 PRO, MH165/146, notes for meeting between Ministers of State, and statutory bodies for nursing, midwifery and health visiting, 23 February 1970.

17 PRO, MH165/149, note of sixth meeting, 13–15 November 1970. Mrs Cooper was replaced by Winifred Eustace in February 1971.

18 This sense of unease was also shared by the general practitioner section of the British Medical Association (BMA) and the Council of the Royal College of General Practitioners (RCGP), who made a number of representations for the addition of a general practitioner (rather than a health visitor or district nurse) to the committee's membership. PRO, MH165/153.

19 For discussion of successive governments' policies on health service integration during the late 1960s and 1970s see Klein, R., *The New Politics of the NHS*, London, Longman, 1995, pp. 82–90.

20 *Report of the Committee on Nursing*, preface, v; paras 1–3.

21 For more details of the Committee's methods see *Report of the Committee on Nursing*, preface, v; appendices I–III, pp. 220–88.

22 *Report of the Committee on Nursing*, paras 5–7.

23 PRO, MH165/153, 'The role of the nurse', Education sub-committee, n.d., c. June 1970; PRO, MH165/154, second meeting of Briggs Committee, 10 July 1970, pp. 2–4. Also see the wide discussion of the role of the nurse, the boundaries between her responsibilities and those of others, and the various images and realities of modern nursing in *Report of the Committee of Nursing*, paras 11–46; 81–174.

24 *Report of the Committee on Nursing*, para. 179. See also paras 175–90.

25 PRO, MH165/149, sixth meeting of Briggs Committee, 13–15 November 1970. The nursing registers in England and Wales and Scotland were divided into separate parts – general, sick children's, mental illness and mental handicap.

26 PRO, MH165/168, CN (71), 'The Future of Nurse Education', seventeenth meeting of the Briggs Committee, 3–4 December 1971.

27 PRO, MH165/163, CN (71), fourteenth meeting of Briggs Committee, 10 September 1971, discussion of CN (71) 173, 'The role of the nurse'; Davies, C., 'Continuities in the development of hospital nursing in Britain', *Journal of Advanced Nursing*, 2, 1977, p. 489.

28 PRO, MH165/157, C (70), seventh meeting of Briggs Committee, 4 December 1970, pp. 10–11. See also *Report of the Committee on Nursing*, para. 253.

29 *Report of the Committee on Nursing*, para. 198.

30 PRO, MH165/163, CN (71) 173. Too much stress upon high qualifications, the committee felt, would be more likely to polarise ward staffing on the American pattern of ward sisters supported only by auxiliaries. This was contrary to the committee's preference for the broad-based nursing team.

31 See, for example, PRO, MH165/163, minutes of fifteenth meeting of Briggs Committee, 8–9 October 1971; PRO, MH165/157, C (70), 11. Dingwall *et al.*, *An Introduction to the Social History of Nursing*, p. 207.

32 *Report of the Committee on Nursing*, paras 270–302.

33 *Report of the Committee on Nursing*, p. 166.

34 PRO, MH165/158, CN (70) 103. Dingwall *et al.*, *An Introduction to the Social History of Nursing*, p. 201. For comparable but not identical earlier moves in Scotland, see *Social Work (Scotland) Act*, 1968. Also, the Health and Personal Social Services Order (Northern Ireland), 1972 brought a more far-reaching integration of health and social services under a single administrative authority.

35 National Board for Prices and Incomes, *Pay of Nurses and Midwives in the National Health Service*, para. 122.

36 PRO, MH165/160, CN (71), ninth meeting of Briggs Committee, 12–13 March 1971. A similar discussion arose over the future of mental handicap nursing. The committee felt that the projected increase in community-based care for the mentally handicapped would open the possibility for the development of a new caring profession. This line of thinking was later pursued by the Jay Committee, *Report of the Committee of Enquiry into Mental Handicap Nursing and Care* (Jay Report), Cmnd 7468, London, HMSO, 1979.

37 Evidence from the Association for District Nurses had advocated the re-allocation of health visitor duties between district nurses and social workers, but considerable evidence was also received for the continuation of distinct health visitors. The Panel of Assessors for District Nurse Training, for example, felt that the primary function of the district nurse was, and should remain, clinical care. They did not advocate assimilation with health visitors and, indeed, suggested that the role of the health visitor could grow as more began to work from GP practices. The evidence of the RCGP echoed this viewpoint, as did that from the DHSS and Welsh Office.

38 PRO, MH165/156, CN (70), fourth meeting of the Briggs Committee, p. 3. By the early 1970s, the midwife had all but lost her position as an independent practitioner. Most were employed in the NHS, and their work was shaped by many of the same influences which affected nurses. Dingwall *et al.*, *An Introduction to the Social History of Nursing*, p. 172.

39 See PRO, MH165/157, CN (70) 85, evidence from the Central Midwives Board for Scotland, December 1970; CN (70) 86, evidence from the Central Midwives Board for England and Wales, December 1970; MH165/160, CN (71) 32, evidence from the Royal College of Midwives; PRO, MH165/156, CN (70) 39, evidence from the Royal College of Obstetricians and Gynaecologists.

40 *Report of the Committee on Nursing*, paras 246–9 and 303–7.

41 The regulation of midwives covered not only professional discipline and education, but also practice. The CMB, for instance, required annual notification of intention to

practise and all practising midwives to complete a statutory refresher course at intervals of not more than five years. (See chapter 7).

42 PRO, MH165/167, CN (71) 262, paper by Miss Auld and Miss Frost, 'Points to be considered about midwifery'; CN (71) minutes of sixteenth meeting of Briggs Committee. See also *Report of the Committee on Nursing*, paras 616–29. The fact that the main nursing bodies were strongly in favour of integration and hoped that in the future midwifery would not need a separate committee, perhaps increased the potential for tension.
43 PRO, MH165/168, CN (71) 292, M. Auld, W. Frost, and S. Collins, 'Further thoughts on midwifery'.
44 PRO: MH165/170, CN (72), minutes of the twentieth meeting of the Briggs Committee, 18 June 1972; see also *Report of the Committee on Nursing*, paras 626–9.
45 PRO, MH165/157, CN (70) note of seventh meeting, 4 December 1970, p. 4.
46 See Davies, C., 'Policy in nursing education: plus ça change? . . .' in *The Politics of Progress. Proceedings of 19th Annual Study Day*, Nursing Studies Association, University of Edinburgh, May 1985.
47 PRO, MH165/157, CN (70) 85, evidence from the CMB for Scotland; CN (70) 86, evidence from the CMB for England and Wales; PRO, MH165/161 CN (71) 62, oral evidence from GNC for Scotland. The GNC for England and Wales gave support to amalgamation but argued that 'the main priority was the setting up of one statutory body in the first instance in relation to specialities; geographical unification could come later'. PRO, MH165/160, CN (70) 28, oral evidence from the GNC for England and Wales, 15 April 1971, pp. 5–6).
48 PRO, MH165/170, CN (72), minutes of nineteenth meeting of Briggs Committee, 28–29 April 1972, p. 2.
49 *Report of the Committee on Nursing*, paras 618–9.
50 PRO, MH165/208, memo on Treasury reaction, c. September 1972.
51 Dingwall *et al.*, *An Introduction to the Social History of Nursing*, p. 208.
52 Webster, *The Health Services*, p. 442.
53 Ibid.
54 Ibid., pp. 686–7; PRO, MH165/80. Also see PRO, MH165/84, 24 March 1974.
55 *Report of the Committee on Nursing*, paras 39 and 151.
56 PRO, MH165/204, comments from Health Visitors' Association, 15 January 1973. The CETHV and Society of Chief Nursing Officers (Public Health) held similar concerns, but were less dogmatic in their opposition. See also PRO, MH165/206, brief for Secretary of State's meeting with health visitors, 10 May 1973, for the health visitors' reactions and the department's response.
57 PRO, MH165/206, comments from Royal College of Midwives (Scottish Board).
58 Following the publication of Royal Commission October 1973, and especially after the success of nationalist parties in the general elections of February and October 1974, devolution occupied a significant place on the political agenda. See *Royal Commission on the Constitution*, London, HMSO, Cmnd 5460, 1973. The strength of the nationalists in a precariously balanced Parliament encouraged Labour to develop proposals for Scottish and Welsh devolution.
59 The issue was not simply a matter for government consideration, but was also discussed widely among the nursing and midwifery professions in Northern Ireland.
60 Although the Northern Ireland Council for Nurses and Midwives had only been set up in 1970, joint regulation of nurses and midwives had been in existence in Northern Ireland since partition in 1922.
61 PRO, MH165/208, memorandum from F. A. Elliott, 13 February 1973.
62 PRO, MH165/208, letter from F. A. Elliot to R. Mayoh on the position of Northern Ireland, 25 October 1973.
63 PRO, MH165/79, note of meeting with statutory bodies, 24 June 1974.

Representatives from the two GNCs, the two CMBs, and the CETHV were invited to this meeting, with officials from the DHSS, the SHHD, and the Welsh Office. An observer from Northern Ireland was also present; PRO, MH165/79, note of meeting with statutory bodies, 29 October 1974.

64 PRO, MH165/79, letter to DHSS from the CMB for Scotland, 26 November 1974.

65 PRO, MH165/84, sub-group meeting with statutory bodies to discuss disciplinary procedures, 16 July 1974. At the sub-group meeting, a proposal was put forward that in cases of professional conduct, the investigation be carried out by a committee of the national board, chaired by a board member who was also a Central Council member, thus maintaining a Central Council presence but allowing the initial disciplinary process to be carried out on a national basis.

66 PRO, MH165/84, notes for meeting with statutory bodies, 29 October 1974; PRO, MH165/79, note of meeting with statutory bodies, 29 October 1974; PRO, MH165/85.

67 PRO, MH165/80, letter to R. B. Hodgetts, DHSS from I. Sharp, SHHD, 5 December 1974.

68 Ibid.

69 It should be remembered that Scottish midwives had been particularly upset by the Briggs proposals for a unified statutory structure.

70 PRO, MH165/80, draft letter in reply. Officials at the DHSS were clearly getting frustrated with their lack of progress at this time, even to the point of suggesting a complete change of tactic: pressing ahead with a limited bill for educational reform, while temporarily leaving the statutory framework intact. PRO, MH165/85, memorandum by R. Mayoh, 'The present position on Briggs', 11 December 1974.

71 PRO, MH165/85, letter from R. H. Jones, Welsh Office, to I. Sharp, SHHD, 13 December 1974.

72 PRO, MH165/85, letter from I. Sharp to R. B. Hodgetts, DHSS, 20 December 1974.

73 Consultation with local interests had produced, with virtually complete unanimity, an affirmation of the government's proposals. PRO, MH165/85, letter from F. A. Elliott to R. B. Hodgetts, 13 January 1975.

74 PRO, MH165/85, letter from I. Sharp to R. B. Hodgetts, 13 January 1975.

75 PRO, MH165/85, response of the GNC for England and Wales to government proposals, 5 December 1974.

76 See Webster, *The Health Services*, pp. 694–7.

77 PRO, MH165/80, memorandum by the Chief Nursing Officer, P. Friend, 7 July 1975. Webster, *The Health Services*, pp. 687–9.

78 PRO, MH165/79, notes of meeting with officers of London-based nursing bodies, 19 May 1975.

79 Webster, *The Health Services*, p. 690.

80 In 1975, Raymond Mayoh had warned that delays in obtaining legislative time for the Briggs proposals could lead to greater fragmentation. See PRO, MH165/80, memorandum from R. Mayoh to J. Wheeler of the Nursing Division, n.d.

81 PRO, MH165/80, memorandum by R. Mayoh, 27 March 1974.

82 Ibid. See also PRO, MH165/80, draft paper setting out the government's views on the main recommendations of the Briggs Report, n.d.; PRO, MH165/79, second discussion paper on the constitution of the Central Council for Nurses, Midwives and Health Visitors, and of the national education boards.

83 'Tales of mystery and suspense, or how the Briggs Bill reached the statute book. 1. Personalities', *Nursing Times*, 31 May, 75(22), 1979, pp. 910–11. See also PRO, MH165/111, meeting notes and papers of working group four of the Briggs Co-ordinating Committee.

84 See, for example, the view of Margaret Thomson of the GNC for Scotland, in 'Tales of mystery and suspense. Or how the Briggs Bill reached the statute book. 2. Organisations', *Nursing Times*, 7 June, 75(23), 1979, p. 953.

85 *Parliamentary Debates* [Commons], 958, 13 November 1978, col. 46.
86 'Tales of mystery and suspense. 1. Personalities', p. 908.
87 Webster, *The Health Services*, p. 691.
88 *Parliamentary Debates* [Commons], 958, 13 November 1978, col. 37. See also *Parliamentary Debates* [Lords], 398, 19 February 1979, cols 1643–6.
89 Stacey, M., 'Collective therapeutic responsibility. Lessons from the GMC', in Budd, S. and U. Sharma (eds) *The Healing Bond*, London, Routledge, 1994, p. 110.

2 Legislation and its aftermath
Making a reality of the Council, 1979–83

A completely new framework for the UK-wide regulation of three previously separate professions was outlined, in twenty-four clauses and eight schedules, in the Nurses, Midwives and Health Visitors Act, 1979.[1] This long-awaited piece of primary legislation established the UK Central Council for Nursing, Midwifery and Health Visiting and four National Boards. It made provision for the creation of a single professional register and for the possibility of new forms of education and training. The task of translating outline responsibilities into workable relationships, processes and procedures fell to a 'shadow' Central Council, working in collaboration with colleagues in 'shadow' National Boards and with members of the outgoing regulatory and training bodies.

Thirty-three people were appointed by the Secretary of State to serve on the Shadow UKCC, twenty of whom had been nominated in equal numbers by the Boards. A majority (twenty-seven out of thirty-three) were nurses, midwives or health visitors – many of whom had reached senior posts. A considerable proportion were involved in professional education; others in service management. Some had been members of the outgoing statutory and training bodies, while others came to the Council with limited experience of regulatory processes and legislation. Six members were drawn from outside the professions to be regulated; two of these were doctors and four 'lay' members with either educational or financial expertise. The chairman of the Shadow Council,[2] also appointed by the Secretary of State, was Catherine (later Dame Catherine) Hall, a well-known and respected figure in government circles by virtue of her twenty-year tenure as General Secretary of the Royal College of Nursing. She had recently served on the Committee of Enquiry into the regulation of the medical profession.[3]

Initially, the Council was supported by staff seconded from the DHSS.[4] The first permanent appointees began to take up post in the summer of 1981, starting with Maude Storey, then Registrar of the GNC for England and Wales, as Chief Executive Officer,[5] and Mike Hanson, who had previously been the London Regional Director of the Manpower Services Commission, as Principal Administrative Officer.[6] They were gradually joined by a team of administrators and a small band of professional officers, the majority of whom had worked for the former statutory and training bodies.[7] The Shadow Council started work in November 1980. Legislation allowed a timetable for the handover of functions of no more than three years.

A distinctive form of legislation?

The legislation brought a fresh start. It swept away a series of Nurses Acts and Midwives Acts whose complex modifications over the years proved particularly challenging to understand. There were as many as nine bodies to deal with. The Act dissolved the General Nursing Councils and Central Midwives Boards for England and Wales, and Scotland, the Northern Ireland Council for Nurses and Midwives and the Council for the Education and Training of Health Visitors and disbanded three non-statutory training bodies, the Panel of Assessors for District Nurse Training, the Joint Board of Clinical Nursing Studies and its Scottish equivalent, the Committee for Clinical Nursing Studies. Amendments to a whole series of legislative provisions were made so that now out-of-date descriptions of 'certified midwife', 'state registered nurse' and so on, no longer appeared. The way was paved for familiar acronyms – SRN, SCM, SEN – to be replaced by the new terminology derived from the single professional register.

The purpose of the 1979 Act was 'to make provision with respect to the education, training, regulation and discipline of nurses, midwives and health visitors and the maintenance of a single professional register'. The principal functions of the UKCC were described as 'to establish and improve standards' of both training and professional conduct. Decisions on admission to training and on the kind and standards of training leading to registration were to be made (ensuring consistency with European Community obligations). There was also scope to decide on kinds and standards of further training and to give advice on standards of professional conduct. The remit to 'improve' standards was quite new. The possibility of statutory recognition for a framework of post-registration training and the ability to give advice were equally novel aspects of the legislation.

Council's duty to 'prepare and maintain' a register was more familiar, albeit that it was now to be a single register. There were provisions to add and remove names, to devise parts of the register and allow persons to be registered on more than one part, to devise ways of keeping the register and allowing access to it and verifying registered status. There was provision for registration to remain effective or to be subject to renewal – opening the way to a concept of a more 'live' or 'effective' register, where only those who had demonstrated competence in some way would remain registered. Under the Act a person could be removed from the register 'for misconduct or otherwise', a formula that for the first time allowed provision for removal on health grounds. The Act also followed previous legislation in making it an offence for a person, falsely and with intent, to claim registered status, under penalty of a summary conviction and fine.

The legislation set out how things should be done as well as what should be done. The responsibilities of Council and Boards were in the main sections of the Act and in more detailed schedules. Standing committees for finance and midwifery were prescribed for both Council and Boards, and a Joint Committee for Health Visiting was also required by statute. The Act enabled the new statutory bodies to establish further standing and joint committees if they so wished. There were further detailed provisions relating to midwifery. Financial provisions gave powers to raise fees from registrants, allowed for the possibility of grants from the Secretary of State and set out requirements in terms of the provision of accounts.

With hindsight, three features of the legislation are particularly striking. First, the Act said remarkably little about the rationale, purpose and justification of professional self-regulation. Considerable energies were expended in making sure that groups within the professions to be regulated were represented, particularly those concerned with education, and with ensuring that the professions had a majority. The Secretary of State's appointees were to be drawn from within the professions, from registered medical practitioners and only finally from such others deemed to be 'of value to Council in the performance of its function'.[8] In these ways, the 1979 Act took for granted that a profession could and should regulate itself – there was no sense of the debates about lay representation that were to grow in momentum over the next twenty years. Second, however, the Act built in safeguards. It required Council to consult on all the substantive decisions it made, and to enact the results of its decisions and consultation in the form of rules in an Order in Council. Such Orders must be laid before parliament, before they emerge as statutory instruments through which decisions can be put into effect.[9] Few can have realised as the Shadow Council took up its work the tortuous route that the 'new provisions' for education and discipline that the 1979 Act promised would need to take. Before the 'appointed day' on which the new legislation came fully into force, a total of twenty-three statutory instruments was prepared. The process of consultation, and the meticulous legislative drafting that followed, was to become a permanent feature of the work of the Council. Third, and perhaps most importantly, no details were given about the future of pre-registration education. The professions had been waiting for change since the publication of the Briggs Report in 1972, and for many the Act's silence on this matter was the biggest disappointment.

The Shadow Council set up seven working groups, each comprising a core of Shadow Council and National Board members and supported by the growing number of UKCC staff.[10] Close co-operation with the National Boards and wide consultation with the professions were confirmed as correct in principle and sensible in practice. There was excitement, trepidation and almost a sense of awe among members of the Shadow Council as to the tasks to be undertaken.

Practitioner voices at regulatory body level

The legislation allowed for an elected element at Board level and required Council to devise a scheme to hold elections within two years. On the face of it, this was a largely technical matter. Working Group 1 looked to the experiences of the former statutory bodies for guidance and sought the advice of the Electoral Reform Society.[11] But it was also an issue that encompassed important questions of national and professional representation.

The stated aim was to create an electoral scheme which would provide a representative Board. But representative of whom? One key issue was representation for specialist nursing groups. The possibility of having a number of reserved places for mental health nurses, mental handicap nurses, sick children's nurses, district nurses and occupational health nurses, was considered but ultimately overturned in favour of a single 'nurse' category. Among the decisive factors in bringing the Working Group to this decision was advice from the Electoral Reform Society that, provided each occupational group ensured the active participation of their members, there was no reason why a basic single transferable vote system (already in use by the GMC, the General Dental Council (GDC) and a number of other self-regulatory bodies) should not produce balanced representation.[12] Guaranteeing representation to some occupational groups within nursing and not to others could expose the scheme to the charge of unfairness. As the report of the Working Group stated, 'it has to be all groups or none'.[13] Moreover, the 1979 Act was clearly based on three professional groups – nurses, midwives and health visitors – and to add additional categories could be seen as casting doubt on the legitimacy of this framework.

Ultimately, it was decided that elections should be held in each country to create a body comprised of the three groups named in the Act – nurses, midwives and health visitors – in a ratio of four:one:one. Members of each professional group in each country were to opt into discrete parts of an electoral roll.[14] Elections to the National Boards would be held at five-yearly intervals, and the term of office of all members, both elected and appointed, would be of the same length. Following consultation with the shadow Boards, the Working Group also made recommendations on the size of their memberships. The 1979 Act allowed for each Board to have a maximum of forty-five members, with the exception of the National Board for Northern Ireland where the maximum was set at thirty-five. The Working Group recommended that the English National Board should consist forty-five members (thirty elected, and fifteen appointed), the National Board for Scotland, thirty-six members (twenty-four elected and twelve appointed), and the Welsh and the Northern Ireland National Boards thirty-five members (both with twenty-four elected and eleven appointed).[15] Council membership, too, was agreed at the maximum allowable in the Act – that is forty-five members, two-thirds of whom were to be members of the National Boards, nominated by them in equal numbers and including at least two practising nurses, one midwife and one health visitor, and one person engaged in professional education.[16] Following a meeting with Ministers from the four Health Departments, the relevant statutory instrument was prepared and came into force on 31 July 1982.[17] During the autumn of 1982, around 118,700 nurses, midwives and health visitors had opted in to the new electoral roll and, following the nomination of 441 candidates, the ballot for the membership of the first National Boards took place during April and May of 1983. Over 62,000 ballot papers were returned, and on 17 June 1983 the election results were made public.[18]

The work on the election scheme had provided a first opportunity for generating wider awareness of the new statutory structures among the professions. The drafting of proposals for elections, indeed, was the Council's first exercise in consultation and was felt by members to 'have implications for the long term development of the Council as a representative and participative body.'[19] It also gave rise to a strong supportive statement in the House by the Minister for Health, Kenneth Clarke, who asserted that the 'whole point' of the 'Briggs structure' was to enable the professions to be 'self-regulating and to have control over their training, discipline and development'.[20] Electoral and representation issues were not fully settled at this point, however. It remained for the reconstituted Council to consider procedures for subsequent elections and for Council members to experience the dilemmas and ambiguities of being elected to one body and thereafter appointed to another.

Internal channels of representation

Working Group 5 was given responsibility to recommend the composition and terms of reference of the statutory Standing Committees outlined in the primary legislation. These were a Finance and a Midwifery Committee at both Council and National Board level, and a Joint Committee of Council and the Boards for Health Visiting. The Group was also asked to consider whether further committees should be established to assist Council execute its regulatory functions. The need for new Practice Rules for midwifery to be agreed by the Midwifery Committee and drafted in time for the handover of functions in July 1983 gave a particular urgency to the task.[21]

Remitting the question of the establishment of the Central Council Finance Committee to the Finance and General Purposes Sub-Committee of the Shadow Council enabled the working group to concentrate on arrangements for the two statutory standing professional committees. Complex questions of how far delegation of functions could or should occur, and the precise nature of the relationship between committees and their parent bodies proved difficult to resolve.[22] A number of the decisions taken at this point were later reversed, having been criticised as cumbersome and inefficient by the management consultants appointed to review the working of the 1979 Act (see Chapters 3 and 7). The other principal area of debate was membership of the professional committees. In both cases, the initial proposals of the working group were criticised during consultation with the profession as not containing a sufficient majority for the group in question, and both were subsequently revised.[23] There was more agreement that the professional committees would need adequate professional support. It was agreed that a professional officer for midwifery should be appointed by the UKCC as soon as possible. It was also agreed that UKCC and National Board staff concerned with health visiting matters should meet together regularly to discuss professional developments.

Working on the principle that it would be better to introduce as few committees as possible at this stage, so as not to perpetuate unnecessary divisions, the Group recommended a broad-based Educational Policy Advisory Committee (EPAC). This was to consider all aspects of educational policy across the range of nursing specialties and across the UK as a whole. Reactions from the professions were mixed. While the case was generally accepted,[24] a considerable number of responses indicated the desire for standing committees in specific areas of clinical practice (particularly mental illness and mental handicap) and for a separate committee for continuing clinical education. Other comments showed concern over the relationship between EPAC and the other professional committees and the lack of consensus over membership issues, particularly over the proportion of seats reserved for each occupational and professional group. Although sympathetic to these anxieties, the Working Group affirmed its intention to recommend the establishment of a single committee for professional education.

One area of nursing, though, was felt to be something of a special case. District nursing not only had had its own training body, the Panel of Assessors for District Nurse Training (PADNT), with responsibility for the setting of standards across the UK, but in September 1981 possession of the Panel's Certificate was made a mandatory requirement for those wishing to practise as district nurses. 'After years of some uncertainty and scarce resources', the Working Group suggested, real achievements were being made. It was 'imperative' that this 'momentum' should not be lost with the handover of statutory responsibilities.[25] In particular, expertise in district nurse education needed to be harnessed. Not all within the Shadow Council were convinced that the case for a separate district nursing committee was sufficiently strong. Some felt that a single primary health care committee might offer a better way forward. After further consideration, the Working Group maintained its original stance: for the time being, at least, district nursing would benefit from the support of a standing committee.[26] The proposal was finally carried in Council, with the proviso that the work of the District Nursing Joint Committee (DNJC) be reviewed before the end of the first full term of office. The necessary statutory instruments were duly prepared for the EPAC and the DNJC, with both coming into force in June 1983.[27]

Establishing a single professional register

The establishment of a single professional register of nurses, midwives and health visitors for the whole of the United Kingdom was remitted to Working Group 2, which over the period 1981–82 identified two broad issues. The first concerned the mechanisms of the registration process and the physical assimilation of the registers, rolls and records of the nine bodies which the Central Council and the National Boards were to replace. The second concerned the concept of registration itself.

Assimilation of records was a 'formidable task', not least because of the huge scale of the documentation, amounting to around 1.25 million individual entries. Moreover, since there had not been a common basis for recording information and since in a mainly female profession there were changes of name on marriage, there were considerable difficulties in reconciling data held by the different bodies. Some of the extant bodies recorded only names and not registration or enrolment numbers, and not all changes of name were notified to the statutory and training bodies. Individual nurses, midwives and health visitors registered with one statutory body, therefore, had to be 'matched' against the entries of another.[28] Each body also used sequential registration numbers, so that the same number reference could refer to a different person and a different qualification.[29] To make matters worse, some of the records of district nurses had been lost. During the summer and autumn of 1982 a special exercise needed to be undertaken to collect and update information about district nurses to supplement the records held by the PADNT.[30] Assimilation also raised a number of technical questions, including the exploration of the best available computer technology. The GNC for England and Wales had already computerised its records and its system was taken as the starting point for the new single register.[31] Following discussions with the National Boards it was agreed that a jointly developed and managed system incorporating the registration requirements of the Central Council and the training records of the National Boards was the best way forward. This became known as SPRINT-UK – 'Single Professional Register and Index of Training'.[32]

Consideration was also given to the division of the register into Parts to indicate different qualifications and kinds of training. Existing training arrangements meant that entry to the profession could be made through a number of 'gates' – through general nursing care, nursing for the mentally ill, nursing for the mentally handicapped (each at first and second level), nursing of sick children and midwifery. These were confirmed by the working group and a total of eleven parts was agreed (these were later to be extended, see Appendix 2). Criteria for the recording of additional qualifications, such as certificates in district, occupational health and school nursing, and in professional education, were also agreed.[33] Discussions on these issues were punctuated by expressions of disquiet from the district nursing lobby. The former training body for district nursing, the PADNT, in particular, expressed concern over the decision not to introduce a specific part of the register for those with the Certificate in District Nursing or its equivalent.[34] The Parts of the Register Order (SI 1983 No 667) was signed in April 1983, enabling the Council to assume responsibility for registering all nurses, midwives and health visitors in the United Kingdom and also for evaluating applications for registration from practitioners educated overseas from July of that year.

Developing the idea of 'effective' registration

Working Group 2 did not confine its interests solely to the mechanisms and processes of registration; it also considered just what registration should denote. While the prime function of the register was 'to protect the public by providing a means of verifying that a person holds a specific qualification or qualifications',[35] there was an important distinction to be drawn between 'current competence and a competence once achieved'.[36] An 'effective' register, the Group argued, should be one that ensured that those registered were currently fit to practise. The new legislation, with its separation between qualification (the business of the Boards) and registration (the business of the Council) opened up new possibilities. The registering authority could not deny anyone the professional qualifications they had once earned, but it could stipulate additional conditions for maintaining eligibility to practise. The Working Group's proposals included the introduction of an upper age limit for registration, the possible extension of midwifery's 'notification of intention to practise' process to nurses and health visitors, the imposition of a mandatory period of re-orientation or refresher training for those returning to practice after a period of prolonged absence and the need to undertake updating courses (both of these were also already statutorily required of midwives). Since this enlarged concept of registration would require additional resources, the introduction of a system of periodic fees was proposed.[37]

Consultation undertaken during the shadow period revealed broad support for such ideas in the professions (though concern about practicalities). There were doubts, however, from the Council's legal advisors as to whether these attempts to draw a distinction between registration and entitlement to practise could be incorporated within the terms of the Act which, after all, provided for only one statutory register.[38] Council handled this by treating the ideas offered by the Working Group favourably, but as part of a longer-term agenda. The Working Group's deliberations marked an early commitment by the UKCC to a set of issues that were to take up considerable time later in its lifetime (see Chapter 6). This matter, moreover, was to rise up the regulatory agenda, not only in the field of nursing, but more generally in health and social care as issues of competence and performance came more to the fore.[39]

Professional discipline and conduct

Although the 1979 Act allocated the preliminary investigation of potential misconduct to Boards, it gave considerable scope to Council to rethink both the procedures of professional conduct work and the underlying rationale. First, the legislation gave Council the power to remove names from the register for reasons of misconduct 'or otherwise'.[40] The 'or otherwise' clause paved the way for removal on the grounds of unfitness to practice owing to ill-health. Second, both in the fitness to practise area and in the area of misconduct hearings more generally, it was left to the statutory body to decide its own procedures and rules of evidence. Thirdly, Council was explicitly required to 'improve' standards of professional conduct, and given new powers to advise registrants on the standards expected of them. Working Group 4 of the Shadow Council seized the opportunities afforded by these legislative provisions, building on steps taken by the former statutory bodies, particularly the GNC for England and Wales, and on recent debates within the medical profession.[41]

Establishing a basis for a Health Committee created an entirely new strand in the professional conduct process. The former statutory bodies for nursing and midwifery had 'all too often' found themselves 'in possession of reports about practitioners who were clearly dangerous but about whom they could do nothing' or, alternatively, using 'the awesome power of the statutory body's disciplinary machine and a public hearing to deal with someone whose basic problem was their illness'.[42] Members of the Shadow Council (and, as far as consultation responses indicated, the wider professions) were happy to use this opportunity to introduce an entirely new dimension to the regulation of their professions.[43]

Appraising existing conduct procedures and creating a new set of Professional Conduct Rules gave an important opportunity to reflect upon the broad principles of professional discipline.[44] The purpose of the disciplinary machinery, Working Group 4 stressed, was public protection and the maintenance of public confidence in professional standards. Thus, although the exercise of professional discipline might carry the penalty of removal from the register, it was not to be regarded primarily as a punitive process.[45] This approach to professional discipline was also reflected in the decision, later ratified by Council, to continue the statutory bodies' association with the Nurses' Welfare Service, a charitable organisation created under the auspices of the GNC for England and Wales in 1972 to provide support for practitioners involved in disciplinary proceedings. While some reservations were expressed, members generally felt that the service provided a useful function and could help to reinforce the message that the prime function of professional discipline was not the punishment of the individual practitioner but the broader aim of public protection.[46]

The group's focus upon public protection gave rise to the question of whether a complainant, aggrieved by a decision of the investigating committee of a National Board not to forward a case to a disciplinary hearing at the UKCC, should be allowed the right of appeal. Granting a right of appeal, the group argued, would indicate to the wider community that the statutory bodies were determined to give 'paramount consideration to the interests of the public' in all elements of the disciplinary process. Negative reaction to the proposal from the former statutory bodies, the National Boards and a wide range of staff organisations, however, encouraged the Shadow Council not to press the issue, and interest subsequently faded.[47]

Working Group 4's proposals were endorsed by Council in October 1982. The remaining period was spent on the complicated task of preparing draft Rules which could accommodate both Council's decisions and the requirements of the 1979 Act. The relevant statutory instrument was passed less than a month from the 'appointed day'.[48] Although allegations of professional misconduct had continued to be investigated and heard by the former bodies during the shadow period, a heavy backlog of cases had accumulated by the point of handover. This meant an immediate and extremely heavy professional conduct workload for the new members – a problem that was to cause considerable concern both within and beyond the Council for a number of years.

Creating a Code of Professional Conduct

The principal outcome of the new power to 'improve' standards and give advice, was the publication of a Code of Professional Conduct, the prime purpose of which was to inform and advise practitioners of their duties as professional nurses, midwives and health visitors. The former statutory bodies, over time, had responded to individual requests for advice, and in some instances had even produced advisory material on specific topics such as advertising. These *ad hoc* developments, however, had not been based on explicit legislative provision. The new opportunity was quickly appreciated by the Shadow UKCC, not least by its new Director of Professional Conduct and Registration, who was given lead responsibility for the drafting of the first edition of the Code.[49] The production of such a document, however, also reflected a more limiting aspect of the new legislation. The absence of a specific power to reprimand or deprecate the conduct of a practitioner whose actions, though inappropriate or undesirable, were not considered by the Preliminary Proceedings Committee of the National Boards as constituting a possible case of professional misconduct serious enough to warrant removal from the register was felt to be a worrying omission.[50] Drawing attention to a Code of Conduct was deemed to be a useful tool to fill this gap.

The first edition of the *Code of Professional Conduct for Nurses, Midwives and Health Visitors* was issued to all those admitted to the Register after July 1983. Copies were also widely distributed to established practitioners through nurse educationalists and senior managers in the NHS and the private sector. By 31 March 1984, over 300,000 copies of the pocket-sized document had been issued.[51] Representatives of the Council addressed meetings, seminars and study days on the aims and purposes of the Code. It was not, they insisted, an attempt to define misconduct (this was to be evaluated on a case-by-case basis) but rather a back-cloth against which allegations of misconduct made against nurses, midwives and health visitors could be judged. The Code sought to move nurses in particular away from a view of themselves as carrying out assigned tasks, encouraging them instead to be more questioning. It also put a considerable onus on them to report circumstances that might endanger safe standards of practice – including inadequate resources and work overload.[52] A note at the end of the first edition stated the Council's intention to review the Code annually, and members of the professions were asked to submit their comments. Reg Pyne has recalled that over 4,000 comments were received and that the second edition, coming out the following year, was the subject of a meeting 'running deep into the night' with Council Chairman Catherine Hall and four other Council members.[53] It was an important and innovative step and was to continue to give a high profile to the Council.

Entry to the register and the reform of pre-registration education

For many of those inside as well as outside the statutory structure, the question of training for entry to the single professional register was the most pressing issue of all. Primary legislation now not only required the UKCC to determine, through Rules, the conditions of entry to pre-registration training, and the kind and standard of such programmes of education, but to work to improve standards in this area. The matter had now been on the table for approaching a decade.

Since the Training Rules of the former statutory bodies were due to lapse on the 30 June 1983, the most immediate requirement was the drafting of a new set of Rules which, at the very least, would maintain the status quo in nurse, midwife and health visitor training. In the event, Working Group 3 was able to suggest a number of significant innovations which began the process of building greater flexibility and freedom into Training Rules. Two new and broadly defined Rules were proposed. The first concerned the objectives to be achieved by a course of preparation for registration. Training was now 'described in terms of outcomes rather than processes through which a learner must pass'.[54] The UKCC circular announcing the changes explained that nurse training should now 'provide opportunities to enable the student to accept responsibility for her personal professional development and to acquire a specified set of competencies relating to the care of the particular type of patient with whom she is likely to come into contact when registered in a specific part or parts of the register'. This change in style was intended to reflect developments already occurring in many programmes of nursing education, especially the move away from a 'task-oriented' approach to nursing.[55] The second change related to the criteria to assess suitability for training. In large part this reflected the need to assimilate the different arrangements for entry existing in the several parts of the UK, but it also indicated a growing interest in additional methods of selection. The new Rules allowed the existing practices in each country to continue until 1 January 1986 when the minimum requirement for all first level entrants would be either five 'O' level GCE passes at A, B or C, or equivalent, or success in the Council's new entrance test. Two other specific changes were also made to the Rules. The minimum age of entry to training was set at 17½ years, and in certain circumstances, at 17 years, and it was agreed that the terminology used to differentiate between 'registered' and 'enrolled' nurses should be 'first' and 'second' level nurse.[56] How far this went towards meeting Briggs's vision of flexibility and accessibility is a moot point.

The activities of the Working Group, however, went further than this. While Council had agreed that the changeover to the new statutory bodies 'should be managed with as little disruption [as possible] to existing educational schemes', Working Group 3 was also encouraged to consider the philosophy that might govern the future direction of professional education.[57] This was particularly important given the legislation's silence on this matter and the high expectations that had built up since Briggs. Two main problems were encountered. First, the exploration of a future framework for education and training meant that the Group was working at the sensitive and still unclear interface between Council and Board responsibilities. Working Group 3 accepted that the National Boards needed maximum flexibility to develop training programmes that were responsive to local conditions. On the other hand, legal advice indicated that Council had to set clear overall standards and could not simply delegate functions to the National Boards. Attempts to walk this tightrope at times led to tension between the two tiers. The English National Board (ENB), in particular, felt that the Shadow Council had insufficient appreciation of the boundaries between central and national functions in this area. Second, the Working Group found that its decision to issue two wide-ranging consultation documents outlining its preliminary thoughts on the future of nursing and midwifery education had the result of increasing anxieties far more than inspiring hope in the possibilities of reform.[58] Particular controversy surrounded its tentative proposal for a single standard of entry to the profession through qualification as a 'registered' nurse. Enrolled nurses were quick to see this as evidence of an uncertain future in the profession. Controversy and confusion also surrounded the Group's exploration of the introduction of a 'common core' for all kinds of pre-registration nurse training and its rather ambiguous statements on the status of the nursing student. In the light of all this uncertainty, the Working Group declined to make any firm recommendations to Council but rather chose to present its report as the first step in an on-going process of discussion. The Shadow Council agreed that it would be inappropriate for an all-appointed body to determine policy on issues that were of such importance to the future direction of the professions. It would be for the reconstituted Council to decide the best way forward.

The wider organisation

Alongside this substantial array of professional issues, the personnel and accommodation needs of the new organisation needed to be planned, and steps had to be taken to follow through on decisions made. The responsibilities of Working Group 6 included monitoring the progress of the subordinate legislation, management of the single professional register and associated computer developments, and making arrangements for the transfer and recruitment of staff.[59] Discussions were held with the Health Departments and with the existing bodies whose staff would be affected. A Joint Staff Consultative Committee, with trade union, professional associations and employee representatives, together with a Management Policy Advisory Group comprising members of both the new and old bodies, helped facilitate this.[60]

Working Group 7, a small group containing representatives from the Council and Boards and the Chief Officers of the existing bodies, was responsible for estimating the accommodation needs of the new bodies and identifying the assets that would be transferred to them on the 'appointed day'. A largely inconclusive round of discussions took place between June 1981 and July 1982, when the former bodies decided to exercise their right to dispose of their assets directly. The Central Council, however, did arrange to take over the property of the GNC for England and Wales at 23 Portland Place. Although a major renovation was necessary, with no fire certificate on the building and surveyors' reports indicating that most of the essential services – heating, plumbing, lighting – needed complete overhaul, the location and the long lease on the property made it the best option, as well as one of the cheapest.[61] The Council took possession of its premises on 30 June 1983.

While the costs of establishing the Central Council were met by the four Health Departments, members and senior officers regarded long-term financial independence from Whitehall as essential for a regulatory body. Achieving this, however, was not going to be straightforward. Apart from a single payment of £60,000 (a proportion of the financial assets of the GNC for Scotland) the UKCC inherited no financial assets from the former bodies. The organisation inherited the net liabilities of the GNC for England and Wales (about £30,000), and the Council and the National Boards became responsible for payments to the pensioners of former bodies, for which no continuing financial provision had been made.[62] During its first year, the Shadow Council examined the future financing of the organisation, and work continued on this crucial issue throughout the shadow period and into the first full term.

Conclusion

Creating a new framework for the shared regulation of nursing, midwifery and health visiting across the UK was no easy matter. The sheer scale of the administrative task of assimilating records and procedures was formidable. The matter of designing systems and establishing new roles and relationships was complex. The demands of work within statute was challenging even for experienced officers and a novel experience for some of the members. The Working Groups of the Shadow Council did not 'solve' all of the issues that came before them. But, in a relatively short period of time, they had indicated the intention of the new regulatory bodies to take their statutory responsibilities to establish and improve professional standards extremely seriously. Many of the matters raised during this important period of transition were to reverberate through the following three Council terms of office as outside forces brought new challenges to health care professionals and as different constituencies within and beyond nursing and midwifery came to view the structures and processes of professional self-regulation in new ways.

Notes

1 The Act was passed in April 1979. A general election held the following month brought the Conservative party to power for a period of 17 years.
2 The term 'chairman' was in use at this point at the UKCC and thus it is used here (see Chapter 1, note 7).
3 *Report of the Committee of Inquiry into the Regulation of the Medical Profession* (Merrison Report) London, HMSO, 1975, p. ii.
4 Two people were seconded from the DHSS but, from the outset, Catherine Hall insisted that the Council should be able to appoint its own members of staff. A skeleton staff was built up gradually between 1981 and 1983.
5 Maude Storey took the additional title of Registrar from the date of handover of functions. The position has remained a combined one of chief executive and registrar though the terminology has varied slightly between the different incumbents.
6 UKCC, *The First Twelve Months*, London, UKCC, 1981, p. 7.
7 The shadow Council and its staff were initially accommodated at the offices of the Queen's Nursing Institute at 57 Lower Belgrave Street, London. In May 1982, the staff moved to 110 Euston Road. The final move, to 23 Great Portland Street, took place on 30 June 1983.
8 *The Nurses, Midwives and Health Visitors Act, 1979*, Section 1 (4).
9 The opportunity for parliament to debate statutory instruments is limited. Under the negative procedures a statutory instrument has the force of law unless either House votes to annul it within forty days. Under the less usual affirmative procedure statutory instruments require positive approval of both Houses. The times during which motions can be debated are very restricted and very few are debated in the Commons at all. Furthermore, statutory instruments cannot be amended: they must either be accepted

or annulled. Commentators have pointed to the need for such mechanisms in order to speed the business of government, but they also suggest that the increasing volume of this secondary legislation might diminish Parliament's role in lawmaking very substantially: Silk, P. and R. Walters, *How Parliament Works*, London, Longman (third edn), 1995, p. 149. These authors point out that there has been unease in both Houses over bills with a Henry VIII clause, that is enabling primary legislation to be repeated by secondary legislation without further parliamentary scrutiny, over skeleton bills, and over the extent of use of the weaker, negative procedure.

10 These were Working Group 1, Elections to the National Boards; Working Group 2, Single Professional Register; Working Group 3, Education and Training; Working Group 4, Professional Conduct; Working Group 5, Standing and Joint Committees; Working Group 6, Handover of Functions; Working Group 7, Accommodation and Property. Details of their activities are covered below.

11 The former statutory bodies with an elected element, the GNC for England and Wales, the GNC for Scotland, the CMB Scotland, and the Northern Ireland Council for Nurses and Midwives, utilised a number of different electoral schemes, UKCC, Elect 1.1, 'Proposals in respect of an electoral scheme – Consultation paper', May 1981, pp. 2–6. For the experiences of the GNC for England and Wales, see Bendall, E. and E. Raybould, *A History of the General Nursing Council for England and Wales, 1919–69*, London, H. K. Lewis and Co., 1969, pp. 29, 65–7, 165.

12 UKCC, Elect 1.1, 'Proposals for an electoral scheme. A consultation paper', 1981, p. 16.

13 UKCC, Elect 1.1, CC/82/6, 'Proposals for an electoral scheme. A report by Working Group 1', 1982, p. 13.

14 An opt-in procedure was necessary as there was no single up-to-date list of registrants. See later for the UKCC's work on assimilating and updating registration information.

15 UKCC, Elect 1.1, CC/82/6, 'Proposals for an electoral scheme. A report by Working Group 1', 1982, pp. 14–15.

16 *Nurses, Midwives and Health Visitors Act, 1979*, Sect.1.(3) (a), Sch. 1, Part 1 (1). See also MIN 21/82 (4–8), 1982.

17 SI 1982 No. 1104.

18 *Annual Report 1983/84*, p. 15–16. The numbers opting in to the electoral roll and then voting were very small compared to what was later shown to be half a million on the register.

19 UKCC, Elect 1.1, Elect/81/11, 'Presentation of the electoral scheme', 1981.

20 *Parliamentary Debates* [Commons], 27 July 1982, cols 1019–31, contained in Elect 1.1.

21 See chapter 7 pp. 145–6.

22 UKCC, COM1.1, Working Group 5, 'Standing and Joint Committees. A first consultation paper', January 1982, p. 4; notes of second meeting of Working Group 5, 13 August 1981; notes of ninth meeting of Working Group 5, 31 March 1982.

23 CC/81/70, p. 11.

24 Notable exceptions from this consensus were the GNC (Scotland) and the Committee for Clinical Nursing Studies. In addition, the National Board for Nursing, Midwifery and Health Visiting for Scotland (NBS) expressed doubts as to the feasibility of setting up the committee in the immediate term. See UKCC, COM/82/26, 'Working Group 5: response from the profession to the second consultation paper', pp. 2–3.

25 UKCC, COM1.1, Working Group 5, 'Second consultation paper', May 1982, p. 2.

26 UKCC, COM1.1, notes of thirteenth meeting of Working Group 5, 1 November 1982.

27 Nurses, Midwives and Health Visitors Act (Educational Policy Advisory Committee) Order 1983 SI No. 726; Nurses, Midwives and Health Visitors Act (District Nursing Joint Committee) Order 1983 SI No. 724.

28 *Annual Report 1983/84*, pp. 17–18.

29 This, of course, was the reason for the use of the Professional Identification Number (P.I.N.).

30 Coping with applications for restoration was another problem, given the manner of how the information was kept. To this day, the UKCC receives applications for restoration from people who had been removed from the registers of the former bodies.

31 UKCC, L2.1.1, 'The formation of the single professional register. A report from Working Group 2', April 1982, p. 1.

32 The contract for developing and managing the system was awarded to EDS computer bureau. The arrangement lasted until 1988, when three of the Boards decided to withdraw from the shared system.

33 Details of the qualifications which the Central Council agreed should be recorded on the register can be found at *Annual Report 1983/84*, Annex 4.

34 Although, as a non-statutory body, the PADNT had not defined a set of statutory rules for district nurse training, detailed regulations concerning entrance to courses, course content and duration, competencies to be achieved and the type and form of the qualifying examinations had been in place for some time. Moreover, since September 1981, possession of the certificate had been mandatory for those wishing to practise as a district nurse. It appears that the PADNT had been under the impression that this arrangement would be cemented under the new regulatory arrangements by the introduction of a specific district nursing part of the single professional register. The question of district nurse registration returned to the agenda in 1984. See CC/84/C16 and MIN 98/84, July 1984.

35 UKCC, L2.1.1, 'The single professional register – Consultation paper', November 1981, p. 2.

36 UKCC, L2.1.1, 'The formation of the single professional register. A report from Working Group 2', April 1982, p. 6.

37 Ibid. See also notes of tenth meeting of Working Group 2, 20 May 1982.

38 UKCC, L2.1.1, notes of eleventh meeting of Working Group 2, 21 June 1982. DHSS lawyers also felt that difficulties might be encountered with the EC. The introduction of refresher courses for nurses it was argued, could be seen as an infringement of the EC's Directive on the General Care Nurse.

39 Interestingly, the Merrison Committee had stopped short of recommending similar strategies for medicine in the mid-1970s, on the ground that it was too great a change of approach to regulation. Re-licensure was felt to be 'sufficiently important and complex' a matter 'to warrant a separate inquiry of its own'. The medical profession duly conducted its own examination of the issue through a committee consisting of representatives of the specialist Royal Colleges and Faculties in England and Scotland, the RCGP, BMA, Councils of Postgraduate Medical Education, and of Community Medicine, which was set up to look at the issue of re-licensure. Its terms of reference were 'to review the present methods of ensuring the maintenance of standards of continuing competence to practise and of the clinical care of patients, and to make recommendations'. Interestingly, the committee was chaired by Mr E. A. J. Alment, a medical practitioner who was one of the Secretary of State appointees to the Shadow UKCC. See *Report of the Committee of Inquiry into the Regulation of the Medical Profession*, paras 162–5.

40 *Nurses, Midwives and Health Visitors Act, 1979*, Section 12(1).

41 For developments in medicine see *Report of the Committee of Inquiry into the Regulation of the Medical Profession*; the Medical Act, 1978. See also Stacey, M., *Regulating British Medicine. The General Medical Council*, Chichester, John Wiley and Sons, 1992.

42 Pyne, R., *Professional Discipline in Nursing, Midwifery and Health Visiting* (third edn), Oxford, Blackwell Science, 1998, p. 70. Reg Pyne was the UKCC's first Director of Professional Conduct and Registration, having taken up post in February 1982. He had previously been Deputy Registrar at the GNC (England and Wales).

43 MIN 78/82, October 1982, p. 2. Medicine had been required to establish a 'fitness to practise' process under the terms of the 1978 Medical Act. Primary legislation for the regulation of nursing, midwifery and health visiting was far less restrictive, however.

44 UKCC, M2.1.1, notes of first meeting of Working Group 4, 10 July 1981.

45 UKCC, M2.1.1, 'Working Group 4 – Professional Conduct. Consultation paper', April 1982; 'Working Group 4 – Professional Conduct. Proposals in respect of removal from and restoration to the register and allied matters. A report to Central Council with recommendations', October 1982.

46 UKCC, M2.1.1, notes of second meeting of Working Group 4, 15 September 1981; third meeting, 6 November 1981; fifth meeting, 19 February 1982; seventh meeting 15 April 1982. See also Pyne, *Professional Discipline* (second edn), 1992, pp. 52–9.

47 UKCC, M2.1.1, Working Group 4, 'A report to the Central Council with recommendations', October 1982, p. 7; MIN 78/82. Interestingly, the question was later to be revived in a late 1990s legislative review, which concentrated on public protection as the rationale for redesigning regulation (see chapter 9).

48 The Nurses, Midwives and Health Visitors (Professional Conduct) Rules 1983 Approval Order 1983, SI No. 887; The Nurses, Midwives and Health Visitors (Professional Conduct) Rules 1983 Approval Order (Northern Ireland) 1983, SI (Northern Ireland) No. 153.

49 Pyne's interpretation of the new power can be found in his *Professional Discipline* (second edn), 1992, pp. 25–32; (third edn), 1998, pp. 48–53. In drafting the Code, Pyne found inspiration in the 1973 *Code for Nurses* produced by the International Council of Nurses, and in the American Nurses Association's *Code for Nurses with Interpretative Statements*, published in 1976. Pyne's draft text was discussed by the Shadow Council and circulated to the National Boards for their comments. Following further Council discussion, the revised draft was remitted to a six-member group for final drafting. See CMIN 27/83; MIN 29/83(d); MIN 45/83(a); CC/83/C24; CC/83/15.

50 The previous statutory bodies did have the power to criticise a person's conduct and to reprimand or warn him or her for particular conduct. See UKCC, M2.1.1, notes of the ninth meeting of Working Group 4 on Professional Conduct, 5 August 1982 and Working Group 4, 'Proposals in respect of removal from and restoration to the register and allied matters. A report to Central Council with recommendations', 11 October 1982, pp. 8–9. See also Howie, C., 'New code, old problems', *Nursing Times*, 1 June, 79(22), 1983, p. 14.

51 *Annual Report 1983/84*, p. 32.

52 See Pyne, R., 'Grasping the legal nettle', *Nursing Times*, 28 September, 79(39), 1983, pp. 36–7; *Annual Report 1983/84*, pp. 56–7.

53 Pyne, R., 'Foreword', in Heywood Jones, I. (ed.), *The UKCC Code of Conduct: A critical guide*, London, NT Books, 1999. See also MIN 60/84(b); CC/84/62; CC/84/118.

54 This is seen, for instance, in Rules 18 and 18(2) of Part III of the 1983 Nurses, Midwives and Health Visitors Rules, SI 1983, No. 873. It was an approach that was to be further embedded during Project 2000. See chapter 4 for further discussion.

55 UKCC, PS&D/83/02, Nurse Training Rules, 1983.

56 *Ibid.*

57 CC/80/10, pp. 4–5.

58 UKCC, K3.1, Working Group 3 Consultation Paper, 'Education and Training: The development of nurse education', 1982; Working Group 3, 'Education and Training: Report to the UKCC following consultation with the professions', 1982.

59 For details of the activities of this group see CC/81/70 and CC/81/36 p. 4.

60 CC/82/C7.

61 *Annual Report 1983/84*, p. 39.

62 *Ibid.*, p. 40. See also UKCC, *Account 1983–1984*, London, HMSO, 1984.

3 Three Councils, 1983–98

There was much to do to follow up the ambitious programmes of activity initiated by the Working Groups in the shadow period. Creating a new framework for pre-registration education was perhaps paramount, but there was also an urgent need to deal with the backlog of professional conduct cases. The question of UK-wide midwives' rules was also particularly pressing. Furthermore, establishing a single professional register with up-to-date information on all those in practice in the UK, was going to be feat of immense proportions. Once that was in place, and once the process of collecting periodic fees started, not only would Council be on a stronger and more independent footing, but more effective communication between Council and those on its register could begin. In all these activities, everyone was aware of two major challenges. One was ensuring that the voice of 'minorities' was heard. The other was the question of just what the relationship between Council and National Boards was to be. Neither of these issues was to be resolved quickly or with ease.

This chapter gives an overview of the three Councils between 1983 and 1998. This serves as a preliminary map, pointing to some of the well-known landmarks as well as introducing issues that are often less well known by those who have not participated in the statutory structure.

Foundation-building: The First Council, November 1983–September 1988

The group of members attending the first meeting of the re-constituted Council on 18 November 1983, forty-five people in all, was considerably larger than the Shadow Council of thirty-three. There was now an elected component – albeit that members had been elected to Boards and not directly to Council itself. Yet there was also a significant amount of continuity in that just over a quarter of the members of the new Council had also been members of the shadow bodies.

Over the next five years, Council was to meet formally on more than thirty occasions, usually for both an open and a closed session of business. Extraordinary, special and private meetings were held in addition to this, often for a period before formal business started. An extraordinary meeting could be very brief. It took just ten minutes on 19 July 1987, when the new statutory instrument came into effect that enabled Council to elect its own chairman, to decide to ask Dame Catherine Hall to remain in the chair until her appointed term of office ran out at the end of October. Extraordinary meetings, however, could also take up more time and be of great significance for debates about the overall direction of the work. This was the case when it came to discussing the objectives and overall strategy for the First Council, as will be seen below.

From the outset, it was clear that demands on the time of Council members were going to be high. Papers had to be digested and Council meetings attended every two months. There were also other committees to attend, all with their own timetables and business to cover. All members were involved in professional conduct business and hearings were often stressful as well as time-consuming. Work on the EPAC became doubly onerous once the decision was taken that the whole committee would act as the project group for Project 2000 (see Chapter 4). Council members could also find themselves commenting on drafts of documents or on occasion submitting papers for discussion themselves.[1]

The structure of committees and sub-committees had already been established in the shadow period. The Finance Committee and the Midwifery Committee were standing committees as specified in the Act. Joint committees for health visiting and district nursing had been agreed, and terms of reference set for these and for the professional conduct, health and educational policy committees. To complete the picture, the Registration Committee met as and when there was business to carry out, and a Committee on Research was established.[2] The exact membership of Council and of committees, both of which, of course, changed somewhat through the five years through resignations and replacements, can be traced through the Annual Reports.

To service these committees and to carry out the business of the Council, the UKCC had an agreed establishment of 112. This was a smaller figure than the 151 originally estimated by the Health Departments, and the total staff for most of the period of the First Council was 100 or less. Staff were organised under three directors, each reporting to Maude Storey as Registrar and Chief Executive. Professional Conduct and Registration, under the professional leadership of Reg Pyne, managed all matters associated with the machinery of deciding on cases of professional misconduct and ill-health. Professional Standards and Development, under Peta Allen, included Professional Officers for Midwifery, Health Visiting and Nursing. Later a grade of professional adviser was added to cope with the range of work in the nursing area and in particular the volume of requests for advice. Staff reporting to Mike Hanson as Director of Administration included the finance officer and personnel officer (this post having responsibility for committee services and establishment matters). By 1985, there had been some adjustments, in particular moving the registration department's line of account-ability to Director of Administration.[3]

'Into the 90s' – a difficult passage

A three-day meeting was hosted by the King's Fund Staff College early in March of 1984 where the overall strategy for the five years of office of the Council began to be discussed. The end result was *Into the 90s – A Plan for Action for the UKCC*. It included four broad objectives to be achieved over the first five year term (see Figure 3.1).[4]

Behind these objectives lay a period of intense debate which was to exemplify the uneasy relationships which had been set up in legislation between the National Boards and Council. At the three-day meeting, it had been clear that all bodies needed to work closely together. Collaboration was written into the Act, but it was also essential if the legislative arrangement whereby Council was to 'establish and improve' standards was to function properly. It was also important to avoid duplication of effort and, not least, to let the professions know and understand the new arrangements. The paper that came to an extraordinary meeting on 30 March set out, as its first objective, the strengthening of the statutory structure. It was noted that the five bodies already shared work in relation to professional conduct (Boards having the duty to undertake the investigatory function). They were also co-operating in a shared computer system which provided both the individual training records necessary for the Boards and the data for the register. It was not intended, the paper was quick to stress, that Council would dictate to the Boards, but rather that the five bodies should work in harmony.[5] But difficult questions were raised. Was there enough cross-membership? What was the role of the officers? Should Boards be able to exercise a veto? Ultimately, the specific objective of strengthening the overall structure was set aside. The final introduction underlined that that Council and Boards were committed to developing the new statutory arrangements. It stressed a philosophy of 'unity but not necessarily . . . uniformity',[6] and was presented as a strategy largely for the UKCC rather than for the five bodies as a whole.

Between the changes of text there had been a great deal of discussion at Council, in its Committees and at the four Boards. Prior to a formal session of Council on 30 March, members split into small groups for a whole morning of discussion of the draft document. They agreed to send in proposed changes within a week

- to determine an education and training policy and programme to ensure that nurses, midwives and health visitors who are trained and registered meet the needs of society in the 1990s and beyond;
- to promote a heightened awareness amongst nurses, midwives and health visitors of (i) professional standards (ii) the responsibilities and opportunities of being members of professions;
- to develop perceptions of professional conduct positively and to improve standards of professional conduct, and in dealing with matters of professional misconduct to ensure a consistency of approach throughout the UK;
- to make the Central Council financially viable and a cost-effective and efficient organisation.

Figure 3.1 Strategic objectives of the First Council

before the document went out to the four Boards for their comments. For the Council meeting in June, they then received a substantial package of material.[7] The ENB had set detailed comments alongside specific paragraphs and had suggested redrafts throughout the whole of the document. It also made clear that it wished to comment on any redrafts. The Boards from Wales and Northern Ireland provided shorter and perhaps more positive comments, though they too were raising further issues. NBS comments were to be made available on the day. In addition to these contributions, there were papers from the two joint committees, from the Midwifery Committee, a particularly wide-ranging set of comments from the Committee on Research, as well as material from EPAC and the Finance Committee.[8]

The biggest single area of controversy centred on educational reform. Against that part of the text which proposed that EPAC should conduct the education and training review, the ENB outlined six areas of its work that it already had in hand under section 6 of the Act. 'There is concern', the Board stated, 'that the work of EPAC should not either restrict or be restricted by the work of the Boards'.[9] It was hard to see how this could be accomplished unless one body gave way to the other. This question of who was to carry out the pre-registration education review exercised all four Boards. Some comments were positive – there were offers, for example, from the Welsh Board to help and share resources on the review – but overall there was a definite thread of wariness about how collaboration was to work out, who would attend which meetings, and what papers needed to be shared. Other issues too were causing concern. The National Board for Scotland's tabled paper brought up the matter of professional conduct, putting the view that arrangements between Council and Boards needed to be 'harmonised not unified'.[10] And it was not just a matter of Boards. Each committee added its own comments. The amount and tone of these showed how very alert every interest group remained to the question of what the new statutory structure meant. It must have been a disheartening start for officers and particularly confusing for quite a number of members. Elected to the one body and appointed to the other – where should their loyalties lie?

On 26 June 1984, the Director of Administration wrote to each of the Chief Executive Officers of the Boards enclosing a revised draft.[11] The document had been shortened and now incorporated its comments on the five-body statutory structure in the introduction. On the matter of the education review, which was clearly causing so much disquiet, the letter set out options and asked for comment. Following this letter, *Into the 90s* was finalised and its text incorporated in the first Annual Report. It was now possible for senior staff to take and examine the agreed objectives and put forward plans for how each of their departments would seek to achieve them over the period of office of the First Council. That meeting took place at the end of February 1985.[12]

If anyone thought at that point that the question of the relationship between Boards and Council was beginning to settle, they were very soon proved wrong. A progress report on Project 2000 came forward for discussion at Council later in the month.[13] A proposal that the Project Group should now invite comments from the Boards was agreed. But what was the status of these comments? What indeed was the status of the ENB's report that had already set out a structure for future education, sought the opinion of the profession and had been forwarded to the Department of Health? It was quite clear from the debates that some still felt that Council was exceeding its powers by undertaking this work. Invitations to consult and collaborate had borne some fruit but something more had to be done if the work of the professions were to go forward more smoothly. With the agreement of the Chairmen of all the Boards, a formal legal opinion was sought by the UKCC, and it was reproduced in full at the May meeting together with a covering introduction and proposed way forward by the Chairman.[14]

Counsel's opinion described the UKCC as having an 'overseeing and initiating function and power' as far as education and training was concerned. The interpretation endorsed the concept of a hierarchy of function, whereby Council set standards UK-wide and the Boards 'subsidiary in the hierarchy of functions, should have the duty and the obligation of following those standards'.[15] This, it was immediately added, did not preclude the widest possible consultation and co-operation nor did it mean that there should be no variation of practice between the Boards. Council powers were widely drafted, setting out principal functions and implying that other powers may be adopted in order to carry these out; regarding Board powers the legal drafting was more narrowly defined. Circumspect as these comments were, however, the parting shot warned against trying to take this legal route further.

> I would not recommend proceedings of any kind except in the most extreme circumstances. The field with which I am concerned here seems to me, if I may respectfully say so, to be classically the one in which there should be the widest possible consultation and the most active collaboration. It is to be remembered that there is an intense public interest involved.[16]

A protracted process ensued. A joint working group including the five Chairmen, the five Chief Executive Officers and other members of both Council and Boards took on the task preparing a statement on roles, functions and operational policies. This eventually emerged, however, not as a landmark policy paper of Council but as a joint statement giving an account of points of agreement between Council and National Boards.[17] The statement affirmed that Council's approach in drafting Rules broadly enabled Boards to respond to the needs and opportunities of their countries. It was clarified that National Board members were not delegates – they would bring a Board perspective to Council discussions but debates at Council would be 'likely to be a determining influence on their vote'.[18] The bulk of the document however, was devoted to ways of working between officers.

Those who had faith in the power of the law as effecting a once and for all settlement had had that belief shaken by the progress of events through 1985 and 1986. The last-minute compromise drafting of the 1979 Act was taking a severe toll. Later, the conviction was to come that the law itself needed to be changed.

An 'eventful and successful term'?

Notwithstanding these protracted debates, many matters were taken forward in the term of the First Council. By 1988, the Project 2000 report had been issued and the proposals had been accepted in principle by Ministers. Other educational issues were also taken forward during this busy period. Council, for instance, had reached agreement on common and UK-wide alternative academic entry require- ments. In May 1985, Council adopted the DC Test (developed by Professor Dennis Child at the University of Leeds) as an entry gate to first level training. A UK-wide policy on the recording of nurse, midwife and health visitor teaching qualifications was the subject of consultation in late 1984, and the matter was further explored during the first term by a working group.[19] The situation of existing enrolled nurses also occupied the attention of EPAC and the wider Council. Two issues, in particular, were considered alongside the review of pre- registration education. The first concerned the provision of courses enabling second level or enrolled nurses to convert to first level status. By the end of the first term, approval had been given to a number of new programmes offered by the National Boards and Council had determined that conversion was to be regarded as a flexible process, based on an individual assessment of educational and professional needs and allowing for the accreditation of up to 50 per cent of the additional preparation needed to become a first level nurse.[20] Secondly, the inclu- sion of the Enrolled Nurse (EN) qualification among the entry gates to first level training was agreed by Council in July 1985, and implemented through statutory instrument in March 1987.[21] Work on professional conduct had been time- consuming and although procedures were reviewed and seemingly operated well, the continuing backlog was cause for concern. Revision of the Code of Conduct[22] was an important early achievement, and further work on elaborating its clauses on advertising and confidentiality was undertaken.[23] The work of integration and consolidation which had gone on in relation to Midwives Rules in the shadow period, was brought to fruition with the *Midwife's Code of Practice* and the *Hand- book of Midwives Rules*, both issued in May 1986. Deliberation on a framework for post-basic education was necessarily delayed, given that decisions on the shape of the future pre-registration programme had to come first. It also became clear that neither the professions themselves nor employers were necessarily ready to imple- ment standard procedures in nursing on matters of maintaining eligibility to practice or mandatory return to practice schemes. A set of guidelines on good practice in implementing return to practice schemes was issued,[24] and in March 1988 a questionnaire was prepared and sent to health authorities across the UK to explore current practice and help determine ways forward.[25]

Members were only too aware of growing change in the circumstances of day- to-day practice. They noted the lack of support and resourcing that were some- times key factors in professional conduct cases. What was the Council's remit here? The strongly stated position from Dr Donald Irvine, a Secretary of State medical appointee to the Council and later to be the President of the GMC, was that Boards were closely associated with management issues but that Council as 'a standard-setting body' should not be 'concerned with service provision'.[26] Not everyone agreed. Two principles later emerged in the context of a discussion of the Griffiths Report on management changes in the NHS. One was that implementation of the new policy should not put nurses, midwives and health visitors at risk in fulfilling their professional responsibilities. The other was that any such change would need to be of concern to Council were it to put arrangements for education and training in jeopardy.[27]

Further issues of policy change began to come onto the agenda at the clear instigation of Health Departments and Ministers. At its meeting in March 1984, Council considered an invitation from a House of Commons Select Committee to submit evidence concerning 'an enquiry into community care, with special reference to the adult mentally ill and mentally handicapped'.[28] Draft circulars from the Health Departments and European Community (EC) consultation documents also started to be regular items as Council's term progressed. There was no extended discussion of this stream of work during this first term of Council. Unease surfaced from time to time as to matters that were in essence 'personal views' as opposed to what could be thought of as Council policy.

The business of creating and maintaining a live register of practitioners across the UK should not be forgotten. While the largest part of the mammoth task of reconciling the records of the previous statutory bodies was completed for handover, a massive updating campaign was put in hand in 1985–6 to bring in the information previously held on district nursing and by the Joint Board for Clinical Nursing Studies (JBCNS). This helped to transform the register into a 'live' one – it became clear that of the 1.25 million names first added to the newly integrated register only around 500,000 were currently practising. Introducing a periodic renewal of fees for all those in practice was a crucial step if the UKCC was to become financially independent. It had inherited few assets and a number of liabilities from the former bodies. It was working with a transitional grant from the Department of Health and an income drawn largely from registration fees. It had no assets against which to borrow and a major overhaul of the building in Portland Place was imperative. A consultation in 1983 had shown broad support from the professions for periodic fees. Students in particular welcomed it since it enabled the cost of registration – which had risen to £65 for those newly joining the register – to be reduced to £10. Practising nurses, however, were not necessarily appreciative of it; the registration department received many abusive phone calls from nurses who argued that they had paid a fee for life and the matter was taken to judicial review.[29] The target date for having the periodic fee structure in place, 1 January 1987, however, was met. The deficit for the year ending 31 March 1984 was turned into a surplus once the fee structure was in place and income rapidly increased.[30]

Day-to-day contact with the UKCC operated and continues to operate on a substantial scale. The registration department employed a total of 36 staff to deal with the volume of queries being received at the height of its work on updating and periodic registration. It receives applications from overseas trained nurses and midwives, quite a number of which need to be considered on a case by case basis, verifies registration status for regulatory bodies in other counties and issues confirmations of registration for employers.[31] The volume of telephone queries concerning day-to-day work-practice issues handled by professional officers also began to mount after the first couple of years. Invitations to speak, seminars and study days were also ways in which officers stayed in touch with problems being experienced in practice. Access to a rather different perspective on regulatory matters was afforded by the UKCC's position as the UK Competent Authority for nursing and midwifery in the EC.[32] From the outset, members took part in discussions and officers held positions as representatives on the EC Advisory Committee on Training in Nursing and (from its inception in 1984) on the EC Advisory Committee on the Training of Midwives. Though it was not ultimately progressed, work was in hand during the First Council exploring the possibility of sectoral directives on paediatric nursing and later on mental health.[33]

At its meeting in May 1987, with another eighteen months to run, the feeling was that considerable progress had been made in relation to each one of the objectives. Staffing reviews had been carried out and the work of several areas was reorganised. Those working at Portland Place were now enjoying the refurbished building, many of them having attended the official opening by the Queen on 18 December 1986. One further move that was to make a great difference to working lives was in hand – exploration of the economics of providing a restaurant in the basement. As the First Council came to an end, a five-year review concluded that it had been an 'eventful and successful' first term, in which firm foundations had been laid. Referring in particular to the improved financial position with periodic fees, the UKCC claimed that for the first time in the history of the nursing and midwifery professions 'self-regulation and independence have been achieved'.[34] If it was an overstatement, it was an understandable one in view of the difficult context in which Council had had to work. A year later, a more independent assessment was to come in the shape of the delayed review of the five bodies commissioned by the Department of Health. This was to come to a different conclusion.

Towards a realignment: The Second Council, November 1988–March 1993

Before the First Council ended its term, changes were afoot. Following the retirement of Maude Storey in June 1987, Colin Ralph, the new Registrar and Chief Executive, had taken up post in September and an internal organisation review was in train. The outgoing Council had bequeathed its predecessor a new Standards and Ethics Committee which was to have its first meeting in the same month as the new Council.[35] Just one month after the Second Council held its first meeting in November 1988, Peat Marwick and McLintock began a review of the whole statutory structure – including both the Council and the National Boards – on behalf of the four government Health Departments.[36] Everyone was aware that this could have major repercussions, and there were rumours that one or other tier, Council or Boards might be disbanded altogether. With a Government strongly committed to curbing public expenditure and showing doubts about the performance of a wide array of professions, at least some of the members who filed into the Council Chamber in November 1988, to start a new term of office, must have wondered what was to come.

There were important continuities. Audrey Emerton, who had been elected as Chairman of Council in 1985 following the resignation of Catherine Hall, was continuing in office. She had been the only nominee, unanimously elected at an extraordinary meeting on 18 November. A further thirteen of the other forty-four members were also continuing, some of whom, having been members through the shadow period, were about to embark on a third term of office.[37] Criticism appeared in the nursing press from several groups – midwives and occupational nurses, for example. The composition of the new Council, thought Trevor Clay, General Secretary of the RCN, had an educational bias, which was unsurprising given the attention that had been and still needed to be paid to Project 2000.[38] The Secretary of State, however, had departed somewhat from previous practice, in that the non-nurse appointments – previously doctors, educationalists, and those with a management and finance expertise, now included two people who would bring more of an outsider perspective. One was Julia Cumberlege, who had chaired the Community Nursing Review, the other was Judith Oliver, President of the National Association of Carers.

New objectives for a new Council

Much as in 1983, Council members were given a first opportunity to think about the strategic direction of the UKCC and objectives for the new term at a residential meeting. A Strategy Conference was planned to start on the 19 January 1989, feeding into the formal Council meeting on the 21st. In March, a final document incorporating work from a sub-group on post-basic education and results of the Registrar's internal review was presented. It was agreed that the Chairman and Deputy Chairman of Council and the Chairmen and Deputy Chairmen of all the committees would work with officers on the plan. This done, the full document received assent in May.

Compared with the strategic objectives of the First Council, those of the second had a smooth passage. There was no detailed cross-referencing between Council and National Boards, nor were there comments from committees in the way there had been previously. The differences were not only procedural, however. In content and in approach the strategy started to take a different direction (see Figure 3.2).[39] A public interest objective now headed the list. It was followed through in the reference to meeting changing health needs in objective 2 (an echo, of course, of the terms of reference of Project 2000). It also emerged strongly in the rationale for developing the register. *Into the 90s*, by comparison, had had much more of a focus on members of the profession and on the potential of the 1979 Act for improving education. In addition to this, there was a new separation between the four overall objectives and the more internal matters – termed 'core objectives'. The ongoing goal of long-term financial viability was brought together now with a stronger emphasis on internal management.

The Public Interest

- to ensure that Council's policies safeguard and improve standards in the public interest and are sensitive to the changing social climate and health needs.

Standards of Education and Practice

In order to meet effectively the changing health needs of society:

- to monitor and improve the effectiveness of education leading to registration;
- to determine an education and standards policy and a framework for the education and practice of registered nurses, midwives and health visitors.

Standards of Professional Conduct and Practice

- to encourage, promote and maintain high standards of professional conduct and practice;
- to ensure that the arrangements for dealing with allegations of misconduct are simple, speedy, fair and effective;
- to ensure that the arrangements for dealing with alleged impaired performance through ill-health are simple, speedy, humane and effective.

The Register

- to review and develop the professional register for the recording and interrogation of appropriate data relevant to the role of Council for the benefit of the public, health services and professions.

Core objectives

- to achieve long-term financial viability in order to provide the resources necessary for Council's planned developments;
- to achieve quality standards for UKCC activities through a well-organised and well-managed structure, which is responsive to the needs of both the professions and the public.

Figure 3.2 Strategic objectives of the Second Council

The change of emphasis became more strongly embedded as the details of the plan were clarified.[40] Under the public interest objective, the term 'consumers' was used for the first time. There was a commitment to monitor consumer views, engage in opinion-sampling on the effectiveness of policies and standards, to consult with consumers on Council policy and – most specific of all – there was to be an annual conference between Council and representatives of consumer bodies. Under the educational objectives, there were new commitments to explore the effectiveness of education and to develop research that would ensure education was relevant to developments in practice and health care. The move that was to take pre-registration education into higher education – something that was not envisaged when the original proposals were formulated – was prefigured in an action plan to monitor and interpret educational policy changes in general education and further and higher education. Work on the post-registration education and practice project (PREPP) now gathered speed and was to take the lion's share of member and officer time. On professional conduct, the main targets were about creating a smoother, speedier and cost-effective operation. The backlog of cases had remained, despite heavy involvement by members in professional conduct business. There was therefore to be a review conducted by Council members and regular twice-yearly reports each year.

Though not explicitly mentioned in the plan for the second term, the difficulties experienced by second level nurses remained an issue of concern to Council, as well as to the wider profession.[41] Building on the efforts of the previous Council, in 1989 members agreed that enrolled nurses who had been unsuccessful in a first level examination on more than three occasions should be given a further three attempts.[42] The employment problems of enrolled nurses, particularly in the light of the growing deployment of health care assistants, were also debated. Attention focused on whether Rule 18(2), listing the competencies required of second level nurses on completion of training, was hampering the professional practice and employment prospects of enrolled nurses. In April 1989, the Registrar of the UKCC made a statement to the RCN Congress, that the competencies in Rule 18(2) were not to be regarded as the limits of the capabilities of enrolled nurses. They were the minimum required and a basis for further development after qualification. The issue was by no means resolved at this point, however, and was to return to the agenda during the third term.

During the period of the Second Council, debate about the position of the UKCC in relation to vocational qualifications also took up considerable time. Back in 1987, with the formation of the Care Sector Consortium (CSC) as lead body in the care field, Council, liaising closely with the four National Boards, had opted into membership of the CSC. The aim was to influence and support work that would result in a programme of training for health care assistants. In the summer of 1990, when this work was completed, a shift to observer status was made. By the time the Second Council came to an end in 1993, a number of other professions, law, engineering and architecture for example, were involved in pilot projects exploring the potential alignment of professional and vocational competences, and a new Occupational Standards Council was in the offing.[43] The regulatory bodies in the health field, however, remained cautious. They were not entirely mollified by Department of Employment's reassurances that the government 'recognises and respects' the distinctiveness of the professions.[44]

New thinking about standards of practice was starting to crystallise during this period. In January 1988, as the First Council was coming towards a close, the

Director for Professional Conduct had introduced a paper arguing that more definite attention to questions of professional standards was needed, in the face of growing complexity in the delivery of health care and the experience of practitioners. Council then agreed that a new Standards and Ethics Committee should take responsibility for reviewing the Code and associated documents, that it should consider all matters of ethics and standards remitted to it by Council or by the Registrar and that it should identify new issues. In an important departure, but one in line with the emerging emphasis on the public interest, it was agreed that in addition to its eight Council members, the Standards and Ethics Committee would have four others appointed for the contribution they could make – particularly where it was felt that they could make a contribution in the public interest. A list would be drawn up of further experts on whom they could call.[45]

Interestingly, the objectives for the structure and management of the staff and the daily business of the UKCC were also couched in a new standards vocabulary. This echoed the managerialism that was pervading the NHS in the 1980s. An appraisal system meant staff had to grade their priorities and rehearse exactly how their objectives for the year meshed with the strategic plan. Some were suspicious of this, especially of the element of performance-related pay. Others judged it to be good – they could see how they fitted into the overall picture and gained more of a sense of where the UKCC was going. Communications, not only with the professions but with the public and other bodies, came to the fore. A plan to hold some of the Council meetings in Edinburgh, Belfast and Cardiff, and to combine the meeting with clinically focused seminars and conferences for the professions at large, was outlined at the first meeting of the new Council. This it was felt would underline the UK-wide remit and help forge better relations with the National Boards.[46] Targets in terms of using new media, new networks and tailoring publications to their different audiences were outlined. A notable inclusion was an international dimension. There had always been international visitors to the UKCC building in Portland Place, but at this time, there were regular items on Council agenda that encouraged comparative thinking. Owing largely to the initiatives of the Registrar, Colin Ralph, a first International Standing Conference on the Regulation of Nursing and Midwifery was held in Madrid in June 1993. A list of actions to improve relations with the National Boards completed the detailed work of the strategic plan.

All in all, it seemed clear that the focus, image and style of the UKCC were in process of change. The Second Council – in its paper objectives at least – seemed determined to be more outward-looking and more oriented to the public than its predecessors and was going to question its own effectiveness.

By early 1990, and after much consultation with staff, new internal organisational arrangements were in place.[47] On the professional side, Heather Williams, Professional Officer for Health Visiting was appointed to a new post as Deputy to the Registrar and Assistant Registrar, Policy and Planning. Three further assistant registrar posts were created and, following an interview and selection process, three existing staff took these up – Assistant Registrar for Standards and Ethics (Reg Pyne), for Professional Conduct (Jane Macdonald) and for Education

Policy and Registration (Maggy Wallace). In recognition of the workload associated with PREPP, taking half the time of the Deputy Registrar and the Assistant Registrar, Education Policy and Registration, additional staff were recruited to the Professional Unit. On the business side, a Business Manager reported directly to the Registrar, co-ordinating personnel, registration activities and committee services. The new Head of Communications, though of middle rank, also reported directly to the Registrar. Changes on the professional side were particularly significant. The new structure brought professional staff together to form a new professional unit; they found themselves involved in all professional matters not education or practice or professional conduct, and they met regularly, jointly working up papers for Council. They began to share thinking about how best to collect information and intelligence about trends needed for strategic planning and how better to analyse the voluminous responses to consultation documents.

The Quinquennial Review and moves towards legislative change

While all this organisational development and goal-setting was being finalised, Council also needed to come to terms with and respond to the results of the Health Departments' review, available in March 1989. This was not only a review of Council. It was a review of the five statutory bodies in their internal working and in their relations with each other. Two items were off the agenda. Staffing and grading (which had been recently reviewed) was not to be covered. Also – a factor that must have given not a little comfort to all of those involved in statutory body work – the principle of self-regulation itself was to be taken as given.[48]

None of this prevented far-reaching questioning of current ways of working. The reviewers challenged the efficiency and effectiveness of the structure. Procedures were cumbersome and slow; cross-membership duplicated discussions; there was too much emphasis on formal ways of working and nothing to encourage informality and speed. These weaknesses were attributed to the 1979 legislation and its blurring of roles of Council and Boards. The division of responsibility over professional conduct was singled out, prompting criticism of a position where Council handled funds for investigations but was not able to control the process or assure itself that there was a proper uniformity of approach across the UK. The review team was also unconvinced that Council should have the job of managing elections to the Boards.

A new kind of split between Council and Boards was recommended. Council should be the elected body. It should deal with all matters relating to standards and should take over the whole of the professional conduct process. Boards should work through officers rather than committees. They should become smaller executive agencies with strong lines of annual accountability to the Health Departments. On this model, Council needed fewer and different committees. The joint committees could be replaced by a primary care committee. It should also work differently – being clearer about what had to be enshrined in rules (a complex legalistic time-consuming process) and what was more properly the province of guidance. Council should also be smaller, using co-option, drawing people from the register to help to carry out its business. The reviewers recommended piloting a jury system to help reduce the burden and backlog of professional conduct work and to involve registrants in the work of the Council. As far as Boards were concerned, the review team questioned the way approvals had developed in relation to larger and more educationally based institutions and programmes. It did not feel that institutional visits involving large numbers of members as well as officers were cost-effective. It suggested officer approvals, and it went on to recommend that Boards should have managerial and financial control of educational institutions. These latter would then sever their links with the NHS and staff would be directly employed by the Board.[49]

The reviewers recognised that Council needed to be independent of government in its work, not swayed by NHS service pressures – though at the same time there was an onus on it to be realistic in its decisions.[50] They went on to reason that since the UKCC was funded by the professions not by government, it should be more *directly accountable to the professions*.[51] Their recommendation for elections and for short-form annual reports stemmed directly from this. This was an interpretation of professional regulation that emphasised self-regulation of the profession by the profession through the UKCC. It meant that the trickier questions of how to be accountable both to the professions and to the public[52] were largely left for another day. Later, with a stronger emphasis on the regulatory task as protecting the public, these issues were to come up for discussion more directly.

Once in the public arena in March 1989, the report was widely discussed within the statutory structure. It became the basis for the work of a Legislative Implementation Group, where the relation between Council's officers and Department officers was a close one as proposals for what was to become the 1992 Act began to take shape. The eventual legislation was significantly to alter the role of the Council along the lines that the reviewers had envisaged. Council became a largely elected body, taking over the whole of the professional conduct process. While a vision of co-option and involvement of lay participants and practitioners in its processes did slowly emerge, energetic lobbying reversed the recommendation to create a smaller Council. One way or another, however, thirteen years on from the legislation which brought the UK structure into being, its dimensions were about to be drastically altered.

A broadening set of activities

Notwithstanding changing internal structures and time devoted to issues of drafting the new legislation, a great deal was achieved in relation to the strategic objectives of the Second Council. Under the theme of working in the public interest, contact had been made with a number of consumer organisations to gain their views about the standards of practice education and conduct that Council was trying to achieve. A preliminary meeting was held in February 1991 and the first Annual Standing Conference of Consumer Bodies was inaugurated seven months later. By the end of the term of the Second Council, contacts had been made with further voluntary bodies, and the circulation list for UKCC materials had expanded and diversified. A regular joint liaison meeting with the GMC had begun, its first meeting being held in the year 1989–90. As the Standards and Ethics Committee got under way, statements were issued on controversial topics: HIV and AIDS was a particular concern. Nor did members ignore wider changes in health policy. A working group of members was set up to consider the NHS and Community Care Bill as it passed into legislation in 1990 and a further group of members met on community care more generally. Towards the end of Council's term, comments were made on government documents on health strategy for England and for Scotland, on government policy on mentally disordered offenders, on the prison nursing services as well as on themes and initiatives being pursued by other bodies – for example, the Association of Community Health Councils for England and Wales and the National Institute for Social Work.[53] Following the trend of concerns arising in professional misconduct hearings, Council took the initiative in holding a meeting with representatives from nursing homes in August 1990. All in all, Council was beginning to be more outward-looking and also more critical on questions of health policy.

New-look Annual Reports epitomised many of the changes. Introducing the 1988–9 Annual Report, the first of the new Council, Audrey Emerton drew attention to the new 'user-friendly' style. A regulatory body, she felt, had a special duty to communicate effectively with practitioners.[54] Two years later, matters went further. The explicit aim now was that the report should be attractive and appropriate not only for the professions but for the public too. Council should not see professional affairs in isolation and 'the contribution of the professions must be relevant and responsive to the needs of society'.[55]

Staff at this time were busy getting new information bases set up – on the implementation and impact of Project 2000, for example – and were feeling their way towards methods of monitoring both the impact of Council policies and of wider change through feedback and through more systematic research. Meanwhile, notwithstanding considerable work to streamline procedures, professional conduct cases were still taking up large amounts of time on the part of members and officers. A great deal of time too was consumed by PREPP. This was the period in which the complexity and range of issues involved in establishing a post-registration framework began to be appreciated. The report of the project group, sent out for consultation in October 1990, marked the beginning of a new phase, where an implementation group handled responses and took matters forward and goals and targets were frequently revised.

The new work of the Standards and Ethics Committee on the nature of the Code of Conduct, was particularly important and was to mark a watershed in more flexible thinking about professional responsibilities. The third edition of the Code, published in June 1992, and building on experience of professional conduct cases and of the advice service, was a departure in several respects. It addressed the practitioner directly with the words 'you are personally accountable'. It separated out and gave more prominence to the importance of maintaining and improving professional knowledge and competence. The onus was on individuals to acknowledge limitations and to decline duties unless they felt able to perform then safely. Also new were clauses requiring working in an open, co-operative and involving way with patients and clients and their families and fostering teamworking.[56] The extent of the reorientation was underlined by the simultaneous publication of *The Scope of Professional Practice*. No-one was to expect a detailed blueprint from the UKCC as to which new roles were acceptable and which were not – instead they had to think things through themselves and be prepared to be accountable for the decisions they made. The UKCC was offering guiding principles and questions to ask – whether change was in the interests of the patient or the client, whether their own knowledge was sufficient for what was proposed, whether there were elements of delegation that would compromise care assistants, and so on.[57]

With the implementation of periodic re-registration, the financial position had already dramatically improved. Income from fees rose to over £7 million by 1993. Grants from Health Departments ended in 1991 and it proved possible in that year to repay the £3 million bank loan taken out for the refurbishment of 23 Portland Place and still show a healthy surplus. The Health Departments' review of the statutory bodies at the start of the second term had scrutinised finances, finding those of the UKCC considerably more straightforward than those of the Boards and had given the Council a fairly clean bill of health. The largest out-goings were the costs, principally in legal fees, of professional conduct work. The Annual Report for the first year of the Second Council showed these to be running at some £900,000 per year, a figure that was to rise to £1.5million by the end of the second term.[58] The other substantial item was the cost of maintaining the register, which the consultants noted, had reached £570,000.[59] Even with these outgoings, the UKCC was starting to gain an investment income and build its reserves.

New ways of communicating with the professions at large, and new initiatives to work with representatives of health service consumers were now bringing feedback and challenges in ways that had not occurred earlier in the life of the UKCC. Looking back at the end of Council's term, Audrey Emerton felt that the Second Council had seen a highly significant shift in thinking and practice. She referred to the recent extension of duties that had come with the 1992 Act as an affirmation of the trust placed in the Council to regulate the professions in the public interest.[60] All were looking forward to work under a new statutory basis and for the first time with a directly elected Council. Clearly things were set to be different yet again.

New members, new approaches: the Third Council, April 1993–March 1998

A new electoral scheme had been devised for a Council of sixty rather than the previous forty-five members. Lobbying by the UKCC on the grounds of the volume of its professional conduct work had persuaded government of this move, notwithstanding the consultants' view that Council should be smaller. With two-thirds of its sixty members now directly elected, the change was substantial. Only eight members had previous experience of the work of the UKCC. UNISON took a particular interest and for the first time had a clear presence on Council, though unions were reported to be critical that the Secretary of State's appointments had included people who had been unsuccessful on the first vote and included no clinical nurses at all.[61] Government appointments on this occasion included at least three who could perhaps be thought of as offering a voice for the consumer.[62]

Following also from the 1992 Act, there were opportunities to make changes to the committee structure. The joint committees, subject of such strong feelings in the run-up to the 1979 Act, were removed and this was the point at which Council established what were to become known as the two practice committees. One was the Midwifery Committee (named in the 1979 Act as one of two statutory standing committees, alongside the Finance Committee). The other was the entirely new Nursing and Community Health Care Nursing Committee.[63] These committees were to deal with all matters relating to establishing and improving standards. They would be aided by an Education Committee drawn in important measure from the practice committees themselves. The Standards and Ethics Committee continued. The Council now had a President rather than a Chairman and Mary Uprichard, who had served continuously since the shadow period in the capacity of a midwife from Northern Ireland, was elected.[64] A President's Advisory Group – drawn from chairmen of committees – was put in place to advise the President on issues requiring urgent attention between Council meetings.[65] The new Council largely accepted the proposals as put, but was keen that a review of this structure be carried out in due course, and that a review of the President's Advisory Group should occur within a year.

For many of those taking their places in the Council chamber for the first time, the UKCC's remit and the way in which it pursued its business were new. One of the new members, attending the RCN congress two months later, met plenty of questions as to what Council was doing and tended to agree with what she saw as disappointment at the UKCC's narrow interpretation of its role. She felt that the goal – to regulate the profession in order to protect the public – was clear. But, she asked: 'does this mean it should simply issue edicts and act as the nursing police or should it also support practitioners who are struggling to maintain acceptable standards of care?'[66] This was a sign of what was to come, when the UKCC moved into the objective-setting process in its September conference for Council members.

Rethinking objectives

On September 13–16 1993, Council members met to start to formulate overall objectives, with the intention that the results of their strategic planning conference be formally agreed at the October meeting and ratified after drafting amendments at the November Council. Work on the detailed implications, involving the President and an Advisory Group, was then to get under way, so that in February 1994 the objectives and business plan could be finally agreed with reports on progress then coming forward in February of each year of the Council's term of office.

Figure 3.3 sets out the objectives as agreed at the Council meeting of 23 February 1994.[67] The theme of establishing standards was more prominent in the objectives of the Third Council. The way in which the objectives were formulated in terms of protection of the public through maintenance of the register, through establishing standards of practice, education and conduct was in a form that could be more readily appreciated by outsiders. In a new departure, Council also agreed a 'statement of purpose' which ran

> The Council's key duty is to establish and improve standards of nursing, midwifery and health visiting care. The principal purpose of the Council's work is to serve and protect the public and to influence policy and practice for the benefit of patients and clients.[68]

Presented with such a statement and with the new objectives, many of those involved with the UKCC earlier might be tempted to say that there was nothing unremarkable. Looking at the evolution of the work, however, these formulations could not have come in the early years. They encapsulated the growing sense of purpose that had been evolving in the period of the Second Council. There was a shift away from improvements *per se* (especially improvements of education) and away from establishing the machinery to deal with misconduct and unfitness to practise, towards identifying and supporting relevant standards of practice and towards an increasingly direct and insistent attention to what was in the public interest.

In reaching this position, there had been a great deal to explore concerning just what the remit of Council was and how it was going about its business. At the strategy conference, new members had been vocal in raising an array of questions as to exactly what Council was prepared and able to do. Just what powers did it have when it was concerned about standards of practice? Could Council provide real and overt support for practitioners in situations where standards could not be met? If it were a matter of lack of clinical leadership, for example, how far could Council go in trying to insist that employers provide clinical support or perhaps clinical supervision in order to facilitate standards improvement? And what about care assistants acting beyond their role with consequent risk to standards – could and would Council be prepared to press for legislation here? Officer replies were circumspect. Council, it was explained, has the power to investigate the conduct of individual registered practitioners and 'may wish to influence practice and standards where necessary in a broader context'. The nature of any support provided 'would need to be investigated carefully'.[69] Responsibility for and control of support staff was accepted as a key issue for Council and an objective of reviewing and revising Council's position in respect of support staff was written into the business plan. Also in the business plan was an objective of developing a model of clinical supervision (though later, and notwithstanding a great deal of

The Public Interest

- to ensure the Council's register, systems and policies safeguard the health and welfare of the public;
- to ensure that Council's policies improve standards in the public interest and are sensitive to changing expectations and demands of consumers;
- to enhance relationships with consumer organisations in the field of health and welfare and the health and welfare services.

Standards of Practice

- to develop standards and frameworks for practice which secure, as a minimum, safe care for individual patients and clients and for groups of patients, clients and communities;
- to develop policies for effective supervision and support of nurses, midwives and health visitors to enable competent and compassionate care;
- to ensure that current and future standards and policies are relevant to contemporary and changing health need and for practice to be patient/client-centred;
- to promote standards that encourage innovation and provide a framework for ethical practice and sound professional judgement and for the improvement of standards of care.

Standards of Education

- to ensure that standards of pre- and post-registration education are relevant and responsive to the changing needs of patients, clients, society and the health and welfare services;
- to ensure that policies for post-registration education promote and assist the continuing professional and personal development of nurses, midwives and health visitors.

Standards of Professional Conduct

- to ensure that the systems for dealing with complaints of professional misconduct and for dealing with cases of ill-health are just, fair and efficient and command public trust and confidence;
- to develop initiatives to promote high standards of professional conduct by nurses, midwives and health visitors using case material and other evidence.

Figure 3.3 Strategic objectives of the Third Council

Core objective

Communication

- to improve the level of understanding of the role and work of the Council and actively promote its policies;
- to influence relevant policy consistent with the Council's duty to protect the public interest;
- to improve relationships with representatives of public, government, professions and the health and welfare services.

Influence

- to develop initiatives to influence national and international policy for the improvement of standards and the positive contribution of regulatory systems.

Intelligence

- to improve national and international networks to promote greater understanding of policy and development and to gather intelligence to inform decisions.

Organisation

- to ensure an effective and efficient organisation to support the Council across the range of its duties and actively promote its policies and position.

Figure 3.3 (continued)

consultation, the exact status of this model was to be the source of much misunderstanding).

Alongside these questions and listed separately were the 'organisational issues' that had emerged at the conference. One array of questions concerned the conduct of business: how often would Council meet, what was the policy on open closed and private sessions, what were the powers of committees and the status of their reports to Council? Another set of issues related to publications – who was deciding what was published, and how user-friendly was the material? Then there were questions about where research fitted, what the European dimension was and what the UKCC's relationship was with the Occupational Standards Council – this last was a particularly fraught issue, raising as it did questions about the relationship between professional qualifications and vocational qualifications.[70]

The Annual Report for the first year of the Third Council gives a sense of how important it had become for the UKCC to comment on what the report called

'Health and Social Policy Affairs' and how much new work was under way in all the committees. Those with longer memories of the UKCC were justified in feeling that a significant cultural change was under way before the Third Council came on the scene. New members with no statutory body background, however, wanted the Council to speak out even more as far as the matter of improving standards for the public and for the professions was concerned. This was to happen dramatically in the following year, when, following a review of professional conduct cases involving nursing homes, Council published a statement on standards that attracted national publicity.[71] But the year 1994 was a watershed for a second reason, when a very different source of tension made a sudden appearance on the horizon.

A management crisis and a total organisation review

On 18 May, the news broke in the nursing press that eight senior officers had lodged a collective grievance with the President against the Registrar and Chief Executive.[72] The press reports highlighted two issues, one concerned the manner in which an appointment was made; the other had to do with overall management style. By the time this news broke, the matter was already in hand. Over a weekend – on 24 April – officers had taken the unprecedented step of faxing a letter of complaint to the President at her home. The allegations were taken seriously and a procedure was set in motion to deal with the issues as internal matters of UKCC management. The first matter was resolved but, following an attempt at external conciliation, the formal grievance procedure was set in train and a sub-committee of the Finance Committee was established to investigate and make recommendations on the second. A task force was then created to take the recommendations forward. The Registrar, however, was not suspended for the period of the investigation and the hope was that the business of the Council and UKCC would continue as usual.

This hope was dashed. Throughout the summer of 1994, the UKCC's report dealing with standards of care in nursing homes was in the headlines of both the national and the professional press. This report, stemming from an analysis of cases which had come before the professional conduct committee, attracted the most remarkable level of media coverage that Council had ever received. It was coverage, furthermore, that was largely sympathetic to the UKCC and supportive of the criticisms that could be inferred of government policy. It could have been a moment of strong unity and an opportunity – particularly for the professional press – to explore and discuss the concept of a regulatory body and the way its actions in the public interest and in support of professionals could work in the same direction. The professional press, however, kept up weekly reporting on Council's management crisis.

Two particular problems were apparent. First, while a letter had been sent informing Council members of the matter and the steps being taken to resolve it, not all had received this letter by the time that the press came to them for comment. Some were content about how things were being handled, others were putting on repeated pressure for an immediate discussion in Council.[73] Second, the content of the task force reports and the recommendations, instead of closing the matter, only fuelled further controversy. From May until November, the issue continued to attract attention in the professional press. Matters also went further. Questions tabled in the House of Commons brought a reply from Health Minister Tom Sackville that it was for Council to decide its internal ways of working. Shadow Health Secretary David Blunkett gave the *Nursing Times* his opinion that the Registrar should have been suspended for the duration of the investigation.[74] What had largely been fairly brief news items in the professional press began at this point to be supplemented with editorials and with full-length articles and with the beginning of interest in the correspondence columns.[75] The issue even reached *Private Eye*. Although the Registrar left the UKCC on 2 November 1994, and a formal statement on the mutual agreement that had led to this was given to the press, the issue rumbled on, with questions still being asked about the nature of that agreement and about the financial settlement involved.[76]

Catherine McLoughlin[77] was appointed as Chief Executive and Registrar for an interim period. Action was already in train to carry out an organisational review of the workings of the whole of the UKCC. Consultants from the Office of Public Management were appointed and their work was given top priority. There was wide consultation with outside stakeholders as well as with those involved. The aim of the review was 'to find ways of establishing an identity for the UKCC of the future, shared by Council members and the Executive, and to identify the organisational structures and processes needed to support it'.[78]

Whatever the assessments that history makes of these events in the life of the Third Council, they galvanised the 'fresh start' that the nursing press by then was urging. There was a complete rethink of the role of Council members and their relations with officers. There was also a clear commitment to make Council more open and transparent in its dealings with the outside world. Most important of all, it is from this point that one can trace a much stronger articulation than had emerged previously of the role of the UKCC in protecting the public. The newly appointed Chief Executive and Registrar, Sue Norman,[79] formally took up her post on 1 June 1995. Prior to that date, she had taken part in a number of events discussing and developing the new organisational arrangements.

The new organisational structures which came into effect fully in April 1996 brought the term 'governance' into UKCC vocabulary.[80] Governance meant a focus on the role of Council in setting the strategic objectives and direction and the role of the executive and senior managers in putting it into place. It was agreed that Council members needed to focus on outputs and hold managers to account, rather than be concerned with operational detail. One important recommendation in support of this was for a Management Board. Another was that a set of guidelines for Council members be drawn up, clarifying their corporate role, setting out how sectional interests could make a positive contribution and more generally spelling out expectations of them as 'ambassadors' and in respect of the conduct of business.[81] There was clarification of the roles of President and Chief

Executive, with a particular emphasis on the need for the President to keep in touch with members' interests and concerns through more informal contact and direct and open access.[82] There were amendments to committee structures. The two practice committees were charged with establishing a proactive annual programme of work, sensing trends and identifying implications for developing new education and practice standards.[83] It was felt to be particularly important to link education and practice more closely together and a new Joint Education Committee, with equal numbers from each of the two practice committees, was designed to facilitate this. A Policy Development Directorate would aid in analysing trends in health and social care delivery and co-ordinating the research programme of the Council. It was to work closely with a Standards Promotion Directorate, tasked with ensuring that standards were understood, workable in practice and subject to evaluation. The period was also marked by a number of new faces. Sue Norman had already arrived as Chief Executive and Registrar in June 1995. Mandie Lavin took up the post of Director of Professional Conduct in April 1996. A new Director of Policy Development, Angie Roques was also appointed in June 1996, and in September 1997 Sarah Waller took over the position of Director of Standards Promotion. Above all, however, the organisational review set out a new vision of working together. It recommended use of task groups and a project management process to facilitate this. It recognised that Council members and officers had areas of expertise that could and should be used in the development of particular areas of policy and standards setting.[84]

Finance had been examined in detail as part of the organisational review, but emerged unchanged. An Audit Sub-Committee had been added in 1994 and, as in the NHS, proved to be a vehicle for a wide range of investigations into practice and procedure. By the end of the third term, the income from periodic fees was running at over £7.5 million, and the annual investment income was around £1.5 million. The three largest areas of expenditure were professional conduct work (£3.8 million), registration – more complex and costly now with the implementation of PREPP (£2.8 million) – and the growing volume of communications and publicity work (£1.7 million).[85] The UKCC had a reserve in excess of £20 million. Council had taken a decision in April 1995 that it no longer needed to charge for publications or for its confirmations service to employers.

It is ironic perhaps that it was the departure of the Chief Executive and Registrar that galvanised so much change. A close look at the organisational changes that had been put in place as the result of his arrival, and at the plan of work that emerged, suggests that a good many of the new ideas were already present in embryonic form. New committee structures were all but in place as the Third Council started work and the proposals made by the consultants developed and extended these. The proposals were subject to an intense debate.[86] What was important was that the review had given an opportunity for frustrations to be aired and new ways of working to be put into words. There was a renewed belief in the possibility of working together and doing so with greater openness and transparency. The whole process had had a strongly unifying effect.

A new style and pace of activity?

The organisational review inaugurated a more satisfying and productive period for the Third Council. From late 1995 onward, Council found itself uncomfortably in the public eye concerning its decisions on restorations to the register (see Chapter 5). But it deliberately opened its activities to public scrutiny too, conducting listening exercises and setting up consultative conferences before bringing out its policies and guidelines. It was also asking more direct questions about the evidence base for its policies and about monitoring and evaluating their impact and making adjustments in the light of research.

Council was already committed to tracking research evaluating Project 2000 programmes and finding ways of enhancing the effectiveness of pre-registration education. A formal review of the emerging research in this area commenced in the summer of 1994 and a consultation on teacher standards, prepared jointly with the Boards, went out to the profession in July 1995. By 1997, a considerable programme of work under way exploring multidisciplinary education, comprehensive nursing and midwifery training and the feasibility of an all graduate entry. June 1998, shortly after the Fourth Council took office, was to see the establishment of an Education Commission, under the independent chairmanship of Sir Len Peach, charged with carrying out a fundamental review of pre-registration education and its fitness for purpose. In the later stages of the Third Council, a research programme managed within the Directorate for Policy Development through a new Research Advisory Panel began. Projects on midwifery supervision and on how the Scope of Practice document was being received in practice settings were all set in train and had borne fruit by the time the third term was over.[87] No doubt wider movements – such as the stress on evidence-based care that was by now a strong theme in the NHS – had an influence on all this.

The situation of enrolled nurses continued to occupy the attention of members and officers. For one thing, it seemed that there were still insufficient opportunities for conversion to first level. For another, there was much concern about jobs and job prospects of those who wished to continue as enrolled nurses. Despite Council advice against a narrow interpretation of Rule 18(2), employers were using it to limit the practice of second level nurses.[88] There was also growing amount of evidence reaching the UKCC that employers were actually redeploying second level nurses as health care assistants.[89] The issue came before Council in May 1995, at the request of one of its members who had herself had experience as an enrolled nurse, Jackie Furlong.[90] A task group was established to explore the issues. It was agreed that it would report back regularly and ultimately result in a public statement on the matter.[91] At the same time, the Institute of Employment Studies was commissioned to conduct a survey.[92]

Findings presented to Council in summer 1997 confirmed a very unsatisfactory state of affairs. A summary outlining the results and the UKCC's agenda for further work on the issues was to be sent to every second level nurse, their employers, commissioners and providers of professional education, professional organisations and other key stakeholders.[93] *Enrolled Nursing – an agenda for action* was published in October 1997. A new task force, working jointly with the National Boards then took the matter forward. By the final meeting of the Third Council in March 1998, it had concluded that one of the key tasks was to disseminate a clearer understanding of Rule 18(2), to employers, the public and nurses themselves. Enrolled nurses were registered nurses who, with further training and experience, could expand their practice in the same way as their first level colleagues. They were accountable for their activities in the same way. Things, it seemed, were coming full circle. The complaint that ENs were used as first level nurses had now been replaced with a practice of using them as care assistants. Respecting them for what they were and what they could do, often seemed as distant as ever.

The Third Council declined to take up an invitation to pursue membership of the Health Forum of the new CSC/Occupational Standards Council.[94] Working alongside the other regulatory bodies in the health field, however, the UKCC continued to raise questions with the new body and civil servants, as to exactly what government's policy intentions were. In 1995, considerable attention was paid first to an official consultation document on higher level vocational qualifications and then to a review of the CSC.[95] From the regulatory bodies' perspectives, fundamental questions remained unanswered. Was it feasible to bring together professional and vocational education in the way the government seemed to want? Could vocational competence as it had developed ever encompass professional knowledge and skill? Was the system not altogether too narrowly skill-focused and led too much by immediate employer needs? The Department of Health seemed more sympathetic to the regulatory bodies than the Department of Employment, but even here the messages seemed mixed.[96] The government's later position paper on higher level vocational qualifications did much to acknowledge concerns about the distinctiveness of professional knowledge and skill.[97] Links with the CSC were maintained at officer level and, though boundaries continued to cause concern,[98] a further relationship was established with the new Qualifications and Curriculum Authority when, in 1998 the CSC ceased to exist.[99]

By now, registrants were increasingly being drawn in to the work of the UKCC.[100] The first consultative conferences, on mental health nursing and on nursing homes, had been held before the Organisational Review was completed and in October 1995 there was a further conference on the theme of clinical supervision.[101] The publication in June 1996 of *Guidelines for Professional Practice* – culmination of work by the now disbanded Standards and Ethics Committee – and of *The Council's Proposed Standards for Incorporation into Contracts for Hospital and Community Health Care Services* also had the benefit of consultative conferences prior to their publication. The guidelines document set out to help practitioners with the difficult day-to-day decisions that many were telephoning the UKCC about. Patient advocacy, informed consent and complementary therapies, as well as research and audit, were some of the topics now covered. The appointment of two additional professional officers, in the mental health and learning disability field and in the field of paediatric nursing, signalled a new determination to focus on standards across the spectrum of practice.[102] So too, for example, did the programme of work culminating in a position statement on 'The Nursing and Health Visiting Contribution to the Continuing Care of Older People' in November 1997. The work which resulted in consultations around a higher level of practice[103] was taken forward with a direct invitation to interested parties to join a mailing list and give their views. In all these instances, it was being more clearly acknowledged that Council needed to demonstrate to its many audiences how standards were developed, what kinds of information were used and how modifications would be introduced.

PREP legislation came into effect on 1 April 1995. There was much satisfaction on the part of Council concerning the landmark nature of its approach to continuing professional development and the admiration it attracted for an approach that was more than a matter of merely adding 'points' for courses attended.[104] PREP brought a substantially added workload for the registration department with every registrant now renewing registration every three years. Since each practitioner now also notified the UKCC of present practice, it also gave an opportunity to produce practice statistics and extend information which, until then had only been available for midwives.[105] A major listening exercise was carried out on the vexed question of specialist and advanced practice, something that had dogged the PREP project from the very start (see Chapter 6). New thinking that was to culminate in the idea of a higher level of practice rather than the delineation of spheres and roles began to take firmer shape.

Participation of lay members in the activities of the UKCC was also quite clearly growing. The Annual Standing Conference with Consumer Organisations, instituted in November 1991, continued to grow over the remaining years of the Second and during the Third Council terms. The Standards and Ethics Committee, established in 1989 broke new ground by specifically including the consumer members of Council and representatives of consumer interests from outside in its membership. Changes following the passage of the 1992 Act further increased consumer participation in the work of the Council. New primary legislation enabled Council to establish a consumer panel for the Professional Conduct Committee. By 1994, indeed, all committees, except the Health Committee contained members representing the consumer interest. By the end of the Third Council, measures were afoot to extend consumer participation to the closed preliminary proceedings committee. In July 1997, the first leaflet designed specifically for the general public to enhance understanding of the role of the UKCC and its public protection role was issued.[106]

The UKCC's position as Competent Authority in respect of education and training of the professions in Europe was becoming higher profile, with increasing amounts of discussion about the content and assessment of educational programmes. In October 1995, Jane Winship, Professional Officer for Midwifery and European Affairs, was elected President of the Advisory Committee on the Training of Midwives. At home, too, the Council's reputation was improving. One sign of the new times was the commissioning of an attitude survey in 1997 to explore what registrants thought of the UKCC. Over 10,000 questionnaires were returned in the main part of the study and levels of satisfaction with contacts with the UKCC, and the proportion describing the UKCC as 'helpful' (around 60 per cent), were heartening. Given other possible adjectives to choose, however, as many as 45 per cent viewed the UKCC as 'remote' and 37 per cent as 'bureaucratic'. Council could not afford to be complacent, but it was certainly clear that, by the late 1990s, the UKCC was no longer the unknown body it had been back in 1983. An interim telephone follow-up in 1999 showed good responses to new publications and a jump in awareness of 'Meet the UKCC events' that were now a regular part of the annual programme. Detailed survey findings were to be integrated into the communications strategy and another full-scale survey was scheduled for January 2000.[107] In its ethos and style, said Mary Uprichard in her final remarks as President at the last Council of the Third Term, the Council had become more open and accessible. All key policy documents were now drafted with the involvement of practitioners, employers and consumers.[108]

Late in 1997, as the term of the Third Council began to draw to a close, another departmental review had loomed. In Council's submission,[109] the emphasis was on how the UKCC had developed in the period since the previous review. The stronger thread of public accountability and the growing role of consumers in Council's policy deliberations were both underlined. So too was the theme of standards in practice. New powers in relation to professional conduct were requested – these were seen as important in fully delivering on public protection. Council was also looking, at this point, for a 'unitary system', an overall structure that would be clearer and simpler, more economical and more effective.[110]

Conclusion

In the lifetime of three Councils, the UKCC had made a series of important transitions. It had moved from thinking focused largely on improvement of education to thinking focused on standards of practice. It had made the shift from dealing solely with individual episodes of misconduct to carrying out a positive preventive role and addressing the wider issues that cases represented. Underpinning its activities was a more flexible and less prescriptive notion of the role and tasks of a practitioner, witnessed in the way the Code developed and in documents such as *The Scope of Professional Practice* and *Guidelines for Professional Practice*. It had become more outward-looking and perhaps more confident in its role of criticising developments in health policy. Most importantly, it had made much more explicit its role in protecting the public. It was not in business simply to safeguard and improve standards in the professions (as stated in the 1979 Act), it was doing these things in order to protect the public. It was also doing all that it did in the context of a scale of everyday work that few really recognised. But was it enough? One year on from the end of the Third Council, in March 1998, however, the government accepted the key recommendations of the new review team. There was to be a new-style Council, much smaller and with wider stakeholder membership. What did this mean? Was self-regulation now at an end? These questions will be taken up in the final two chapters.

Notes

1 The legislation recognised that members needed to be reimbursed for expenses incurred in carrying out Council business, but it offered neither the members themselves nor their employers any direct recompense for their time. These factors, as well as the sheer level of workload, were to surface from time to time causing member resignations.
2 The Research Committee was established on the recommendation of an Informal Research Group formed in the Council's shadow period. See UKCC, *Nursing Research. The Role of the UKCC*, London, UKCC, 1983, p. 1.
3 A detailed organisation chart was produced as part of the Annual Report for 1985/86, p. 49.
4 UKCC, *Annual Report 1983/84*, pp. 43–6.
5 CC/84/C4.
6 UKCC, *Annual Report 1983/84*, p. 43.
7 CC/84/C11.
8 The Chief Executive Officers Group also submitted a paper outlining the arrangements they had set up in the shadow period for a carefully planned schedule of meetings to inform each other of agendas. They challenged a suggestion that each Chief Executive Officer should attend the meetings of the other four bodies. They judged that 80 per cent of the agendas was unique.
9 CC/84/C13. The areas of work of the ENB included a review of the examination system and the syllabus in general student nurse training, a study of the future of paediatric nurse training and examinations of the possibility of supporting pilot schemes for basic education in higher education and of the concept of a foundation course for nursing, midwifery and health visiting.
10 Ibid.
11 CC/84/C14.
12 UKCC, 55/11, 'A Strategy for the Statutory Bodies, 1984–5'. Also see UKCC, 1/9/2, 'Strategy Document – Into the 1990s and Beyond', 1984.
13 See Chapter 4, p. 77.
14 CC/85/C10. Dame Catherine Hall saw the situation as a very grave one for the professions and her hope was that authoritative legal opinion would solve the matter once and for all.
15 In some ways, Counsel's interpretation went further than those who hoped it would defend the UKCC themselves envisaged. The advice suggested, for example, that the UKCC had the remit to determine the content as well as the standard of education and training, something that even the staunchest defenders of UKCC's overarching role had not proposed and something those working on Project 2000 were being careful to avoid. It also suggested that Council, in pursuit of its principal functions, might, for example, wish to ensure that the standards of examinations conducted by the Boards were suitable. This again had not been on the agenda.
16 CC/85/C10, p. 8.
17 The joint statement went through a number of drafts before the final version was sent to the National Boards, under the title *UKCC, ENB, NBS, WNB and NBNI: A Joint Statement*, on 23 December 1985. See UKCC, 4/6/1. Council noted the support of all the National Boards at its meeting of 21 March 1986 and agreed its support. C MIN 3/86.
18 Ibid., p. 3.
19 See EPAC/84/7; CC/84/100; EPAC/87/15 for further details of this work.
20 See EPAC MIN 17/85; EPAC MIN 44/85; EPAC MIN 39/86; EPAC MIN 30/87; EPAC MIN 35/87; EPAC MIN 23/88; UKCC, PS&D/88/05, 'The Enrolled Nurse and Preparation for Entry to a First Level Part of the UKCC's Register'.

21 Nurses, Midwives and Health Visitors (Entry to Training Requirements) Amendment Rules Approval Order, 1987, SI No. 446. See also UKCC, PS&D/87/04, 'Enrolled Nurse Qualification as Entry to First Level Training', n.d. A useful resumé of policy decisions relating to second level nurses can be found at UKCC, RPG/92/59, para. 3.

22 UKCC, *Code of Professional Conduct for the Nurse, Midwife and Health Visitor*, second edition, London, UKCC, 1984.

23 For details of UKCC publications see Appendix 4.

24 UKCC, PS&D/96/06, 'Guidelines for Good Practice – Return to Practice Programmes for Nurses and Health Visitors', 1986.

25 UKCC, *Annual Report 1987/88*, p. 5.

26 MIN 21/84(vi).

27 The paper for the meeting was prepared by Stan Holder, who had taken a lead in previous discussions. CC/84/95.

28 This time, as was often to be the case in future, there was a clear invitation to Council to make comments. The position as far as inviting comments on Griffiths was concerned had been something of a muddle. Comments had been invited on specific aspects by the Secretary of State, but the UKCC was not on the list. The Secretary of State for Wales, however, had invited UKCC comment.

29 In March 1987, a nurse attempted to record against her name in the register the successful completion of an approved course in school nursing. She discovered that her registration had become ineffective owing to non-payment of the new periodic fee. She took the matter to judicial review, arguing that registration with the GNC had given her an entrenched right to remain on the register and that notice to pay had not been adequately served. The entrenched right argument was dismissed although the notice matter was upheld and a small procedural change was made. [*UKCC ex parte Susan Bailey*, (1989)]. The year 1989 also saw the dismissal of a case taken to industrial tribunal by a nurse first registered in New Delhi, who argued that requirements for further experience training and references before she could be admitted to the UKCC register breached the Race Relations Act 1976. Preparations were also made in 1989 for a judicial review of a case of a nurse converting from EN to RGN whose Director of Nursing Education refused to give the necessary declaration of good character. This case, however, was withdrawn.

30 The fees until December 1986 were £65 for an initial registration and £45 for subsequent registrations. From January 1987, the initial registration fee was £10, the subsequent registration fee was £15 (reduced to £14 in 1989) and the periodic fee £10 paid tri-annually in advance. After six years, the periodic fee was increased to £12 and there have been no increases since this time.

31 For more details on the process of registration and the workload, see Appendix 2.

32 The UKCC is unusual in this, as the Competent Authority in other countries is usually the Ministry of Health.

33 See Appendix 2.

34 UKCC, *The First Five Years, 1983–1988*, London, UKCC, 1988, p. 18.

35 An additional change to the committee structure had come in 1987 with the standing down of the Committee on Research, which had increasingly found it difficult to achieve its quorum of five.

36 Formally this was the health departments' first quinquennial review, postponed to allow work on Project 2000 to progress.

37 These were: Miss C. A. Asher, Mr R. Holland, Mr C. McCullough, and Miss M. E. Uprichard.

38 'Criticism for the New UKCC', *Nursing Standard*, 19 November, 3(8), 1988, p. 17.

39 CC/89/C12, Annex 1.

40 The final Plan for Council's Strategic Objectives was presented and agreed at the Council meeting of May 1989, CC/89/C27.

41 See, for example, 'Enrolled, endangered and enraged', *Nursing Times*, 7 June, 85(23), 1989, p. 28–31, issued as a Council paper, CC/89/52.

42 Nurses, Midwives and Health Visitors (Registered Fever Nurses Amendment Rules and Training Amendment Rules) Approval Order 1989 SI No. 1456. Schedule 2, Section 2(12), Rule 19.

43 The CSC formally ceased in April 1993, being replaced by the Occupational Standards Council for Health and Social Care. The original name stuck as the first part of the title of the body, and common usage thereafter was to retain the title CSC.

44 Letter from N. Monck, Permanent Secretary at the Department of Employment to Colin Ralph, 17 February 1993, reprinted as Annexe 2 to CC/93/C05. The letter was a response to a request for clarification by Colin Ralph, prepared in behalf of the GMC, the GDC, the General Optical Council, the Council for Professions Supplementary to Medicine (CPSM) and the Royal Pharmaceutical Society of Great Britain.

45 By the time of the 1989/90 Annual Report, four non-Council members were on the committee. Two had nursing qualifications, and two did not. Of the latter, Dr R. Chadwick was Lecturer in Philosophy at University of Wales College of Cardiff, and Mrs Jean Robinson was the nominee of the Association of Community Health Councils.

46 CC/88/78.

47 Two longstanding senior members of staff had left prior to this: Peta Allen, Director for Professional Standards and Development, and Hilary Pincott who had succeeded Mike Hanson as Director of Administration.

48 Peat Marwick McLintock, *Review of the UKCC and the Four National Boards for Nursing, Midwifery and Health Visiting*, London, Department of Health, 1989.

49 This recommendation was not realised. The model that ultimately prevailed was of nurse education moving into higher education and higher education institutions competing for contracts with the service.

50 'Obviously, the Council must be aware of the resource situation when setting standards – there would be little point in setting standards that produced high quality education for a very few people. In other words, standards cost money and Council has a responsibility to temper professional idealism with realism.' Peat Marwick McLintock, *Review of the UKCC and the Four National Boards*, para. 7.8.

51 The review team stated that Council was 'the professions' body, funded almost entirely by practitioners, and it must therefore, in principle, be accountable to them.' Ibid., para. 4.92.

52 These words actually appeared in the terms of reference at the point where the review team was instructed to accept the principle of self-regulation. Note also that the review team did envisage non-nurse members on its smaller Council, suggesting representatives from an array of organisations, including the GMC, the Institute of Health Service Management, client/patient organisations and health authorities. A stronger emphasis on consumer organisations as a way of involving 'the public' was already beginning to be under consideration at the UKCC, as the text of the next section shows.

53 See UKCC, *Annual Report 1992/93*.

54 UKCC, *Annual Report 1988/89*, p. 1.

55 UKCC, *Annual Report 1990/91*, p. 1.

56 UKCC, *Code of Professional Conduct for the Nurse, Midwife and Health Visitor* (third edn), London, UKCC, 1992.

57 UKCC, *Scope in Practice*, London, UKCC, 1997, gave examples of some of the innovative care regimes facilitated by this.

58 It did not prove possible, given the nature of the records, for the consultants to analyse further or to make recommendations.

59 Their study of this concluded that while the cost was high and the system probably had more capacity than was needed, given the disaggregation of SPRINT, there was also

the potential for recording place of work and of thus being highly useful in planning numbers.

60 UKCC, *Annual Report 1992/93*, p. 1.
61 'Appointments to UKCC announced by Bottomley', *Nursing Standard*, 31 March, 7(28), 1993, p. 6.
62 These were Dr Eva Jacobs, Mrs Rita Lewis and Professor Sheila McLean.
63 At the first meeting of the new Council, on 28 April 1993, the matter of whether there should be such a committee had to be put to the vote.
64 The opportunity was taken to ensure that employers were recompensed for the time taken up by presidential duties, a move that brought the UKCC into line with the GMC. This was enabled under Schedule 1, 8(1) of the 1992 Nurses, Midwives and Health Visitors Act.
65 For the standing orders of the President's Advisory Group see CC/93/30, Annexe 7.
66 Turner, T., 'Tunnel Vision', *Nursing Times*, 16 June, 89(24), 1993, p. 21.
67 CC/94/12.
68 Minute 10/94(2), February 1994; CC/94/12, Annexe 1.
69 CC/93/C27, Annexe 4.
70 CC/93/C27, Annexe 5. Some might argue that these questions were rather more than 'organisational' matters and, like the previous list, were raising fundamental issues about the powers of Council rather than only about its style of working.
71 UKCC, *Professional Conduct – Occasional Report on Standards in Nursing Homes*, London, UKCC, 1994.
72 'UKCC Officers in Revolt Against Colin Ralph', *Nursing Times*, 18 May, 90(20), 1994, p. 5. 'Management Crisis Erupts at UKCC', *Nursing Standard*, 18 May, 8(34), 1994, p. 5.
73 The issue was not formally discussed at the June Council. In September, normal business was suspended and Council stayed in private session for the whole day to discuss the matter.
74 'Blunkett Calls for Ralph Suspension', *Nursing Times*, 6 July, 90(27), 1994, p. 6. 'Questions in the House over UKCC Turmoil', *Nursing Times*, 24 July, 90(26), 1994, p. 5.
75 On editorials, see for example, *Nursing Standard*, 14 September, 8(51), 1994, p. 3; *Nursing Standard*, 9 November, 9(7), 1994, p. 3; *Nursing Times*, 21 September, 90(38), 1994, p. 3, *Nursing Times*, 8 November, 90(45), 1994, p. 3. Articles include Pink, G., 'Heads in the Sand', *Nursing Standard*, 27 July, 8(44), 1994, pp. 48–9; Rowden, R., 'Gloom at the Top', *Nursing Times*, 12 October, 90(41), 1994, p. 66.
76 See 'IHSM Questions Bonuses Paid to former UKCC Chief', *Health Service Journal*, 10 November, 104, 1994, p. 7.
77 Catherine McLoughlin was a Secretary of State appointee to the UKCC in 1995 and was re-appointed for a further five-year term in 1998. Her background had been in nursing management and general management posts. She spent a brief spell as Director of Nursing at the NHS Management Executive in 1989–90 and from 1991 was Chair first of Bromley FHSA and then of Bromley Health.
78 UKCC, *Organisational Review*. London, UKCC, n.d., p. 3.
79 Sue Norman came to the UKCC from a post in the Personnel Directorate at the NHS Executive where she was responsible for policy on non-medical education and training and workforce issues. Prior to this her background included nurse teaching and practice in the fields of acute psychiatry, community nursing and oncology.
80 UKCC, *Organisational Review*, p. 6; CC/95/C08, Annex 1.
81 UKCC, *Code of Best Practice for Members*, London, UKCC, 1996.
82 The President's Advisory Group was disbanded at this point.
83 The Standards and Ethics Committee was stood down, much of its work going to the practice committees, though an Ethics Advisory Panel was established in its place. See Chapter 8, page 181.

84 In November 1995 Council agreed a new set of eleven strategic objectives, and in March 1997 it approved the first annual business plan. For a review see CC/98/12.

85 While the major expenditure headings are broadly similar to those in earlier years, no easy comparisons can be made, given the changing legislative remit and alterations to accounting conventions.

86 There was a particularly strong view that midwifery should be handled differently. See Chapter 7.

87 For details of publications see Appendix 4.

88 UKCC, RPG/95/06.

89 Minute 6/94(3) 1994; CC/94/06. See also Minute 17/94.

90 CC/95/34.

91 Minute 31/95.

92 CC/95/10; CC/95/44. See also commentary in the nursing press, for example, 'A benchmark not a barrier', *Nursing Standard*, 15 November, 10(8), 1995, pp. 48–9. Delays in getting the work under way led to some adverse publicity. See UKCC press statement 57/1996, 6 November 1996.

93 Minute 15/97(7); CC/97/18; UKCC press statement 30/1997, 5 June 1997. See also 'Enrolled nurses: a bright future?', *Nursing Standard*, 30 July, 11(45), 1997, pp. 22–3.

94 See note 43.

95 Department of Employment, *A Vision for Higher Level Vocational Qualifications*, London, DoE, 1995. This document is reprinted in full Appendix 1 to Annexe 4, RPG/95/07. It was debated at a seminar for Council members held on 2 May 1995, immediately prior to the Council meeting. Department for Education and Employment, *Review of the CSC; Report for Consultation*, London, DfEE, November 1995. The Departments of Employment and Education had been merged to form the DfEE in July 1995.

96 A letter from the NHS Executive gave assurances that the NHS would 'not promote alternatives to programmes of education and training which lead to registration with a Statutory Body'. But it also underlined the centrality of vocational qualifications to the government's agenda and encouraged exploration of occupational standards to underpin existing professional curricula. NHSE EL(95)84.

97 DfEE, *Higher Level Vocational Qualifications. A Government Position Paper*, London. DfEE, 1996.

98 There was some correspondence, for example, querying the coverage of the project that was to result in the report from the CSC in May 1997, under the title *National Occupational Standards for Health Care Practitioners*.

99 In 1992, Council had recognised NVQ 3 and GNVQ Advanced and their Scottish equivalents as meeting the educational entry requirements to pre-registration nursing and midwifery courses. This decision was implemented in 1995 by Registrar's Letter 11/1995, The Council's requirements for entry to pre-registration nursing and midwifery programmes using vocational qualifications, 8 March 1995.

100 The creation of a panel of practitioners to help with the work of professional conduct was agreed in principle in March 1996, but did not come into operation until later. See Chapter 8, p. 182.

101 This followed publication of an initial position statement in January 1995, and was followed by a further *Position Statement on Clinical Supervision for Nursing and Health Visiting* in April 1996.

102 See UKCC, *Guidelines for Mental Health and Learning Disabilities Nursing*, London, UKCC, April 1998.

103 See Chapter 6, pp. 132–3.

104 See UKCC, *Annual Report 1995/6*, p. 8.

105 But see Appendix 2 on this.

106 UKCC, *Protecting the Public*, London, UKCC, 1997.

107 For press commentary on the initial survey, see Leifer, D., 'Getting Better', *Nursing*

Standard, 21 May, 11(35), 1997, p. 16. For more on interim results, see UKCC, MG/99/27.

108 Annexe to Council Minutes, March 1998, p. 2.

109 UKCC, *The Future of Professional Regulation – submission of the UKCC for Nursing Midwifery and Health Visiting to the Government's review of the Nurses, Midwives and Health Visitors Act*, London, UKCC, 1997.

110 The growth once again of a debate on devolution was to become significant. While the ENB argued in response to the interim report of the reviewers that there should be a coherent structure with a single mission and accountability to Council, the NBS envisaged and later elaborated a 'federal model'. See ENB *The Regulation of Nurses, Midwives and Health Visitors. Response of the ENB to the Invitation to comment on issues raised by a review of the Nurses, Midwives and Health Visitors Act 1997*. London, ENB, March 1998; NBS *Professional Regulation. Safeguarding the public and protecting the future*, Edinburgh, NBS, n.d.; NBS *Professional Regulation:– safeguarding the public and supporting the future. A further exploration*, Edinburgh, NBS, May 1998.

Part II
The agenda develops

4 The reform of pre-registration education
Hopes, fears and realities

The reform of pre-registration education was one of the principal tasks of the new Council during the first five years of office, and an important testing ground for the new statutory framework. By the time the new statutory bodies were in place, the question of the future of nurse education and training was at the top of the leadership agenda, and hopes and fears on this score were high. Midwifery education too, especially in England and Wales, was regarded as in need of a major overhaul. While clinical preparation was felt to be of a good standard, education-alists had grown frustrated by the peculiarities of the funding arrangements of the CMB and by the Board's restrictions on expenditure on educational development.[1]

Much time had now elapsed since the original Briggs proposals for educational reform, and the extent to which they were applicable still remained controversial. The HVA, for instance, was concerned that hard-won educational gains might be lost in the amalgamation with nursing. Indeed, all types of community-based practitioner were concerned that general hospital nursing would dominate the new statutory structure and thus its education proposals. Midwives were certainly anxious that their distinctive training would be diluted. Many of the broader educational issues were complex and equally controversial. For some time, the most problematic areas had been felt to be the future of the enrolled nurse, the status of the nurse learner and the organisational structure and funding of nurse education.[2] The task of reform, however, was further complicated by the five-body structure created under the 1979 Act and its division of responsibilities. An early warning of tensions came in February 1982 when the 'shadow' ENB issued a document, *The Organisation of Nursing, Midwifery and Health Visiting*.[3] Reform of education was the issue on which and through which the new Central Council needed to establish itself as the authoritative voice on professional self-regulation working in collaboration with the four National Boards. It was a tall order.[4]

The new Council and Project 2000

The establishment of the Project

While there was excitement about what was to come, the experience with Working Group 3 left a lingering sense that the new regulatory body had already scalded its fingers on the hot issue of education reform. What was the best way forward? The first full Council assembled in November 1983 and gave a wide-ranging review of pre-registration education and training priority status. Between January and June 1984 its newly established EPAC discussed a possible pro-gramme of work.[5]

A number of Board members felt that it was inappropriate that EPAC, a Committee responsible to the Central Council, should have responsibility for the review; their preference was for a joint committee between Council and Boards. The ENB was concerned that its educational functions, as outlined in Section 6 of the Act, should not be restricted by the activities of EPAC.[6] Also, there was concern that EPAC had insufficient 'service' representation among its member-ship.[7] At its meeting in July 1984, however, Council formally agreed to remit the work to EPAC. It emphasised that 'irrespective of the mechanism adopted for undertaking the review, the persons concerned in it must be free to function as individuals and must not be, or feel themselves to be, constrained by the views of Council or National Boards.'[8] The most obvious way forward would have been for EPAC to set up a sub-group on educational reform, reporting periodically to the main committee. Professional sensitivities and the position of the Boards precluded this. By September, it had been decided that the whole of EPAC should act as the project group, dividing into 'task-orientated' groups when necessary to investigate specific issues. Margaret Green, Director of Education and Principal of the Institute of Advanced Nursing Education at the RCN and the Chairman of EPAC, was to chair the project.[9] For the duration of the education review, EPAC's agenda had to be divided into two parts. The great majority of its time was spent on the pre-registration education review. The remainder was devoted to routine matters and 'on-going business' such as work on the preparation of teachers of nurses and midwives, the development of alternative entry requirements for nurse training, continuing mandatory education and re-entry programmes.[10]

In the late summer of 1984 the Chairman of the Council secured funding from Nuffield Provincial Hospitals Trust for the appointment of an experienced project officer to oversee the review, analyse reports, synthesise available information and produce the final report in conjunction with the Project Group.[11] The post was not restricted to a qualified nurse, midwife or health visitor, and Celia Davies, a sociologist and formerly a Research Fellow at the University of Warwick, was appointed. This was an unusual move, but bringing in an outsider was perhaps understandable given the intra-professional tensions that had dominated the previous decade.[12]

Both the title of the pre-registration education review, 'Project 2000', and a timetable of two years were agreed at the September meeting of Council. The timetable was intended to give time to explore basic principles and to generate evidence on possible proposals for change. Terms of reference were 'to determine the education and training required in preparation for the professional practice of nursing, midwifery and health visiting in relation to the projected health care needs in the 1990s and beyond and to make recommendations'.[13] The explicit emphasis on health care needs was an encouragement to new thinking. It also acted as a unifying factor – adapting education to meet changing health care needs was something on which all groups within nursing and midwifery, in principle, could strongly agree.[14] By late 1984, organisational arrangements were in place, staff were in post and the work, finally, could start in earnest.

Work under way, but worries remain

Project 2000 did not have a clear field. First, the RCN had decided to set up a Commission on Nursing in March 1984 under the independent chairmanship of Harry Judge.[15] It was clear that this was involving substantial new research – not something that Project 2000 was resourced to do – and its likely impact was uncertain. Second, and causing greater uncertainty, was the decision by the ENB in September 1984 to produce its own strategy document on education and training.[16] Early in 1985, just as the first progress report on the work of the project group was submitted, Council was forced to consider the implications of the imminent publication of the ENB's consultation document on educational reform. It was at this point that legal advice was taken on the respective responsibilities of the UKCC and the National Boards.[17] When the ENB and RCN reports appeared, in quick succession in April and May 1985, there was real concern that these publications would confuse the issues for the wider profession and even perhaps weaken the case for reform in the eyes of government.[18] Given this context, Council agreed that the importance of the UKCC's review should be reiterated, and that the Project 2000 report should be produced as soon as possible. As a result, the Project timetable was effectively cut by six months.

During the first months of the project, the question of consultation also loomed large. National Boards, professional associations and trades unions clearly needed to be approached for comment, but the level of involvement of the wider profession remained unclear. Members agreed that the ideal was to keep the profession informed at all stages of the review process, but there was 'hesitation and fear about getting it wrong'.[19] The publications by the RCN and the ENB made it all the more imperative that the status of Project 2000 was understood. A press release was issued on the communications strategy. Project 2000 was to be open about all stages of its work – it was to be an example of policy-making 'in the sunshine'.[20]

Work on the substantive issues of education and training began in earnest in July 1985, when a weekend meeting was called to clarify the themes that had arisen during the Project Group's discussions of the previous months.[21] Over the summer and autumn, the initial thoughts of the Project Group were set out in a series of 'discussion papers', distributed to the professions and discussed at 'road show' meetings in each of the four countries of the UK.[22] It was immediately clear that considerable interest, and not a little anxiety, were being generated, particularly from midwives and enrolled nurses.[23] Initial discussions with the profession also revealed much about the context into which the proposals were being launched. Considerable concern was expressed about the manpower and resources implications of educational reform, and members of the project team worked hard to argue that the professions should have a 'vision' which looked beyond immediate cost constraints. Yet it was also apparent that many nurses wanted more than just education reform. They wanted the review to bring to the attention of government and employers the difficulties of nursing in a financially stretched health service. The low morale and broad-based discontent of the profession at this juncture was making the statutory body's task especially hard.

From January to May 1986, the Project Group worked to forge a coherent and cohesive report from the varied viewpoints that had emerged. One of the biggest developments was the Group's commitment to a single level of professional qualification: a shift from the position at the end of 1985 when a minority of five members were in favour of retaining a modified second level.[24] As time went on the question of the learning environment was brought into sharper focus and members also began to consider the necessity of including a discussion on the implementation of reforms. In early March, a paper summarising the recommendations agreed to date was produced. One issue, though, remained especially contentious: the balance between generic and specialised training. The majority of the Project Group was in favour of a training model based on a two-year common foundation programme (CFP) and a one-year 'branch' programme in adult nursing, children's nursing, mental illness nursing, mental handicap nursing or midwifery. Midwives, however, remained unconvinced. Mary Uprichard, at the time the only midwife member of the Project Group, felt sure that her colleagues would regard a one-year 'branch' in midwifery as insufficient preparation for an independent, autonomous practitioner.[25] It was finally agreed that these differences of opinion should be made explicit through a recommendation that the eighteen-month post-registration midwifery course should continue alongside experimental one-year branch programmes in midwifery.[26] Added sources of difficulty were the anxieties of district nurses, and the frustrations of a committee formed to deal with education matters that detailed work on the curriculum was more properly the concern of the National Boards.

The Report is published

Project 2000 – A New Preparation for Practice was published simultaneously in the four countries of the United Kingdom on 13 May 1986, following a series of private briefings with members of the four National Boards, colleagues in the Health Departments and the professional press. The report was a 'framework document', outlining the philosophy and approach of future educational programmes, the conditions of the learning environment and the general outcomes of professional preparation. It began with an extensive exploration of the background and the rationale for reform and a consideration of changing health needs. It then presented twenty-five specific recommendations for change. Its overall stance was uncompromising. The existing system was 'fundamentally flawed': it left nurse teachers 'no time for research or professional development', while the student learning experience was regularly undermined in an effort to ensure that wards were staffed.[27]

The report recommended a more flexible and responsive education and training programme, less narrowly orientated towards the hospital and with greater emphasis on community-based care. The pattern of training was to be simpler, with a single registration noting the branch specialism. A two-year common foundation programme, followed by a one-year branch programme in either adult, child, mental illness or mental handicap nursing (with experiments also in a midwifery branch) was recommended. Students were to be supernumerary throughout the entire period of their preparation. The location of education was left open, though the report firmly advocated both the development of stronger links between training schools and institutions of further and higher education and the amalgamation of smaller nursing schools. It also recommended that joint professional and academic validation should be pursued.

In articulating its vision, the Project 2000 report outlined a new model of practice that placed a single level of trained nurse, the 'knowledgeable doer', at the heart of the delivery of nursing care. Supported on the one hand by a non-nurse helper, and on the other by specialist or advanced practitioners in the relevant clinical field, the nurse was to be the linchpin of both the co-ordination and the delivery of nursing care. Existing second level nurses were to be enabled to convert to first level status but protected if they did not wish to do so. Post-registration nurse education had not been regarded as part of the remit of the Project 2000 group, but the report noted the importance of developing a coherent and cost-effective framework of education beyond registration.

There were obviously major staffing implications for the NHS. The report made preliminary comment on this and added recommendations on a helper grade. The Project Group recommended that an 'aide' would be instructed in her role by the employing authority, but not professionally recognised by the UKCC. This was the start of much debate about the nature of the support required and the qualifications needed.

The report was received into a highly expectant arena. The nursing press welcomed its readable style and its clear presentation of the issues. But expressions of puzzlement and notes of caution were also quickly heard: a 'framework document', however clearly argued, could not supply the answers to the detailed questions which surfaced within the wider profession, particularly on the content of the new curriculum and its costs.

Consultation, costing and compromise: May 1986–February 1987

Between the publication of the Project 2000 report in May 1986 and the submission of recommendations to Health Ministers in February 1987, an important period of consultation and costing occurred. Taking the project forward was not simply a matter for the UKCC. It required input from the National Boards and close liaison with the Heath Departments. Council also took the decision to involve management consultants in detailed work on costs and staffing implications. A Project Steering Group was set up to oversee this new phase.[28]

Consultation

Following the report's launch in May 1986, Council officers and members began a new programme of publicity. Communication with the wider profession was maintained through 'link officers' designated by health authorities to receive Project 2000 material from the Council. A summary document, *Time for Change*, two newsletters and a video were produced, and a telephone 'hot line' was put in place.[29] The aim of all this activity was to try to ensure that the debate was well informed and that the recommendations were widely understood. Information supplements were also issued on what were felt to the most complex and controversial topics – the position of the enrolled nurse, the education of midwives and the role of the specialist practitioner.[30] The period of consultation lasted until 3 October 1986. By the time it ended, over 15,000 copies of the report had been distributed, a copy of the report summary sent to over half a million practitioners and meetings of all types and sizes held all over the United Kingdom.[31]

Over 2,500 responses, representing about 8,000 practitioners, were received by the Project Office. There were forty submissions from formal organisations, which included the National Boards, the professional associations and trade unions. Only a very small number of submissions (forty-five) were received from non-nursing bodies or individuals. By the end of the consultation an estimated 50,000 people had contributed in one way or another to the debate.[32] A first analysis of the responses to the consultation suggested that while there was a great deal of support for Project 2000, there was also a 'considerable amount of continuing concern in specific areas'.[33] Particular anxiety was expressed on the proposed cessation of enrolled nurse training. Strong opposition came from the National Union of Public Employees (NUPE), the Confederation of Health Service Employees (COHSE), the National and Local Government Officers Association (NALGO) and from the Trades Union Congress (TUC).[34] The unions' submissions drew attention to the important role played by a 'practical' nurse and indicated concern over the pay and career progression opportunities of existing ENs and the manpower and recruitment implications of a cessation of EN training. Similar worries were expressed in submissions from the Nurses and Midwives Advisory Committees of health authorities and by a small number of groups of clinical nurses working in hospital settings. In addition, the Project Group received well over 500 submissions from enrolled nurses themselves, clearly concerned about the implications of ending second level training. Yet few made a firm case for its continuation, and many gave evidence of their own misuse and abuse as enrolled nurses.

Experimentation in a one-year branch programme for midwifery proved highly controversial. The proposal to retain an eighteen-month post-basic preparation was much more acceptable, but many midwives also indicated their wish to see this coupled with the development of direct-entry midwifery programmes. The Royal College of Midwives (RCM) argued that the deficiencies of midwifery education were not the same as those of nursing.[35] On this basis, experimentation with a CFP and branch was firmly rejected along with the idea of a shared list of 'competencies' to describe functioning at the level of the registered practitioner.[36] The RCM also expressed its concern over the Report's comments on specialist practitioners. Midwives were already specialist practitioners in their own right.[37]

The responses of other specialist groups varied.[38] Children's nurses were generally positive about the recommendations. Mental illness and mental handicap nurses, *Nursing Times'* commentators observed, had been 'unusually quiet' during the early consultation period.[39] Responses suggested that mental illness nurses 'warmly welcomed' many aspects of the report, but were anxious that the gains of the 1982 syllabus should be incorporated and that sufficient time should be available for branch work. Many also favoured a name change to 'mental health'. Mental handicap nurses were doubtful of what was felt to be the narrow conception of their role in the report. Comments from the Welsh and English National Boards also demonstrated anxieties in this area, with the latter appending an alternative statement on mental handicap nursing to its comments.[40] Community nurses, too, had a number of concerns, particularly relating to the question of separate training for different community practitioners. Some rejected the idea of separate recordable qualifications in health promotion and in the 'curative' areas of district nursing, community psychiatric nursing and community mental handicap nursing. Many drew attention to the growing amount of shared learning and what was seen to be the better model offered by the recently published Cumberlege Report.[41] The logistics of providing community placements for students caused concern, and doubts were expressed on the feasibility of offering students a sufficiently comprehensive grounding in community practice. The need for more clarification on the role of the specialist practitioner was a further important theme of the responses. While general support was given to the notion of an 'advanced' or specialist practitioner, the RCN, the District Nursing Association, and the ENB all felt that the proposals were inconsistent and liable to cause confusion.

In all, the professions' responses indicated that the concept of the registered practitioner had been broadly endorsed and the notion of an education programme based on a common foundation programme was acceptable to the majority. Wide support had been received for the introduction of supernumerary status, improvements in conditions for teachers, and partnerships with further and higher education. Fears about the resourcing of such reform, however, remained strong. In all, it seemed that the consultation had demonstrated that educational improvement was 'now very high indeed on the professions' agenda' and that the package as a whole contained 'a great deal' that was acceptable.[42]

The costs and benefits of change

If the UKCC was going to be successful in its quest for reform it had to demonstrate not only that its recommendations were generally supported by the wider profession but that they were feasible.[43] To help with this, Council took the unprecedented step in June 1986 of appointing management consultants, Price Waterhouse, to undertake a costs and benefits analysis of the recommendations.[44]

The analysis had three elements: a review of existing information about the current costs of education and training, the clarification and costing of Project 2000's proposals and an investigation of the manpower implications of the Project's concepts.[45]

The first step was to identify current levels of student service contribution, student recruitment and wastage, recruitment and retention among qualified staff, and the different costs of providing grants or bursaries. It proved a difficult task. Reliable information about nursing in the NHS was extremely difficult to find and had to be assimilated by the consultants, officers and members from a range of sources in a piecemeal manner. Co-operation was sought from the Health Departments, health authorities, professional bodies and individual researchers.[46] The next task was to develop the educational proposals outlined in the Project Report to a level of detail that would allow the consultants to quantify possible costs and benefits of the proposed changes. Working assumptions were achieved through a series of liaison mechanisms: with the Project's Educational Development Group; the overall Steering Group; Council officers; two expert panels of Council members – one for service and one for education – and with the Health Departments. With the 'base-line' data and the key assumptions in place, the management consultants were able to plot how manpower and costs would develop over time both with and without Project 2000.[47]

This examination confirmed that nursing was working on a 'high recruitment/ high wastage model'. While large numbers of students were recruited, high proportions of them left at different stages of the training programme or following qualification. Overall, it was estimated that 30,000 nurses needed to be replaced each year, with the great majority, around 70 per cent, of this replacement coming from the appointment of the newly qualified. Until this point, very little attention had been given to the question of improving the flow of those returning to the profession after a period of absence. However, if this situation could be turned around the numbers entering training could be reduced and extra money could be spent per entrant.[48]

In October 1986 Council, for the first time, discussed the recommendations of the Project 2000 report in detail in conjunction with the costs and benefits analysis and the first wave of responses from the professions.[49] The meeting started with a presentation from Price Waterhouse. The relaxed style of the management consultants did much to ease the understandable tension building in the Council room. The issues, however, were complex and the message was worrying. Council's proposals needed to be both 'feasible' from the point of view of manpower requirements and 'reasonable' in terms of the cost. The assembled evidence indicated that some movement would be necessary to meet these aims.

The consultants' presentation indicated that supernumerary status for students was the single most important factor in costs. For around two hours the debate focused on the question of student service contribution. From an educational point of view, it was argued, the ideal service contribution of students should be nil. In the opinion of some members this was the linchpin of the whole project and should thus be non-negotiable. But these were by no means ideal times and it was finally agreed that 'subject to the safeguards of educationally determined preparation a service contribution of 15–20 per cent [of the full three-calendar-year programme] might be possible'.[50]

Costs were not the only problem. With falling birth rates and a diminishing supply of eighteen-year-old entrants, the profession could not continue to operate a high recruitment/high wastage model. The introduction of supernumerary student status and the cessation of enrolled nurse training would exacerbate the recruitment shortfall, at least in the short term. Members were also reminded that the role of the 'helper' would need to be considered further. On the enrolled nurse question, however, Council reaffirmed its support for a single level of practitioner and for the ending of second level nurse training. This decision made a compromise on the question of student service contribution even more important. Members also agreed that a wider entry gate to nurse training was necessary to help meet the manpower implications of this change, and that the existing educational entry requirements for first level training should be replaced by broader criteria, yet to be determined.

The question of the inclusion of midwifery in the CFP and branch programme framework had been debated in depth at a special Council seminar the previous evening, and Council accepted that a significant revision of the original recommendation was necessary. Members agreed that experiments in the CFP/branch model as proposed in the Report should not proceed in midwifery, though with the proviso that training arrangements should not preclude any experimental programmes being proposed. It was also agreed that the eighteen-month post-registration preparation should be retained, an increase in three-year direct-entry midwifery programmes supported and opportunities for shared learning encouraged.

At the end of the Council meeting, Council asked Price Waterhouse to review their costings in line with the following revised assumptions: a student service contribution of 15–20 per cent; a teacher:student ratio of 1:12; a reduction in second registrations of 70 per cent;[51] and enrolled nurse conversions at a rate of 40 per cent. The team was also asked to undertake further work on the benefits that might be expected to flow from Project 2000.[52] In November 1986, Council again considered the alignment of its educational aspirations with the realities of running the NHS. They considered four 'packages' of possible modifications to the Project 2000 proposals. These ranged from minor changes, boosted by extensive managerial action to reduce wastage and improve recruitment, to the retention of some form of second level nurse training and a revision of the level of service contribution of students.[53] Once again a strong view against the continuation of second level nurse training emerged and the 'options' which were based around the maintenance of a second level were largely discounted. Instead, members focused on the feasibility of an educationally led student service contribution of around 20 per cent, and the possibility of combining this strategy with the development of a wider entry gate to nursing and concerted managerial action to broaden recruitment and reduce wastage of both learners and qualified staff. Members also agreed that the draft ministerial submission should include reference to the manpower difficulties inherent in any reform programme and to the Council's willingness to engage with government in the development of measures that could reduce the gap between supply and demand.[54]

'Final proposals'

Final discussion of these points took place in the open session of Council on 16 January 1987, following a frenetic period during which the UKCC's submission to Ministers was drafted and then circulated to the National Boards. Tensions had been exacerbated by appalling weather conditions and the worry that a quorum might not be achieved. Fortunately, sufficient members had been able to reach 23 Portland Place and the UKCC's strategy for education reform was formally agreed. It was presented as a strategy based upon two interlinked elements. The first was a package of education and training reforms which included the introduction of one level of practice based on a two-year common foundation programme and a one-year 'branch' programme in adult, children's, mental health (as opposed to illness) or mental handicap nursing. Midwifery would remain either an eighteen-month post-registration preparation or a three-year preparation for direct entrants. Students were to be supernumerary and their training under the control of educationalists rather than service managers. Nevertheless a service contribution of 20 per cent (of the three years in training) was considered acceptable, and indeed appropriate, given the high practical content of nursing preparation. The second strand comprised proposals to improve manpower supply and retention.[55]

The formal presentation of the proposals to Health Ministers took place at the Department of Health on 5 February 1987.[56] In addition to the Council's Chairman, Audrey Emerton, the statutory bodies' deputation included the Chairmen of the National Boards, the management consultants, the members of the Project Steering Group and key officers, including the Director for Professional Standards and the Project Officer. The Departmental representatives included the four Health Ministers, their senior civil servants and advisors from the Nursing Division. As the meeting was about to begin, and to everyone's surprise, Audrey Emerton got up and handed out the tea that had been left in the corner of the room, prompting the Minister, Tony Newton, to begin the meeting with a laughing comment about the Chairman of the Council being the most distinguished waitress he had ever met. As serious business commenced, the Council was thanked for its hard work on the proposals. The Minister of Health for England announced, on behalf of all four Health Departments, their intention to consult with health authorities and other interested groups before coming to a decision on the Project 2000 proposals. Since the feasibility of the proposals was heavily dependent on management action by the health authorities, their reaction was to be an important factor in the government's response.[57] Significantly, Newton also indicated the Departments' wish to associate the reform proposals with initiatives of their own on the role and training of the support worker.

Making a reality of reform

With Project 2000 delivered to Ministers, Council recognised the importance of ensuring that nurses, midwives, health visitors and other interested parties remained aware of the unfolding debate. Two further Project Papers – on the manpower and costs analysis of Price Waterhouse and on the final proposals as submitted to Ministers – were circulated among the professions, and a second video was produced. Also, a leaflet was sent to doctors registered with the GMC and followed up with a series of meetings with representatives of the medical profession.[58]

Almost immediately, however, it became clear that a further round of developmental work was necessary, engaging more closely with some of the concerns of both government and the professions. A joint Action Group of the Central Council and National Boards was set up to co-ordinate activity.[59] Work was put in hand on the nature of the common foundation programme, preparation for the specialist practitioner, the 'entry gate' to nurse training and the position of enrolled nurses. The Action Group produced a topic paper on the implications for nursing of the government's Youth Training Scheme (YTS) and the UKCC took part in a feasibility study.[60] During 1986, the UKCC was also represented on a Steering Group set up by the Chief Nursing Officer of the DHSS to examine the role and preparation of support workers.[61] The profession's hesitancy on the issue, and its demand for a sharp distinction between registered nurses and their helpers, however, sat uneasily with the government's pressure for concerted action.[62]

Government consultation with the health authorities on the Project 2000 proposals concluded in September 1987. Early indications remained encouraging for Council, pointing towards support for supernumerary status, the common foundation programme, increased numbers of mature and male entrants and a wider entry gate. Support was also forthcoming (though less so in Scotland) for the extension of the direct-entry training for midwifery. Nevertheless, strong reservations remained relating, in particular, to the manpower and costs implications of the cessation of enrolled nurse training and the restriction of student service contribution to 20 per cent. Doubts were also expressed on the skill gap between the helper and the first level nurse who, some authorities felt, might be too academic and insufficiently 'practical'. Concerns 'that the considerable extra costs involved may not be met from additional new central funding' were strong.[63]

On 11 December 1987 representatives of the Council and the Boards discussed with Departmental officials the outcome of the government's consultation, the results of the developmental work and the projected timetable for a ministerial decision on Project 2000. They were disappointed to learn that an announcement was not likely until April or May 1988. Official concerns had been strengthened by a further manpower modelling exercise (carried out by Price Waterhouse this time on behalf of the Health Departments), which indicated that the targets outlined in Council's proposals – particularly those relating to the expansion of recruitment to first level training – had been over-optimistic. The YTS Feasibility

Study, moreover, had not produced the answers the Departments were hoping for. Given the anticipated shortfall of recruits to first level nurse training, and the lack of firm progress on the future preparation of the support worker, Council's desire for an immediate end to second level training was looking increasingly unlikely.

Project 2000 accepted 'in principle'

On 20 May 1988, the UKCC received the news that the government had accepted the Project 2000 proposals in principle.[64] Later that day, members and officers welcomed the Minister for Health, Tony Newton, to a private session of Council to discuss the terms of the Secretary of State's response.[65] Government acknowledged that existing first level nurse training was 'unsatisfactory' and accepted the concept of an eighteen-month CFP and eighteen-month Branch Programme.[66] Agreement was given to a substantial reduction in students' rostered service contribution, to the payment of bursaries and the development of links with higher and further education. Further discussions with Council were proposed on the number and status of teaching staff, though broad support was given to the expansion of degree opportunities for nurses which, it was felt, would lead to an increase in the number of graduate teachers. Concerns, however, continued to be felt about the manpower implications of the Council's proposals. Recent work by the Department of Education and Science had indicated that 'the future recruitment pool' for nursing would be even smaller than previously thought. As a result, the government felt unable to offer a firm date for the cessation of enrolled nurse training. While the notion of a single level of nurse was accepted in principle, its implementation was subject to still further work being undertaken on widening the entry gate and the role of the support worker. Furthermore, calculations for a skill mix based on 64–70 per cent qualified staff were deemed unrealistic. The Secretary of State's letter stated, quite categorically, 'a professionally qualified workforce of the size you envisage cannot now be achieved throughout the UK in the foreseeable future'.[67]

News of the government's response to the UKCC dominated the professional press in May and June 1988 and also received considerable coverage in the daily newspapers. The reaction of the RCN General Secretary, Trevor Clay, was widely reported. It was, in his view, an 'exciting' and 'historic' time for nurses.[68] The reactions of other staff organisations, however, were more muted. COHSE and NUPE both expressed concerns that the strategy for the reform of nurse education adopted by the government paired an elitist vision of the professional nurse with increasing numbers of unqualified care-givers who would remain outside statutory regulation. It was a view that was to persist within union circles. In 1989 Paul Chapman of COHSE published his analysis of the government's response in the union's journal. It was, he argued, a masterpiece of 'flannel and non-commitment'.[69] With so much detail left to be worked out, Project 2000 arguably remained just that – a project and not a complete package.[70]

As the first term of office of the UKCC and National Boards drew to an end, members looked back to reflect on the enormous achievement that acceptance of Project 2000 represented.[71] The government's 'in principle' agreement to the Council's proposals was an immense boost to the educational content of nurse and midwifery training. But it was not a 'green light' for the new world of practice envisaged in the Project 2000 report. There were no guarantees at all that the Project's vision of an explicitly nurse-centred service was going to be won. Battles remained to be fought on a number of issues, including the cessation of EN training, conversion schemes and the preparation of teachers. How far and how fast Project 2000 education would be funded and implemented on the ground, moreover, was something in the hands of the Health Departments, not the UKCC.

A statutory base for implementation

With the government's 'in principle' agreement received, detailed preparations for implementation could now begin. For Council, the main task was to draft and consult the professions on new training rules. Work began in August 1988. A 'flexible framework of guidance' rather than rigid rulings was sought. This, it was hoped, would give National Boards and training institutions maximum scope for innovation, while enabling reciprocity to occur throughout the United Kingdom and ensuring that the requirements of the European Directives for Nurses Responsible for General Care were satisfied.[72]

Following extensive work with DHSS lawyers, and after consulting with the National Boards, two new statutory instruments were issued in August 1989. The first, SI 1989 No. 1455, created four new parts of the single professional register for those emerging from the branches of the new programme.[73] The second, SI 1989 No. 1456, outlined requirements for new courses of preparation.[74] This second statutory instrument was drafted in such a way as to permit new and experimental branches in the future: an important freedom given the difficulties experienced in coming to agreement on the future direction of midwifery education. In November 1989 the UKCC issued two supplementary circulars. The first gave further information on the content of the CFP and the branches, and identified the standard of the Project 2000 programmes as that of the Higher Education Diploma (DipHE). The second identified the amount of rostered service to be provided by the students during the programme.[75]

In relation to midwifery education, a third new statutory instrument, SI 1990 No. 1624, was issued in 1990. This stated the lengths of the two types of programmes of preparation (three years for direct entry and eighteen months for post-registration training), the supernumerary status of students on the three-year programmes, the need for training programmes to meet the European Directives for midwives and the outcomes to be achieved. In 1991 a UKCC Registrar's Letter was produced, identifying the standard of the programmes as that of the DipHE and requiring programmes to be educationally led and to have links with higher education. The status of the student, the period of practical experience and the requirements for the content of pre- and post-registration midwifery programmes were also stated.[76]

   The position of the second level nurse remained to be finalised. Nevertheless, a number of rule changes affecting enrolled nurses were approved in 1989. SI 1989 No. 1456, for instance, enshrined in rules Council's decision to allow ENs wishing to become first level nurses to have three additional examination attempts. Guidance material was also provided on possible routes to entry to a first level part of the UKCC's register.[77]

   If making a reality of the reforms was now a matter for schools and colleges, it was also importantly a matter for the Health Departments. In agreeing to Project 2000, the government indicated that implementation would need to be phased in over a considerable period of time – possibly as long as ten years – and that the timetable for change would vary in each of the four countries.[78] Given the constraints of the public expenditure planning process, and the fact that the Department would need to bid for Treasury funds each year, it was difficult for departmental officials to establish a firm implementation timetable for the introduction of the new programmes, though it aimed to see at least one nursing school in each region move to a Project 2000-type programme from autumn 1989. In October 1988, the first invitation was issued to regional health authorities to put forward submissions for funding (though the proportion of submissions recommended for approval was to vary each year, depending on the availability of funds and the size and cost of the schemes).[79] The first Project 2000 courses commenced in England in 1989, in Northern Ireland in 1990, in Wales in 1991. Scotland opted to begin all programmes simultaneously in 1992. Pre-registration midwifery (direct entry) courses developed rapidly from 1989, which was the first year the Department of Health provided 'pump-priming' money for the development of pre-registration midwifery education in fourteen sites across England. By 1993 thirty-five courses had been validated, with two Regions left to establish programmes. Pre-registration and post-registration midwifery programmes continued (and still continue) to exist side by side throughout the UK.[80]

In practice – 'continual evolution'

In May 1989, a year after the government first announced its 'in principle' acceptance of Project 2000, firm agreement had finally been given to the reforms. The UKCC formally received this in a second Ministerial letter to the chairman, Audrey Emerton. The letter confirmed the government's position on service contributions and bursaries, the expansion of degree opportunities, midwifery education and training, post-registration education and practice and widening the entry gate; announced the first wave of thirteen demonstration sites for the new Project 2000 education programmes and carried the prospect of an end to enrolled nurse training within five years.[81] Yet the statement also indicated the limits of the government's endorsement of radical change. The earlier expression of general support for improving the educational position of teaching staff, for example, was reiterated but not supported with specific policy. Indeed, the original report's recommendation for a move towards an all-graduate teaching staff was rejected as impractical in the current climate. While the cessation of EN training was tentatively accepted, it was envisaged to be a five-year strategy, linked to the evolution of health authorities' plans for Project 2000 programmes. Further progress on the question of the support worker, too, was a prerequisite: it was time, the Minister stated, for the Council to develop a framework for action and for a title and vocational qualifications to be agreed. The final statement of acceptance of Project 2000 – three years on from the publication of the report – was a careful mixture of reassurance and qualification. Educational reform was seen as being in a process of 'continual evolution'. Government regarded the reforms as a gradual process, moving forward 'in the light of experience', as funds allowed, and in the context of a programme, which was then taking shape, of fundamental change to the management structure of the service, bringing an internal market to health care provision.[82]

Council responded to the government's announcement in September 1989, following consultation with the National Boards and EPAC. It noted with appreciation the level of agreement between the statutory bodies and the government, and informed the Minister of the progress of continuing work on access to nursing education and the support worker. An undercurrent of doubt, however, remained over the government's commitment to the cessation of enrolled nurse training, and the opportunity was taken to reiterate the importance of this matter, and of the related questions of continuing education and conversion courses for existing enrolled nurses.[83]

Over the following months, officers and members kept a close eye on progress. In July 1990 the Chairman and the Registrar met with the Secretary of State and the Minister of Health, and received the assurance that government would re-examine the situation of the enrolled nurse. The subject of the support worker was also discussed, and the Secretary of State agreed to reiterate the statement made to the RCN Congress in 1989 that health care assistants should always work under the supervision of professional nurses.

From this point onwards, discussion of Project 2000 lessened.[84] Stages of implementation continued to be monitored as part of the Second Council's strategic objectives but, with funding of pre-registration education in the hands of the Health Departments and the development of programmes in the hands of the National Boards, the health authorities and the educational institutions themselves, the attention of members and officers could be transferred to other business, particularly the development of new standards for post-registration education and practice (see Chapter 6).

By the time the Third Council assumed office in April 1993, pre-registration education was fast evolving in the wider context of NHS and higher education reforms. Since it sat comfortably with neither the providers nor the purchasers of the new NHS internal market, it had been resolved that higher education would be its future home. The higher education sector, at this point, was undergoing substantial change, with the ending of the binary divide between the polytechnics and the universities, and with pressure to increase fee and grant income. While some in the profession had long hoped for such a move, its arrival in this fashion was unanticipated and its consequences could not be easily foreseen.[85] The uncertainty and the upheaval, moreover, generated confusion and criticism from within the profession. Research undertaken in six of the thirteen first-round demonstration sites in England found that while there was 'a sense of possibilities in the air', there was also 'uncertainty and unease about potential benefits'.[86] Individual nurse teachers were struggling to re-position themselves, not always feeling a sense of belonging to their new higher education institutions, and at the same time being answerable through the market to the unfamiliar ideologies of corporate NHS trusts. For ward staff, too, these were difficult times. The process of replacing the student service commitment proceeded in a locally determined and, in some cases, a largely *ad hoc* manner. Already under pressure from the competing demands on their time, many service staff felt ill-prepared for additional roles as 'mentors' and 'assessors' of the Project 2000 students.[87]

For all these reasons, the context of implementation of Project 2000 in the mid-1990s was radically different from the context of its production in the middle of the previous decade. Doubts began to grow, and with them came the call for an evaluation of just what the new programmes were achieving.

A new review takes shape

Change in the NHS and in higher education was accompanied by new thinking in other areas too. By the early 1990s, there was growing talk about the competencies, standards and performance of professionals, demand (already to some extent reflected in new training rules) for specification of outcomes of professional learning, and a growing movement towards evidence-based interventions in health care more generally. The Third Council, product of revised legislation in 1992, furthermore brought new kinds of member and an altogether new mood of questioning (see Chapter 3). It was not surprising then that questions began to be asked as to whether the educational reforms were producing the kinds of nurse that the service needed. An initial exploration of academic research and evaluation studies on Project 2000 was incorporated within Council's strategic objectives from the middle of the 1990s. Between summer 1994 and November 1995, the UKCC's Joint Education Committee set up a small Task Group, with links with the National Boards, the Health Departments and representatives from higher education, to prepare a preliminary report for Council on the current situation.[88] It found that the reforms were proving workable, although implementation had not been without significant 'teething troubles', many of which related to the speed at which programmes were developed and the limited resources available. Yet, while the new programmes needed time to bed down, issues requiring further attention in the medium and longer term were already becoming clear. The focus of the common foundation programme, shared learning and teaching, and entry criteria were drawn out for particular comment, as was the level of qualification and the nature of practice itself.[89]

By summer 1996 Council had expressed its desire to conduct a detailed examination of the effectiveness of pre-registration nursing and midwifery education to deliver 'fitness for practice' and 'fitness for purpose' in an environment of changing health care and professional need.[90] Recognising the growing momentum from outside for a reappraisal of the structure of health care education and training, Council's Joint Education Committee recommended that work progress through four strands: a review of the literature evaluating pre-registration courses; consideration of developments in multi-professional education; exploration of how the effectiveness of pre-registration education could be enhanced; and consideration of an all-graduate entry to the profession.[91] As the third five-year term of office drew towards its close, the Joint Education Committee went a step further. It recommended that a high-profile UKCC Education Commission should be established to determine a way forward, producing work that could be regarded as 'the authoritative stance on the future of pre-registration education'. This was duly agreed at the final meeting of the Third Council on 4 March 1998.[92]

The UKCC Education Commission began work in June 1998. Sir Len Peach, former Chief Executive of the NHS Management Board, and the first Commissioner for Public Appointments in Great Britain, was appointed as Chair. Its terms of reference stressed an education that produced 'fitness for purpose based on health care need'. Its membership included not only educators and practitioners, but consumer representatives and health and social care providers in all sectors. The work was to be as open as possible, with a deliberate seeking-out of the views of different stakeholders. It was also to be underpinned by research evidence on the performance of educational programmes and on changing health needs. All this underlined how far Council had moved its stance over the years as to how thinking about pre-registration education was to be carried out. Project 2000 had been set up at a time when belief in self-regulation by professions in these matters remained strong; it had been more internal in its membership, and deliberately less concerned with the immediate needs of day-to-day practice. It had also come at a time when financial retrenchment was still in its fairly early days.

The sharpest contrast of all, however, lay in the stance of the government. In 1984 the government of the day had been content, with an observer on the Project Group, to watch and wait until the proposals emerged. Only thereafter, as this chapter has shown, did it vigorously negotiate the form that educational reform would take. This time the government was much clearer about what it wanted from the professions for its new health and health care agenda, and was determined to force the pace. The Commission's report was made available in September 1999.[93] It had been preceded, however, in July by the government's new strategy for nursing midwifery and health visiting in England.[94] A wide-ranging document dealing with recruitment, working relationships and career structures as well as education, this went into considerable detail on pre-registration education. Its priorities were a more flexible system of pathways into and through education, a stronger emphasis on practical skills and greater responsiveness to NHS needs. It stated that it had 'shared with the Commission its plans' (para 4.4) and indicated that it would work in partnership to achieve them. With an annual spend of approaching £800 million, however, and a determination to get full value from it, the message was unambiguous: 'the Department of Health will in future take more direct responsibility for the shape and direction of nurse and midwife education' (para 4.13). Its talk of flexibility and responsiveness to service need, its valuing of access into nursing from a diversity of routes, its concepts of stepping-on and stepping-off points were strangely reminiscent of an earlier era. After nearly thirty years, was it to be back to Briggs?

Conclusion

Establishing a new framework for pre-registration nurse and midwifery education was a major test for the new statutory structure. Many of the fundamental issues explored at the time of Briggs, such as the levels of professional nursing, the balance between generic and specialist training and the special needs of midwives and community-based nursing practitioners, remained contentious and open to debate. The task of the UKCC was to steer a path through this maze. It was a high-profile activity, which tested the uncertain relationship between Council and Boards, required the new body to develop its processes for communication and exposed points of difference between nurses and midwives. Once the report was in the public arena, the challenge of holding the professions together and working with government to make political compromises was all too apparent. In the process of what the government liked to call 'continual evolution', neither the educational reforms nor the context of their implementation stood still. There were mixed evaluations in the mid-1990s, at the point at which the last new programmes had launched their students into practice, when the UKCC began to take stock. Change, entangled with wider NHS reform, had in some ways moved faster than those who coined the term 'Project 2000' had anticipated. But the term had stuck. Well before the year 2000 arrived, there was questioning, inside the statutory structure and outside it, of whether 'Project 2000 nurses' were what the health service and the profession needed for the new century. As we went to press, it was looking distinctly likely that the year 2000 was to see another round of pilot projects adjusting nurse education once again and reflecting the still ongoing debate about where the largest group of professions fitted in the overall division of labour in health care.

Notes

1 See Chapter 7, note 12.
2 The Education Working Group of the Briggs Co-ordinating Committee had failed to reach firm proposals on the question of the status of the nurse learner and had expressly passed the issue over to the new statutory bodies. See Briggs Co-ordinating Committee, Working Group 2, BCC(WG2)13, reclassified as a UKCC working group paper as Educ&Trg/81/4. See also UKCC Working Group 3, Consultation Paper 1, UKCC, K3.1, 'The development of nurse education', 1982; CC/82/28.
3 ENB Information Bulletin No. 4.
4 See UKCC, *Project 2000 – a New Preparation for Practice*, London, UKCC, 1986; Davies, C., 'Policy in nurse Education: plus ça change . . .', *Proceedings of the Nineteenth Annual Study Day*, Nursing Studies Association, University of Edinburgh, 1985; Davies, C., *Gender and the Professional Predicament in Nursing*, Buckingham, Open University Press, 1995; and Dolan, B. (ed.), *Project 2000. Reflection and Celebration*, Harrow, Scutari, 1993.

5 EPAC MIN 11/84; EPAC MIN 47/84.
6 C MIN 25/84, p. 3.
7 The majority of EPAC's nineteen members were in posts in nurse or midwifery education, and a further four were educationalists from outside nursing. For full membership details of EPAC see UKCC, *Annual Report 1984/85*, Annex 2, pp. 17–18.
8 C MIN 28/84, p. 2.
9 MIN 117/84, p. 10. EPAC also decided to invite a representative from the Health Departments to act as an observer, believing that early exposure to the Group's discussions might facilitate the process of change at a later stage. See EPAC MIN 53/84.
10 EPAC MIN 84/24.
11 EPAC MIN 53/84.
12 Funding also enabled the UKCC to establish a project office with the services of a full-time project assistant.
13 EPAC MIN 53/84, p. 2; MIN 117/84, p. 10.
14 Davies, C., 'Project 2000 – A word to tomorrow's historian', *History of Nursing Bulletin*, 2(4), 1988.
15 Dr Harry Judge was Director of the Department of Educational Studies at the University of Oxford. The terms of reference of the Commission were 'to examine the whole field of nursing education in the UK and to make recommendations'. See CC/84/29.
16 For details of this decision see ENB, *Annual Report 1984/85*, 1985, pp. 14–15. See also an article by Audrey Emerton on the Board's activities, 'Opportunity Knocks', *Senior Nurse*, 13 February, 2, 1985, pp. 18–19.
17 For a fuller account, see Chapter 3, pages 43–44.
18 The Report of the RCN Commission on Nursing was published on 17 April 1985 and that of the ENB on 15 May 1985. See UKCC, GrpB.JM/01, paper by Jane Macdonald on the reactions to the two documents. See also Kratz, C., 'The shape of things to come', *Nursing Times*, 19 June, 81(25), 1985, pp. 28–9 and Lathlean, J., *Policy Making in Nurse Education*, Oxford, Ashdale Press, 1989, p. 7.
19 P2000/85/3 'P2000: The task ahead (3) Communication'.
20 P2000/85/14, 'Project 2000 – Communications'; Project paper 1, 'Introducing Project 2000', September 1985, p. 6.
21 A longer account of the process of production of the Project 2000 report, together with more details on implementation, is available in an initial working paper from which this chapter has been drawn. A copy of the Working Paper was shown to Sir Len Peach, Chair of UKCC's Commission on Education and will be found among the Commission's papers.
22 Three of the project papers were published in *Senior Nurse* between November 1985 and January 1986, while the *Nursing Times* serialised one of the papers in December 1985 and carried a long accompanying article on the work of the project. A total of 561 people attended the road-show meetings. Participants from education were by far the largest group, representing 54 per cent of the total attendance. Representatives from practising nurses, midwives and health visitors constituted 7.1 per cent of the total.
23 P2000/85/31, 'An analysis of nursing press reactions to the RCN and ENB proposals'; P2000/86/07, 'Analysis of comments received by 3 January 1986 on Project Papers'.
24 P2000/86/15, 'The case for and against one level of practitioner'.
25 P2000/86/23, 'Length of common foundation programme and the branches'.
26 C MIN 16/86.
27 UKCC, *Project 2000 – A New Preparation for Practice*, p. 10, para. 1.14.
28 C MIN 20/86; CC/86/C10. See also CC/86/C26.
29 UKCC, *The Project 2000 Story*, London, UKCC, 1996, pp. 21–2.
30 P2000, 'Supplement No. 1: Project 2000 and the enrolled nurse', 1986; 'Supplement No. 2: Project 2000 and the midwife', 1986; 'Supplement 3: Project 2000 and the specialist practitioner', August 1986. In July 1986 an Educational Development

Group, whose membership comprised members and officers of the Council and the National Boards, was established to co-ordinate discussion of these difficult questions.

31 See Howie, C., 'Project 2000: Hopes and fears', *Nursing Times*, 16 July, 82(29), 1986, p. 20–1, for a report on the first of the *Nursing Times* series of six Project 2000 meetings. See also Dickson, N., 'Project 2000: Winding up the roadshow', *Nursing Times*, 22 October, 82(43), 1986, pp. 47–8. A number of meetings were also held with medical organisations, with the BMA and with the Joint Consultants' Committee. These showed a discouraging response on the cost and feasibility of the proposed reforms and indicated concern about possible blurring of professional boundaries.
32 *Annual Report 1986/87*, 1987, p. 3.
33 CC/86/C31.
34 COHSE members returning the union's postcards with 6 pre-set questions recorded a massive 85 per cent disagreement with the proposition that 'second level (enrolled) nurse training should end'. Project Paper 7, p.15.
35 The response of the RCM was reprinted in a supplement to *Midwives Chronicle and Nursing Notes* in December 1986. See also Newson, K., 'Project 2000: Disputed territory', *Nursing Times*, 6 August, 82(32), 1986, pp. 42–3.
36 See *Project 2000: A New Preparation for Practice*, pp. 40–1, para. 5.21 on the single list of competencies.
37 Project Paper 7, pp. 18–19.
38 *Ibid*.
39 Dickson, 'Project 2000: Winding up the roadshow', p. 47.
40 For responses of the National Boards see UKCC, K3.2(A5), Consultation with the Profession, section 3. Articles in the professional press also pointed to evidence of a growing mental handicap lobby. See, for example, 'Project envisages too narrow a role for mental handicap nursing', *Nursing Standard*, 21 August, No. 461, 1986, p. 1.
41 DHSS, *Neighbourhood Nursing: A Focus for Care. Report of the Community Nursing Review* (Cumberlege Report), London, HMSO, 1986.
42 Project Paper 7, p. 27.
43 Dickson, N., 'Where do we go from here?' *Nursing Times*, 14 May, 82(20), 1986, pp. 20–1.
44 C MIN 20/86; CC/86/C10.
45 C MIN 29/86; CC/86/C16.
46 Project Paper 8, 'Counting the cost: is Project 2000 a practical proposition?', p. 2; Davies, *Gender and the Professional Predicament*, p. 116.
47 Project Paper 8.
48 M. Hanson and T. Patchett, 'When the tap runs dry', *Nursing Times*, 31 December, 82(52), 1986, pp. 26–8.
49 CC/86/C31; C MIN 46/86.
50 C MIN 47/86.
51 The proportion of general nurses with specialist qualifications (and to some extent vice versa) was and continues to be fairly high.
52 C MIN 47/86; C MIN 50/86. A Benefits Report was drawn up in due course, but Price Waterhouse remained cautious about their own estimate that as much as £80 million per annum might arise from various types of benefit, such as the rationalisation of training, reductions in wastage during training and after registration, and better organisation and quality of care. As Davies pointed out, most commentators continued to see the issues as to do with costs and 'manpower', ignoring the relevant but hard to quantify factor of benefits: Davies, *Gender and the Professional Predicament*, pp. 117–8.
53 CC/8/C31; C MIN 50/86.
54 C MIN 51/86.
55 UKCC, Press release, 'Project 2000: Final proposals safely delivered', January 1987.

56 CC/87/24.
57 Letter from Tony Newton to chairmen of Regional, District and Special Health Authorities, 6 March 1987.
58 Project Paper 8, 'Counting the cost'; Project Paper 9, 'The final proposals', 1987; C MIN 23/87; C MIN 60/87; MIN 82/87.
59 C MIN 12/87.
60 This was sponsored by the DHSS, the National Health Service Training Authority, the Manpower Services Commission and the UKCC, to examine the extended use of YTS in the NHS and the possibility of using YTS programmes as a mechanism of entry into nurse training and as a means to prepare support workers. In November 1987 a report was produced which indicated that there was scope for the YTS to provide training for those interested in working in the NHS.
61 During the first half of 1987 Celia Davies was 'seconded' by the UKCC to the Health Department to help draft a consultation paper on the nurse helper.
62 See UKCC, K3.2 (A6), vol. 1, note of a meeting of P2000 Action Group, 20 March 1987; letter from Roger Holland, Chairman Joint UKCC and National Boards Action Group, to Len Peach, Chief Executive, NHS Management Board, 28 October 1987. A more detailed account of the UKCC's discussions of these issues can be found in the detailed working paper (see note 21 above).
63 MIN 82/87; C MIN 44/87 (b); CC/87/C25.
64 Letter from John Moore, Secretary of State for Social Services, to Audrey Emerton, Chairman of the UKCC, 20 May 1988, issued as part of a press release.
65 This was due to be announced at the RCN Congress on 23 May 1988. C MIN 62/88.
66 CC/87/C22, p. 4; CC/87/C28; C MIN 52/87(c).
67 See note 64.
68 See, for instance, *Nursing Times*, 1 June, 84(22), 1988, p. 5; *Today*, 24 May 1988; *The Guardian*, 24 May 1988, p. 24.
69 Chapman, P., 'Another view of Project 2000', *COHSE Journal*, 1(3), September/October, 1989.
70 See Crail, M., 'Project 2000 off to a shaky start', *COHSE Journal*, 2(4), July/August, 1990, pp. 10–11.
71 MIN 114/88 and C MIN/103/88.
72 EPAC MIN 31/88; EPAC MIN 41/88; EPAC/88/23; EPAC/88/25.
73 UKCC, PS&D/89/04(C), 'New parts of the UKCC's single professional register'.
74 UKCC, PS&D/89/04/(C), 'Project 2000 rules'.
75 UKCC, PS&D/89/04(B), 'UKCC requirements for the content of P2000 programmes'; PS&D/89/04/(C), 'Project 2000 rules'.
76 UKCC, Registrar's Letter 12/1991.
77 See UKCC, PS&D/89/04 (E), 'Additional examination attempts for enrolled nurses'; UKCC, PS&D/888/05, 'The enrolled nurse and preparation for entry to a first level part of the UKCC's register'.
78 AG/88/05, letter from J. M. Rogers, Assistant Secretary, DHSS to Colin Ralph, Registrar and Chief Executive Officer of the UKCC, 20 June 1988. National Audit Office (NAO), *Nursing Education: Implementation of Project 2000 in England*, London, HMSO, 1992, p. 11.
79 NAO, *Nursing Education: Implementation of Project 2000 in England*, pp. 1–2; CC/88/C69.
80 Gilmore, A., *Pre-registration nursing and midwifery education in the UK, final report*, research commissioned by the UKCC, 1998, p. 7.
81 UKCC, *Annual Report 1989/90*, p. 3. The letter was reprinted in full in *RCN Newsline*, 14(6), June 1989.
82 The first signs of change had become apparent with the publication in January 1989 of Department of Health, *Resourcing the NHS: the Government's White Paper: Working for*

Patients, London, HMSO, 1989; Department of Health, *Education and Training Working Paper 10*, London, HMSO, 1989; *National Health Service and Community Care Act*, 1990.

83 CC/89/56; CC/89/58; letter from Audrey Emerton to the Rt. Hon. Kenneth Clarke, Secretary of State for Health, 7 September 1989. CC/90/11; A letter in reply was received by the Chairman in November 1989, and considered by the full Council in January 1990, MIN 7/90 (a), January 1990.

84 The introduction of new courses, however, did receive attention from Council, see MIN 34/90 (e); MIN 48/90 (e); C MIN 56/90.

85 Department of Health, *Working Paper 10*. See also Humphreys, J., 'English nurse education and the reform of the National Health Service', *Journal of Education Policy*, 11, 6, 1996. Stanwick, S., 'The market for education: supply and demand', in Humphreys, J. and F. M. McQuinn (eds) *Health Care Education: The Challenge of the Market*, London, Chapman & Hall, 1994, pp. 102–17; and Meerabeau, L., 'Project 2000 and the nature of nursing knowledge', in Abbott, P. and L. Meerabeau (eds), *The Sociology of the Caring Professions* (second edn), London, UCL Press, 1998, pp. 82–195.

86 Jowett, S., I. Walton, S. Payne, *Challenges and Change in Nurse Education. A Study of the Implementation of Project 2000*, Slough, NFER, 1994, pp. 23–40.

87 Elkan, R., R. Hillman, J. Robinson, *The Implementation of Project 2000 in a District Health Authority: the effect on the nursing service. An interim report*, Nursing Policy Studies 7, University of Nottingham, 1991; R. Elkan and J. Robinson, 'Project 2000: A review of published research', *Journal of Advanced Nursing*, 22(2), August 1995, pp. 386–92.

88 EC/94/18.

89 EC MIN 94/30; EC MIN 95/22; EC MIN 95/46.

90 JEC/96/10(b).

91 JEC MIN 27/96(1); JEC MIN 13/97(1); JEC MIN 97/20; JEC MIN 98/02; JEC MIN 98/03.

92 MIN 6/98(2); CC/98/08.

93 UKCC, Fitness for Practice: The UKCC Commission for Nursing and Midwifery Education, (Chair: Sir Leonard Peach), London, UKCC, 1999.

94 Department of Health, *Making a Difference. Strengthening the nursing, midwifery and health visiting contribution to health and healthcare*, London, Department of Health, 1999. The National Assembly for Wales had also produced a strategy document, *A Strategic Framework for Nursing, Midwifery and Health Visiting in Wales into the 21st Century*, Cardiff, National Assembly for Wales, 1999, and it was likely that further developments would emanate from Scotland in the context of its new devolved powers.

5 Upholding standards of professional conduct

The 1979 legislation gave the statutory bodies a wide-ranging remit to improve both standards of education and training for nurses, midwives and health visitors and standards of professional conduct. The opportunity to treat professional-conduct work in a more positive way – to bring together systems for dealing with misconduct across the four countries of the UK and to develop procedures for dealing with those who were unfit to practise on health grounds – was taken up with alacrity, as Chapter 2 has shown. The workload was heavy, and much time and attention were devoted to finding ways of dealing with this. At a number of points, however, Council chose to reflect on the significance of issues arising from cases coming forward. In doing so, it challenged not only individual practitioners, together at times with their managers and employers, but it also sometimes confronted the government of the day on matters of health policy and resources. New legislation in 1992 concentrated the professional-conduct function at Council level and extended the powers of the UKCC significantly. By the end of the period under consideration – whether led by sheer practicality of an overburdening workload or by conviction of the need for fundamental change – mechanisms for the greater involvement of both lay people and ordinary practitioners in the professional-conduct machinery were in place. A series of high-profile and controversial cases, starting in the late 1980s, had brought an altogether new level of questioning, both of what the decisions should be and of how they were being reached. This chapter, with its close look at the pattern of development over fifteen years, offers the kind of contribution that is often missing when debate focuses on the justice or otherwise of single decisions and is fuelled by high-profile media attention.

A new process in practice

For the first ten years of the UKCC, the machinery of professional conduct involved two tiers. National Boards investigated cases and decided whether they should be forwarded to the UKCC. Where it was a case of alleged misconduct, members of Council, sitting as a Professional Conduct Committee (PCC), would hear the case in public session. They would then come to a decision in private session as to whether the practice of the individual constituted professional misconduct and a sufficient a risk to the public to warrant removal from the register. The legislation also allowed for the UKCC to receive cases dealing with unfitness to practise on grounds of ill-health. The Health Committee, sitting in private session, began to hear such cases in September 1984. At this stage of Council's development, applications for restoration stemming from either route would be heard in the course of a session of the PCC. The Nurses Welfare Service, an independent charitable body, offered help to practitioners preparing for a hearing.[1]

An early objective set for both Council and the Boards was to limit to no more than six months the time lapse between the initial report to a National Board and the eventual judgement by the PCC of the UKCC, unless exceptional circum- stances applied.[2] The workload quickly built up, however. The PCC sat on over 100 days in 1987/8 and the number of persons being considered each year soon exceeded 300. Health Committee cases were fewer, but cases dealt with by health screeners had reached 100 in the last year of the First Council; and the Health Committee, first getting into full swing in 1985/86, sat on sixteen occasions that year.[3]

While this work was going on, the preventive dimension was given promi- nence. Activities carried out by the former statutory bodies, particularly the GNC for England and Wales, were continued and extended during the early years of the UKCC.[4] Practitioners, for instance, were encouraged to attend hearings of the PCC as observers, and the Council and National Boards agreed that considered case material should be 'made known and used in an educational manner' at lectures and seminars. It was felt that not only would this demonstrate the statutory bodies' commitment to their role as protectors of the public, but it would also provide members of the professions the opportunity to learn about professional standards and issues of responsibility and accountability.[5] The *Annual Report* of 1984/85 noted that there had been an average of at least twenty observers attending each of the peripatetic PCC meetings. Feedback was extremely positive, indicating 'that those who do attend not only find it a useful learning experience, but also a stimulus to examine their own practice'.[6] The following year, Council reported a significant increase in the number of representatives from Community Health Councils (or Local Health Councils in Scotland) who attended hearings.[7] It was hoped that a report on a selection of cases considered by the PCC would soon be ready for issue.

One of the most pressing areas of concern was the high proportion of second level (enrolled) nurses among the respondents appearing before the PCC. Council expressed concern at the degree to which second level nurses were being 'placed in positions of responsibility for which their nursing training did not prepare them and was not intended to prepare them'. Chairmen of the PCC, it noted, felt obliged to remind 'those who use first and second level nurses in interchangeable roles' of the specific competencies required of trained second level nurses by the statutory training rules. It was 'sometimes necessary', indeed, to read Rule 18(2) of the Nurses Training Rules 'publicly before the announcement of judgements in respect of Enrolled Nurses so that the background against which those judgements is made is properly understood by complainants and public'.[8] Concerns were also expressed over 'the disturbing evidence of improper delegation to untrained personnel', and at the frequency with which practitioners appearing as respondents before the Committee ('especially those from the less fashionable specialities') had been employed in settings which were 'seriously understaffed or inappropriately staffed'.[9] A similar concern was noted about the high proportion of alleged misconduct cases involving mental handicap nurses which showed evidence of serious staff shortages. At the March 1986 meeting of Council the issue was raised by Tariq Hussain, himself a practitioner from this field, and it was agreed that a letter to the Minister of Health and the NHS management authority should be drafted by the Chairman and Deputy Chairmen of the PCC.[10] In principle, the findings of the Health Committee could be drawn upon for further comment in a similar way. In practice, the confidential nature of the work largely prevented this.[11]

Analyses of the implications of misconduct cases highlighted what might be called the political dimension of Council's regulatory role. The first *Annual Report* stated

> the interests of both public and practitioners must be served by the willingness of the Council and Boards to make representations to Government and to employers in the public and private sector where by virtue of inadequate staffing, resources or premises safe standards of practice are not possible and patients are put at risk.[12]

In the view of Reg Pyne, Director for Professional Conduct at the time, this signified an important new development. Whereas 'in the past, statutory bodies have been by their very nature rather blandly apolitical', the new legislation brought the statutory bodies into 'new forms of activity and a new relationship with government'.[13] Council's ability to draw informative conclusions about standards of professional conduct and practice, however, was limited by the fact that complaints had already been sifted by the National Boards. This situation was to change with the 1992 Act.

For most of the first term, however, the sheer volume of work was the most pressing issue. Council members agreed that delay was neither in the interests of natural justice, nor in the interests of public protection.[14] In an attempt to bring the situation under control, members had immediately assumed a heavy PCC commitment. While this short-term approach to the problem of backlog brought some success, a year later, in September 1985, it was clear that the objective set out in Council's first strategy document *Into the 1990s*, that the majority of cases should be dealt with within six months, was still not being met.[15]

An ever-widening reappraisal

Council's response to the problem of backlog and to the rising costs of professional conduct work[16] was to instigate an exercise of self-examination and appraisal, that was to continue throughout the remaining period of the first term and into the next. Towards the end of 1985 a task force was established[17] and a number of helpful administrative revisions was suggested and later accepted by Council and Boards. The discussions also highlighted more deeply rooted problems. At one level, the deliberations of the task force revealed the wariness that remained between the two components of the regulatory structure: a sense of unease demonstrated most strongly by the ENB, which was unhappy with Council's imposition of cash limits on investigation work. This was, indeed, an important issue: if the costs of the professional-conduct function were not met wholly through registration fees, then genuine self-regulation could not be said to be in place. Yet, the alternative – a closer delineation of the types of case which should be treated as priorities – was also perceived by the ENB as neither practicable nor acceptable.[18] Concerns were also beginning to surface over the varied procedures used by the National Boards in their investigation work, leading to calls for agreement on a common format for presentation of cases to the UKCC and on tentative suggestions for guidelines about closing down insubstantial cases.[19] It was an issue that was to be re-opened, with less reticence, by the first Departmental Review of the five bodies, undertaken in 1988–9.

The activities of the task force went deeper. There were anxieties about whether the statutory bodies had achieved the right balance between the 'negative' dimension of the disciplinary control of the small minority who transgressed, and the 'positive' aspect of improving standards of conduct for the professions as a whole. There was, it was suggested, 'no yardstick against which to judge the effectiveness of the professional conduct work' of the regulatory bodies. How could the Council assess whether the increasing amount of money, and members' time, devoted to professional discipline was being well spent? The group's final recommendation was for a major review of the 'whole concept of professional regulation' to 'consider the most appropriate ways in which the public can be protected and professional standards maintained and enhanced in the future'.[20] For a new organisation, barely three years old and still in the process of developing fresh relationships and processes, this was a deeply unsettling message. Though initially shaken, Council did agree to the establishment of a longer-term review at its meeting in July 1986. By this stage, it was conscious that a review of the working of the 1979 Act was likely to be instituted by the Departments of Health: in this context, a major in-house review of professional conduct work did not seem 'so alarming and inappropriate' as it first appeared to be.[21] Indeed, seen in this light, the tentative meetings of the task force provided both Council and the Boards with an important and timely reminder that many of the difficulties experienced by the new statutory structure stemmed from the limitations of the legislation itself.

Council's attention had already been directed to the deficiencies in the secondary legislation – the Professional Conduct Rules. Earlier in 1985, a detailed study of the operation of the statutory instrument (SI 1983 No. 887) was initiated by Council's officers and its solicitor, David Faull, in the hope that any procedural obstacles delaying the progress of cases might be identified and amendments sought. A lengthy process of negotiation between Council members, the Council's solicitor and the Lord Chancellor's Department (Lord Advocate for Scotland, and Lord Chief Justice in Northern Ireland) ensued, which finally was completed in 1988.[22]

A notable issue discussed during this period was the advisability of reducing the quorum of members on both Conduct and Health Committees from five to three. In September 1985 Council had agreed to this revision, though a significant number of members maintained their concern for the possible effects on decision making of a more limited PCC membership. The matter came before Council again in January 1988, as the amended Rules were about to become operative. By this stage a significant groundswell of opinion had accumulated against it, not least from the RCN and RCM. While it was accepted that the continuing backlog of cases awaiting hearing potentially weakened Council's ability to act in the public's interest, the rights of individual respondents to receive a fair and just hearing had also to be acknowledged. The proposal was rejected.[23] Yet members also agreed that the issue of PCC membership could not simply be ignored. In particular, Council felt that the question of the pool of members from which the PCC could be constituted needed to be examined in greater detail.[24] Under the 1979 Act, membership of the PCC was restricted to Council members, constituted 'with due regard to the professional field' of the respondent concerned and the aim was always to have two drawn from the respondent's specialty. As early as July 1985, Council acknowledged the difficulties experienced in scheduling cases involving mental handicap nurses. Many of these cases were practice-related, and consequently required the presence of at least one of Council's two mental handicap specialists on the PCC. Biannual statistical breakdowns of member attendance at PCC and Health Committees confirmed what members had come to suspect, that within the general backlog of cases certain areas of nursing practice were experiencing particular difficulties.[25] Workloads were not getting any lighter.[26] With the option of a reduced quorum discounted for the time being, members perceived the forthcoming departmental legislative review as a valuable opportunity to review the existing position.

Council's interest in a revised system of PCC membership, however, also stemmed from a growing awareness of the wider advantages of expansion. At its April 1988 meeting, members expressed particular interest in using the newly up-to-date register to select a random, but specified, number of registrants from each specialty to serve on Professional Conduct Committees. The existing quorum of five would be retained, but with three members of Council joined by two members drawn from this supplementary pool. This method, it was argued, would introduce 'a more comprehensive (and thereby possibly more respected) concept of peer judgement, since it would inevitably involve a higher percentage of practitioners in direct patient care than the present system affords'.[27] It would also, the Annual Report of 1987/88 noted, contribute to the Council's desire to explore the educational and preventive dimension of professional conduct work, enabling 'those who had served to take back to their work settings some significant lessons'.[28] Taking this forward would require new primary legislation – a process that would not occur before the Department of Health had carried out its first five-year review of the statutory structure. The issue at this stage was referred to Council's newly established Primary Legislation Review Group for further consideration.[29] As the UKCC moved into its second five-year term, a major overhaul of the processes of professional conduct seemed increasingly necessary.

Preventing cases arising in the first place was another way of looking at the matter. As knowledge of cases grew, so work was done on elaborating particular clauses of the code of conduct so as further to inform practitioners of their responsibilities.[30] Later, in 1992, a third edition of the code was to consolidate these and develop them further. It was clear, however, that a rather different educational task was also needed, one to discourage inappropriate use of the conduct machinery. In the second term of Council, work began on advice targeted mainly at employers on the cases they were bringing forward. Issued in November 1990, a new document set out the stringent conditions of evidence that needed to be met for a complaint to be upheld.[31] It drew a clear distinction between decisions about whether a practitioner should continue in post (an employer matter) and whether a practitioner should continue in practice (a statutory/body matter). It stated firmly that the machinery was not about providing employers with an additional avenue of complaint or with giving them grounds for dismissal of an employee. Nor was it to be used 'when an appeal against dismissal has been upheld'. This message had been running through *Annual Reports* almost since the inception of the UKCC. It was the first time, however, that Council had been so direct about dissuading employers and managers from trying to use the machinery for purposes for which it was not intended. The theme was to recur in subsequent publications.

Could more be done to pinpoint just what misconduct was, and hence to divert cases away from the machinery of professional conduct? Council had always been wary of classifications, underlining the uniqueness of individual cases and the complexity of individual circumstances.[32] The 1990 document gave some guidance on this, listing broad types of conduct likely or not to be seen as misconduct, and explained factors that might be seen as mitigating circumstances when it came to a final decision (see Figure 5.1). The document also stressed, however, that there were always relevant circumstances, including the practitioner's history, present position and previous performance, to be taken into account.

Cases likely to result in removal

- Reckless and wilfully unskilled practice
- Concealing untoward incidents
- Failure to keep essential records
- Falsifying records
- Failure to protect or promote the interests of patients or clients

Figure 5.1 Common types of misconduct case 1990[33]

- Failure to act knowing that a colleague or subordinate is improperly treating or abusing patients
- Physical or verbal abuse of patients/clients
- Abuse of patients by improperly withholding prescribed drugs, or administering unprescribed drugs or an excess of prescribed drugs
- Theft from patients or employers
- Drug-related offences
- Sexual abuse of patients
- Breach of confidentiality.

Cases that are often closed

- Offences related to motor vehicles
- Issues that relate specifically to employment, such as leaving duty early without authority, overtime claims in excess of hours worked, or mistakes disclosed by the practitioner which were made under pressure of work
- Cases where the practitioner's failure was effectively a failure to achieve the impossible in the particular circumstances that applied
- Cases that result from careful and conscientious exercise of professional judgement by the practitioner, and which can be justified as reasonable in the circumstances and at the time the decision was taken
- Situations where the case has been brought by a complainant measuring the actions of the practitioner against outdated practices and norms.

Mitigating circumstances

- The incident was isolated and uncharacteristic and the practitioner appears to have learned lessons from it
- There were, at the time, overwhelming personal problems that led the practitioner to behave inappropriately, and which have since been resolved
- The practitioner has been retained in employment and is the subject of good reports
- The practitioner, having been responsible for an error, has made no attempt to conceal it and has immediately reported it in the interests of the patient
- With hindsight it is clear that the incident was an error in professional judgement rather than a culpable act
- The practitioner was one of a number involved, but the only person to be the subject of a complaint
- Removal is judged to be too harsh a response to the facts that have been established.

Figure 5.1 (continued)

Legislative reform takes shape

The first formal Departmental Review of the five statutory bodies was undertaken by consultants Peat Marwick McLintock in 1989.[34] It was an opportunity for an outside look at systems and practices and at the question of backlog which had so preoccupied Council. A unified structure, whereby Council undertook the investigative stages as well as holding professional conduct hearings, was a key recommendation. Delays were not the only matter at issue here. The consultants took the view that roles and responsibilities were not clear. They were particularly concerned at what they felt to be a judgemental attitude adopted by some investigating committees. The reviewers recommended a standard investigating procedure for all Boards, pending the transfer of the investigation function to Council. Disappointingly, from Council's point of view, the report did not recommend a power of reprimand or caution at the PCC stage, something that had been regarded as a weakness as early as the days of the Shadow Council.[35]

The review also examined the issue of membership of the PCC and the value of an extended pool. Its main focus was the benefits this could bring to the Council's problem of backlog, though it was also acknowledged as a way in which the wider profession could become more closely involved. The consultants recommended that a panel of practitioners could make themselves available for PCC work over a period of two or so years and, after some training, would 'sit with central body members as required – say three members and two jurors to constitute a committee'.[36] Council, as we have seen, already viewed this with some favour. While its realisation in legislation was to come shortly, its realisation in practice, however, took considerably longer.

Once it became clear, early in 1990, that the government was prepared to act on the recommendations of Peat Marwick McLintock, Council sought to use the opportunity to broaden the scope of its disciplinary powers. Something of a battle then ensued, focused in particular on the issue of power to caution. This matter was referred to the newly formed Legislative Advisory Group (LAG) which comprised representatives of the government and the statutory bodies. It was made clear to the Council that it would be extremely difficult to achieve major changes since the government 'hoped that as few amendments as possible would be made to the Nurses, Midwives and Health Visitors Act of 1979'.[37] Council, however, was adamant that both the power to caution and also a power to suspend from the register should be incorporated into the amending legislation.[38] From the UKCC's point of view, the introduction of a power to suspend would bring two distinct benefits. Not only could it be used to de-stigmatise those practitioners whom Council's Health Committee recommended should stop practising on health grounds by 'suspension' rather than removal from the register, but it would enable the Council, in exceptional cases, to prevent a person from practising where an immediate risk to the public was perceived.[39]

Over the summer of 1991, the statutory bodies were advised by government officials that the Health Departments were sympathetic, in principle, to amending Section 12 of the Act to allow UKCC a power of suspension from the register.

With regard to the wish for the power to caution, the Departments were 'willing to be convinced that this was appropriate but would need to be assured that all professional bodies and relevant staff interests were content with the proposal'. In July, the statutory bodies reiterated their case for additional disciplinary powers. The proposed power to caution, it was argued, would help the Council to speed up the processing of cases, and enable it to take definite action in cases which, although not serious enough to warrant removal, were cause for concern. The main stumbling block, however, was the 'clear ministerial remit that all amendments would have to be non-controversial, otherwise the whole bill might be in jeopardy'.[40]

By September, Council seemed to be making headway. The government indicated that powers of both suspension and caution were in train. The manner in which these new powers were to be exercised was to be framed in rules by the UKCC following consultation with interested parties.[41] When the draft Bill was discussed at the end of the month, however, Council was disappointed. The Bill provided an express power to make rules for suspension, but contained no reference to an explicit power to administer a formal caution. Officials explained that parliamentary counsel considered it to be unnecessary, as the greater power to remove from the register necessarily incorporated the lesser power to caution or reprimand.[42] Council now urged members of the House of Lords and MPs to support an amendment to this affect, arguing that it was a public-interest matter to speed up the process and reduce the backlog. Baroness Cumberlege, herself a Secretary of State appointee to the Council, spoke on this issue at the House of Lords Committee stage, noting that only 45 per cent of cases heard resulted in the 'draconian solution' of removal from the register.[43] Lord Meston, at this time a UKCC legal assessor, supported Council's case by pointing out that a power of caution would enable it to be made clear, in cases where the ultimate sanction was inappropriate, that behaviour was still not to be condoned.[44] He also drew attention to the fact that absence of the clause from the Bill was due to a difference of legal opinion on whether specific provision was necessary rather than a division over the desirability of the power.[45] Following second reading, the Department reconsidered the issue, and the Government accepted that the power to caution should be available. An amendment was successfully brought and both the power to suspend and the power to caution were incorporated in the new Act.

By 1993, therefore, the legislative framework for dealing with professional conduct and fitness to practise had been changed in a number of key respects. After much lobbying on Council's part, the process was now a unified one, with a Preliminary Proceedings Committee (PPC) operating at the UKCC. The distinction between removal for misconduct and suspension for unfitness to practise for health reasons had been secured and, in instances where an immediate risk to the public was perceived, Council was able to suspend a person from the register pending further investigation and a hearing. The much coveted power to caution was now available. There was also the potential to write into rules the participation of non-Council members – practitioners and lay people – in the disciplinary process.[46] Furthermore, and again following strong lobbying from the UKCC, Council's membership had been enlarged to sixty. This put it in a stronger position both to provide the members needed to carry the continuing workload and to have oversight and assess and evaluate its own activities. However, an altogether different kind of evaluation was soon to be needed. In face of a changing external environment, professional conduct decisions were about to become very much more controversial.

New developments in the face of controversy

The climate of opinion at this point was changing. During the mid- and later 1980s, the GMC in particular had experienced mounting criticism over the perceived deficiencies of its disciplinary system.[47] Lay voices, especially those representing the consumers of health services, were particularly strong. In October 1988 Health Rights published a sharp critique of the GMC, *A Patient Voice at the GMC*, authored by Jean Robinson, a former Chairperson of the Patients' Association and a member of the GMC since 1979.[48] Her starting point was a case where the behaviour of a doctor was regarded by the GMC Professional Conduct Committee as 'below the standard which can be regarded as acceptable in a medical man', but was not deemed to constitute 'serious professional misconduct'. This pronouncement had led Nigel Spearing MP to introduce a private member's bill seeking amending legislation to enable the GMC to incorporate the lesser charge of 'unacceptable conduct' within its disciplinary process. 'Powers that Parliament gave', Robinson reminded, 'are powers that Parliament can take away'.[49] It was a message the UKCC and National Boards, already perturbed by the apparent structural weaknesses of their own system, and preparing for the forthcoming Departmental legislative review, could not fail to hear.

Robinson regarded the UKCC's disciplinary processes as considerably more healthy than those of the GMC. The Council's charge of 'professional misconduct' (as opposed to the GMC's '*serious* professional misconduct'), open access to the reports of UKCC Professional Conduct Committee hearings, the screening of complaints by a committee instead of by one person and the effective simplicity of the Council's *Code of Professional Conduct* were all points in its favour. Nevertheless, the absence of an explicit requirement to include a lay member (particularly one representing consumer interests) on the Preliminary Proceedings Committees, or even the PCC, was highlighted by Robinson as a serious cause for concern.[50]

When the Second Council assembled in November 1988, a controversial case was in process. The case had attracted considerable publicity before it came to the PCC, and the hearing had been accompanied by noisy placard-carrying demonstrators who remained outside the venue for each of the six days on which the case was heard. It was clear that the respondent would appeal against any decision to remove her from the register, and that an already quite unprecedented level of publicity for the Council's disciplinary work in this case would continue.

Jilly Rosser, an independent midwife, had been called before a PCC, following a patient complaint.[51] Various allegations were made concerning the care of the patient. These were denied. Four of seven charges were found proved and she was removed from the register. The case had taken a considerable time in coming before the Council's PCC.[52] The apparent severity of the decision in face of witness statements supporting the respondent and statements of mitigating circumstances caused comments and some began to question whether Council members were in touch with current practice.[53] Many of the demonstrators, some of the press and some midwives believed the issue was about the principle of home confinements and was calling into question the overall worth of the practice of independent midwifery. This last was a matter of particular frustration to the Council, which issued a press statement to clarify that neither of these issues of principle was involved. Ms Rosser appealed to the High Court against the UKCC. The appeal decision went in her favour and she was reinstated. The appeal centred on whether or not the PCC should have allowed the hearing of rebuttal evidence – and the UKCC conceded that there had been an error.[54] The episode left a number of misunderstandings all round.[55] The careful procedural rules – specifying how evidence was to be used, bringing legal advice in at all key stages, enabling a PCC to deliberate on its decision in camera, disallowing Council as a whole the right to re-open a case – had often been admired. In an instance surrounded by publicity, and where such strong feelings had been at stake, it seemed that the system had not been able to address matters entirely effectively.

To this point most of the professional-conduct business had been carried through without public comment. Very few of the cases that had been brought forward had been questioned on other than points of law. Indeed there were very few indeed that had successfully gone to appeal or where leave had been sought for a judicial review which had been decided against the Council.[56] No other case during the term of the Second Council was to generate the public and professional controversy that had been stimulated by this one. Yet there were signs that controversy was mounting. The Donnelly case – a nurse convicted of indecent assault on two 13-year-old boys and later dismissed from employment after being found alone with a 14-year-old – was an example. The decision of the PCC was that misconduct was proved, but no removal from the register was ordered. This gave rise to a certain amount of protest.[57] Other controversies included an employing NHS Trust questioning a restoration decision,[58] and an aggrieved relative of a patient who had died, who wrote a series of letters questioning the evidence and the decision of the committee to close the case.[59] An appeal (Jhugroo case) caused Council to change its procedure and routinely to consider removal for a specified period as a penalty. This could be seen as a technical matter of interpretation of statute and rules, however, rather than as a fundamental questioning of the decisions made.[60]

The Third Council, like its predecessor, began its work in the face of a controversial professional conduct case. This time, the controversy was just a taste of things to come. Three months after its first meeting, in June 1993, the Council received a report from the Registrar, Colin Ralph, on the wide publicity in the national press given to the Leeming case. The case concerned the restoration of a ward sister who had been removed from the register in 1992, following conviction for perverting the course of justice after lying to the police about the circumstances of the death of a 70-year-old patient in a hospital psychiatric ward. The case had come just a few weeks after the shock of newspaper revelations about Beverley Allitt who, when employed in a children's ward at Grantham and Kesteven Hospital, injured and murdered thirteen children in her care. The implications of the Leeming case were considered by David Blunkett, then shadow Health Secretary, who was already taking an interest in the workings of the GMC. In commenting on the issue in the House of Commons he drew explicit attention to the low level of lay representation on the UKCC as a whole, and especially on the PCC.[61] In Blunkett's view, there was 'an important balance to be achieved between those committed to the interests of nurses or other health professionals and those with an interest in protecting patients'.

Such a view lent weight to the contemporary observation in an editorial in the *Nursing Times*:

> There is no reason to suppose that if there had been a lay member on the conduct committee that restored Ms Leeming's name to the register the decision would have been different. Public perception of the outcome might well have been, though.[62]

The issue, the same editorial noted, went to the heart of the public's confidence in nursing and in the Council's ability to fulfil its statutory role. 'Before it gets too settled in', the *Nursing Times* advised, 'the new Council should look at ways in which it can be sure that it not only does a good job on conduct issues but also is seen to do so'.[63] At its October 1993 meeting, Council agreed to establish a panel of consumer representatives, chosen from nominations made by a wide range of consumer organisations in the fields of health and social care. In May 1994 ten consumer representatives were appointed and soon after began to take part in professional-conduct work.[64] Consumer participation at this time was limited to the PCC. Later, at the end of the Third Council and the beginning of the Fourth, members debated the inclusion of consumers on the closed Preliminary Proceedings and Health Committees, and the trend of greater consumer involvement gathered speed (see Chapter 8).

After Leeming, a series of deeply controversial cases followed in quick succession. Three were concerned with restorations to the register of those convicted of serious offences and two concerned with the new power of caution. These cases threw the Council under the spotlight as never before. 'Killer and Rapist can go back to Nursing' was the headline in the *Sunday Mirror* on 25 June 1995. The *Mail on Sunday* also picked up the story. Subaschan Bundhun, removed from the register after being convicted of raping a frail elderly woman in his care, had now successfully applied for restoration. Owen Winn had served a prison sentence for manslaughter and had similarly gained restoration to the register. Letters expressing shock at these decisions appeared in the nursing press. UNISON drew Council's attention to the severe disquiet on the part of some of its members. There were also letters directly to the UKCC expressing dismay and at times deep disgust on the part of practising nurses about the decisions that had been taken and the message they gave about the profession.[65] The UKCC also received two letters from MPs who had been contacted by their constituents about these cases. Shadow Health Minister Nick Brown demanded an explanation from the Minister of Health, Virginia Bottomley.[66]

In mid-September, the *Nursing Times* took up the story and linked the Bundhun case with that of Thorpe-Price, a drug smuggler who had served a prison sentence and had just been cautioned and allowed to remain on the register. It quoted Philip Darbyshire, a senior lecturer in nursing, as saying that nurses were now asking 'What in God's name do you have to do not to be fit to practise?' In a letter responding to the article, the Assistant Registrar for Professional Conduct, Tariq Hussain, attempted to put the cases in perspective. There had been fifty-eight hearings between April and September and in thirty-seven of these cases practitioners had been removed.[67]

There was worse to come. The Choy case, a restoration hearing taking place in March 1996, became the highest-profile case of them all, and an application for judicial review was made by no less a body than the RCN. Mr Choy had first been convicted in 1972 of theft and of administering drugs in order to obtain sexual intercourse. He had been convicted again in 1984 and sent to prison for rape of a patient. At this point he was removed from the register. A first application for restoration was denied in 1995, but this second application succeeded and he was restored to the register in March 1996. This decision occasioned a greater volume of adverse press commentary than ever before and again the UKCC received letters of protest from individual nurses. Before the judicial review could be held, however, it emerged that Mr Choy had failed to disclose his full history to his referees and that he had made no reference to his convictions in applying for a post. With this new information, the UKCC came to an agreement with the RCN that the decision to restore should be quashed. The court agreed and there was no further hearing. Some indication of the level of nurse outrage at the restoration decision can be gleaned from the reaction at the RCN Congress, where those present voted overwhelmingly to make certain categories of offence a complete bar to practice.[68]

Controversy was still not over. Swaadiq Wallymahmed had served a sentence of five years' imprisonment following a conviction for buggery and sexual assault. The victims were his nephews aged eight and five. His case had been referred in 1991 to the Health Committee who, following favourable reports of rehabilitation, had closed the matter. He then came before the PCC in November 1996 for failure to disclose his convictions to a prospective employer. The committee found the facts proven and judged that they constituted misconduct. The respondent was cautioned. Once again, press coverage of the Council's handling of the case was extensive and critical and there were protest letters to the UKCC. The complainant, moreover, raised the issue with the Department of Health and there was ministerial interest in the case. The following January saw the *Mail on Sunday* take up the matter, an action which led over a dozen nurses, seeing the issue for the first time, to write in protest to the UKCC that a convicted paedophile had not been removed from the register.

Restoration under review

Some swift action followed. In the midst of the debates surrounding the Bundhun and Winn cases, in 1995, Council considered the issue of guidance to members involved in restoration cases. This was the theme of a special Council seminar held the day before the September Council meeting, where it was acknowledged that restoration to the register had to be considered with same degree of care as a decision to remove.[69] Members had to decide whether the practitioner was currently safe to practise and yet, as was becoming abundantly clear, they also needed to consider whether the public's confidence in the practitioner and the professions would be maintained if the practitioner was restored. As with mis-conduct, it was felt that each case should be considered on its own merits, and there was little support for creating a predetermined set of offences to exclude a practitioner from applying for restoration. Such 'life bans' were not allowable under existing legislation. Yet it was also decided that a list of basic guidelines would assist members in reaching decisions. A list of potential questions was outlined, in the hope that this would bring greater consistency between cases.[70]

Members also considered how decisions at restoration hearings should be expressed to applicants. In cases where there remained a good chance that a future application might be considered favourably, the committee might wish to offer comments on the steps that might be helpful to reach the stage where restoration could be agreed. In other cases, where restoration was going to remain unlikely, it might be more appropriate to say very little.

Following the Choy case, and at the explicit request of the President of the Council, UKCC officers set about a more detailed review of current restoration procedures and policies. In introducing a paper to Council, Tariq Hussain stated that procedures in relation to restoration cases had been followed, but 'it was necessary for these procedures to achieve a higher profile' and also to ensure that Council's policies were sufficiently stringent.[71] While 'it was not appropriate for the Council, as a judicial body, to comment on decisions made by its conduct or health committees', it was necessary for it to try to ensure that 'the public and professions have confidence in the process' – even if the public disagreed with actual decisions from time to time.[72]

The discussion resulted in a number of changes. Additional referees would now routinely be sent in advance a summary of the 'facts established' at the original hearing. Hearings would be scheduled not, as had been the practice, along with new cases, but would now be heard regularly on a designated day or days. Further training for members was agreed. Committees hearing restoration cases would from now consist of five members, of whom at least one, and preferably two, *must* be a consumer/lay member. Hearings, furthermore, would normally be chaired by the President, or by the Vice-President in the President's absence.[73] It was noted that the review of press and public responses to recent controversial cases had demonstrated that there are certain offences – such as murder, rape, child abuse and serious physical assault – where restoration would be difficult to defend, however long the individual had been removed from the register. In these types of cases any application for restoration, it was agreed, should be granted only if there is the clearest evidence that restoration is justified. Though life bans were not thought to be permissible under the current legislation, Council took the decision that restoration should henceforth not be made 'if this was likely to undermine public confidence' in registered practitioners.[74] An internal review of the Wally-mahmed case in December 1996 prompted further change.[75] There were new arrangements for de-briefing both chair and committee members after contentious cases, and discussions on the value of including information on the criminal justice system and the standards expected. The forthcoming appointment of a further ten members of the consumer panel for the PCC was viewed with satisfaction.[76]

This had been an extremely uncomfortable time for the Council. Chief Executive Sue Norman noted in a letter to the Chief Nursing Officer that both the Choy and Wallymahmed cases had reminded the Council that however committed it was 'to maintaining the integrity of professional self-regulation in the public interest', contentious decisions had the potential 'to call that integrity into question'. The review of the Council's restoration procedures had now taken the UKCC as far as the law would allow in ensuring that rapists and other serious offenders would never be readmitted to the register. But given the 'deliberately democratic process' that governs the UKCC's Professional Conduct and Health Committee work, further contentious decisions could not be ruled out.[77]

At the March 1997 Council meeting, the President, Mary Uprichard, introducing a further review of the issues that had arisen, reminded members that the UKCC, as the 'custodian' of 'common professional values' was responsible for their enforcement and also for 'ensuring that these values were better understood by the public at large'. At a time of change in the area of professional-conduct procedures, it was especially important for the Council to 'explain the services provided to practitioners and the way in which the professions were regulated, and to ensure the administration of justice in professional conduct' took place in an open environment.[78] But how far could the public's response to recent controversial cases be attributed to a lack of understanding about the Council's role and its powers? Was a more fundamental change to the law itself, or at least to Council's Rules framed under primary legislation, desirable?

Two ideas were now being canvassed more widely among practitioners – one was the idea of a 'life ban', the other automatic removal for certain serious offences. A power of life bans would effectively place the Council in the position of imposing a greater sanction than those available to the criminal courts, and legal advice was that this was not possible.[79] The matter of automatic removal for certain categories of offence also raised difficult questions, in that it would 'fetter the discretion of the committee' and as such could be interpreted as 'detracting from the principle of professional self-regulation'. Again, Council decided to defer making a decision, asking officers to explore the issue further.[80] Members did agree, however, that using the existing power of removal for a specified period in conjunction with an amendment to the Rules requiring individuals so removed to seek restoration through the usual process would have the effect of preventing restoration cases coming 'too early' to a hearing.[81] The rule change was sought and subsequently, in September 1997, it was agreed to test the impact of using this new combination of powers for a period of twelve months before reviewing the situation. It also agreed not to return to the issue of life bans.[82]

Matters of health policy and practice

Over the years, Council had continued to single out issues arising from its professional-conduct cases, regularly drawing attention to what it viewed as inadequate staffing levels and employment practices that put patients at risk. The theme became distinctly stronger in the period of the Third Council. The most notable example was publication of a report on standards of nursing in nursing homes in June 1994.[83] There had been a sharp rise in the proportion of cases coming from the nursing home sector. Eight examples of such cases were set out alongside the statistics. The report was deliberately addressed not only to practitioners but also to matrons and owners, registering authorities, health authorities and educators. An extensive agenda for action covered staffing, training and quality assurance systems. Suggestions for improvement in managing residents' finances, in recordkeeping and in the administration of medicines were identified and there were sharply critical comments on the way commercial pressures could operate against patient interests. The report attracted an immense amount of publicity at its launch and was still having an impact in the professions and media a year later.[84] In September 1995 came guidance for those commissioning and providing health care. This linked Council's work on misconduct with that on standards. It underlined the importance for public protection of enabling nurses, midwives and health visitors to practise safely and continue their own personal development.[85]

Council was at its most trenchant, however, a year later in a document explicitly entitled *Issues Arising from Professional Conduct Complaints*.[86] This contained detailed recommendations to managers on matters such as better workforce planning, systems of support and supervision to identify and tackle poor performance and provision of protocols for dealing with aggressive patients and with restraint. Alongside this were comments once again on the need for better systems for dealing with patients' money and well-understood local policies on sexual harassment, and a plea for a less punitive approach to drug errors.[87] These strong recommendations, addressed very directly to those responsible for service delivery, all stemmed from the experience of the pattern of cases coming before the PCC.

The nursing homes report had proved to be a particular effective way of widely publicising standards of care in a way that the routinely available statistical compendia have not done.[88] Statistical profiles do from time to time have an impact on Council, however. Recognition of the high proportion of cases closed at the preliminary proceedings stage,[89] for example, was a key factor in the decision in 1996 to once again issue advice documents to employers on when misconduct and unfitness to practise should be reported. As the term of the Third Council was coming to an end, research was proposed on the high proportions of men coming to the committee and on the proportion of cases involving the abuse (sexual, physical and verbal) of patients – both with a view to developing guidance.[90] The recent instigation of research scholarships[91] may also prompt some independent study of professional-conduct cases, a topic which to date has been all but ignored by the research community.

In this period of controversy, two pressing issues of professional regulation remained unresolved. The first concerned the possibility of regulation of health care assistants. This had been considered by the Standards and Ethics Committee in 1994.[92] Further outside pressure brought the issue to Council in March 1997, but the practical difficulties of such a large-scale regulatory venture and the array of interested parties made it difficult to decide more than to keep a watching brief on this.[93] The second issue was that of the 'intractably incompetent' or 'poorly performing' practitioner. It recognised that professional-conduct procedures – requiring a single incident, or set of incidents, that can be proved to the criminal standard of evidence in order to remove a person from the register – cannot easily extend to deal with poor performance. Council had certainly been aware of this over the years[94] and the matter was taken up in the 1995 Council seminar, where the difficulty of creating a precise definition of incompetence was noted. There were also fears that employers might well try to shift responsibility towards the statutory body. An employer seminar was held in September 1997. Some felt that reliance could and should be put on the new PREP requirements and that these, set alongside the guidance to employers to provide support and supervision for staff, should be enough.[95] Some were concerned that new procedures would mean that cases that would otherwise emerge into a public forum as misconduct might well be steered into a private one as incompetence. Coming as it did at a time when the agenda was very full and Council had been uneasily in the public eye for its work in the field of discipline, it is perhaps not surprising that matters moved only slowly.[96]

In July 1997 it was announced that JM Consulting were to carry out what, in effect, was the second departmental review of the statutory machinery. In a wide-ranging reflection on what more needed to be prepared for the review team, Council recognised the need to maintain confidence in the conduct and fitness to practise system and the growing public demand for openness.[97] It urged the reviewers to consider not only poor performance and the regulation of care assistants, but also a probationary period after restoration and perhaps conditions on practice prior to full restoration. Council also wished to see stronger protection of title and mechanisms to prevent those struck off returning to work as care assistants or managers of care homes. It urged that a mandatory requirement be laid on employers to check the registration status of employees. Meanwhile, matters were not standing still. At the last meeting of the Third Council, in March 1998, it was agreed to extend the presence of consumer panel members to the PPC, thus, as it was put in introducing the paper, 'extending a voice for the consumer at an early stage'.[98]

Publication of the JM Consulting report did not finally occur until February 1999.[99] In the wider world, the reviewers argued, professional conduct procedures were seen as punitive and hard to understand, and the high-profile cases had shaken confidence in the system. They took on board a number of the UKCC's suggestions but added others of their own. They recommended tighter definitions of professional misconduct tied specifically to clauses of the code; they suggested that mediation would be appropriate to some cases and that pre-hearing reviews could be useful. Conditional registration in face of poor performance and a power of reprimand were advocated.

Conclusion

Deciding on removals from and restorations to the register is a key part of a regulatory body's work of protecting the public and it is vital that public confidence in the procedures and in their operation is maintained. Balancing the public humiliation and loss of livelihood of a practitioner with the need to protect a vulnerable public can be a difficult, demanding and harrowing experience for all those concerned. Throughout, the UKCC has battled with these issues alongside the logistics of a heavy workload. It made a number of efforts both to ensure that a complex, legalistic machinery was better understood amongst practitioners and to take forward some of the challenges to employers and to NHS policy that the pattern of cases seemed to indicate. It accepted the case made by outside reviewers for a unified machinery and successfully pressed for further extensions to its legal powers. In the changed climate of the1990s, the work became higher profile and more controversial, and the question of the conditions under which restorations to the register should be made dominated the debate. Important changes followed and more changes are now in train following the second outside review of the statutory machinery. The sheer complexity of the processes, however, and the paucity of independent analysis has hindered the development of informed debate and contributed to misunderstandings and miscommunication. It may well be, as we argue in the concluding chapter, that the whole question of expectations of professionals and the monitoring of their performance needs an altogether broader consideration than it has to date received.

Notes

1 For further details on procedures, see Appendix 3.
2 UKCC, *Annual Report 1983/84*, p. 55.
3 Appendix 3 gives a brief compilation of relevant statistics. While the number of cases coming before the PCC represented a very substantial workload, with numbers of registrants considerably in excess of half a million, approximately one registrant in 5000 comes before the committee each year.
4 See GNC for England and Wales, *Annual Report 1979/80*, pp. 18–19; *1980/81*, p. 18.
5 UKCC, *Annual Report 1983/84*, pp. 56–7.
6 UKCC, *Annual Report 1984/85*, p. 10. In July 1986, after considering a paper outlining some of the disadvantages of holding PCC hearings out of London, a majority of members voted for their continuation. CC/86/40; MIN 51/86(d).
7 UKCC, *Annual Report 1985/86*, p. 8.
8 UKCC, *Annual Report 1984/85*, p. 10; UKCC, *Annual Report 1985/86*, p. 8; UKCC, *Annual Report 1986/87*, p. 8.

9 UKCC, *Annual Report 1985/86*, p.8; *Annual Report 1986/87*, p. 8.

10 MIN 13/86(b); MIN 43/86(b). A response was received from the Minister of State for the Scottish Office and related to the forty-seventh meeting of Council on 15 May 1987. See MIN 35/87(d). Tariq Hussain was a member of the first and Second Council. He resigned in 1991 to take up the post of Director for Professional Conduct (1992–6).

11 To protect the practitioner, no statistics on the work of the Health Committee are included in the professional conduct volume of the annual *Statistical Analysis of the UKCC's Professional Register*. Pyne regards this practice as unhelpful and comments that release of figures would enhance public confidence. Pyne, R., *Professional Discipline in Nursing, Midwifery and Health Visiting*, Oxford, Blackwell Science (third edn), 1998, p. 77. In practice, however, some statistics have always been included in the text of the Annual Report, with the exception of the year 1996/7. No Health Committee records were consulted for this chapter, although some minimal statistics are given in Appendix 3.

12 UKCC, *Annual Report 1983/84*, p. 57.

13 Pyne, R., 'Grasping the legal nettle', *Nursing Times*, 28 September, 79(39), 1983, p. 37.

14 MIN 16/84.

15 CC/85/72.

16 For detail of how costs of legal fees rose over time, see chapter 3, pp. 55 and 62.

17 MIN 89/85(b). The task force was composed of one representative of the Council and one representative from each of the National Boards. After the first meeting, the Chief Executives were invited to join the group. The group met on three occasions and reported in March 1986.

18 Cash limits to the Boards' investigation work were imposed by the UKCC from 1984/85. Additional funding had to come from the Boards. The measure was accepted reluctantly by the Boards, and the ENB, most affected by the change, expressed strong reservations. The task force felt that cash limits would need to continue throughout 1986/87. For the ENB reaction, see CC/86/C15, Annex 1b.

19 CC/86/C6.

20 CC/86/C6, p. 23.

21 CC/86/C15, p. 4. A second review group was established towards the end of 1986, comprising two members of the UKCC and two officers and either one or two representatives from each of the National Boards. Papers for this group could not be traced.

22 This painstaking process was in part prompted by the difficulty of interpreting the relationship between Rule 9 (5), which stated that the validity of a conviction proved in the courts should not be challenged by the PCC, and Rule 18 (1) which related to part of the Civil Evidence Act of 1968 and provided an opportunity for a person to deny guilt in relation to a conviction. Council took the matter to the High Court for judicial review. The ruling confirmed that the Rules did indeed give respondents the right to seek to prove that they were not guilty of the offence. An amendment to the Rules was approved in December 1987, taking effect in February 1987.

23 The voting was thirty in favour of retaining the present position, one against and one abstention. See also the reporting of the meeting in the *Nursing Standard*, 23 January, 2(16), 1988, p. 12.

24 MIN 11/88(3), p. 8.

25 CC/86/64; CC/87/64.

26 CC/85/56. The proportion of allegation cases within the Council's workload compared with those stemming from 'true convictions' had also increased. More cases in which direct evidence had to be given by witnesses in public and under oath, inevitably impinged upon the Committee's ability to process new cases: Pyne, *Professional Discipline*, p. 72. Whereas the Disciplinary Committee of the GNC was

hearing an average of over five new cases each committee day in the statistical year of 1979/1980, the UKCC's PCC was able to hear an average of only 1.3 new cases each committee day in 1989/90.

27 CC/88/32, pp. 2–3.

28 UKCC, *Annual Report 1987/88*, p. 8.

29 MIN 11/88 3(c); MIN 48/88(b). The Legislative Review Group comprised both members and officers.

30 See UKCC, *Advertising by Registered Nurses, Midwives and Health Visitors*, 1985; *Administration of Medicines*, 1986; *Confidentiality: An Elaboration of Clause 9 of the second edition. of the UKCC's Code of Professional Conduct for the Nurse, Midwife and Health Visitor*, 1987; *Exercising Accountability: A framework to assist nurses, midwives and health visitors to consider ethical aspects of professional practice*, 1989.

31 UKCC, *With a view to removal from the Register . . .*, 1990.

32 Misconduct is defined in the Rules as 'conduct unworthy of a registered nurse, midwife or health visitor, as the case may be . . .' Current guidance for members still quotes the words of Dame Catherine Hall in an address of 1983, where she explained that the standard should be 'not the highest standard which a professional person might attain, but the standard which can reasonably be expected of an average practitioner', UKCC, *Conduct and Health Manual*, 1998, Section 1, p. 4.

33 The lists in Figure 5.1 have been drawn up from *With a View to Removal from the Register . . .*, issued in 1990. The same lists appeared in *Complaints About Professional Conduct*, issued in 1993, though the 1998 edition made a number of changes.

34 Peat Marwick McLintock, *Review of the UKCC and the Four National Boards for Nursing, Midwifery and Health Visiting. Commissioned by the Department of Health, Scottish Home and Health Department, the Welsh Office and Department of Health and Social Services Northern Ireland*, London, Department of Health, 1989.

35 The GNC had been able to issue a 'reprimand'. During the shadow period considerable concern had been expressed that this had not been carried over into the 1979 Act.

36 Peat Marwick McLintock, *Review of the UKCC and the Four National Boards*, p. 75.

37 Note of the meeting of the LAG held on 19 March 1991, LAG: MIN/1.

38 Note of meeting of LAG, 16 April 1991.

39 Although the removal/suspension distinction was an important one, it was a difference of terminology only, suspension on health grounds being for an indefinite period. It required to be followed, as with removal, by an application for restoration.

40 LAG:Min/4.

41 Cited in UKCC, *Briefing document re. to Section 12 of the Nurses, Midwives, and Health Visitors Act 1979* and *Clause 7 of the Nurses, Midwives, and Health Visitors Bill* (n.d.).

42 It was suggested that the Council's ability to make rules regarding caution may have been masked by the two-tier system. Government officials argued that Council, in setting up its own Investigating Committee, would be able to make rules enabling a caution to be issued at an appropriate stage. Council's experience of appeals, however, cast some doubt on this.

43 *Parliamentary Debates* [Lords], 532, 26 November 1991, col. 1294. It is not clear how this statistic was calculated. See Appendix 3, Table A3.5.

44 Ibid., 12 November, 1991, cols. 501–2.

45 Ibid., 26 November, 1991, col. 1296.

46 No immediate action was taken to include lay people in the disciplinary process but the matter was soon to take on a higher profile.

47 Stacey, M., *Regulating British Medicine. The General Medical Council*, Chichester, John Wiley and Sons, 1992, ch. 13; Green, D., *Which Doctor? A Critical Analysis of the Professional Barriers to Competition in Health Care*, London, Institute of Economic Affairs, 1985. See also Allsop, J. and L. Mulcahy, *Regulating Medical Work. Formal and Informal Controls*, Buckingham, Open University Press, 1996, pp. 84–6

48 Robinson, J., *A Patient Voice at the GMC: A Lay Member's View of the GMC*, Health

Rights, Report 1, (London, 1988). Jean Robinson came to the GMC as a nominee of the Association of Community Health Councils for England and Wales.

49 Ibid., p. 41.

50 Robinson, *A Patient Voice*. Jean Robinson was one of four co-opted members on the UKCC Standards and Ethics Committee from 1989 to 1993, following nomination by the Association of Community Health Councils.

51 Brief details of the named cases in this section can be found in Appendix 3.

52 Ms Rosser was suspended and without pay for over a year while her case was awaiting hearing.

53 A wide-ranging review criticising the machinery of professional conduct in relation to midwifery emerged at this point, not mentioning the case by name but seemingly influenced by it. See Association of Radical Midwives, *Professional Conduct Machinery for Midwives: some necessary changes*, Omskirk, Lancs, ARM, (n.d.). It was discussed by Council, CC/89/C17.

54 During the initial hearing, the specialist members of the PCC, finding that the expert evidence given in defence of Ms Rosser's practice was at variance with their own experience, had taken an unprecedented step of calling for rebuttal evidence. Although such evidence was allowable under the rules [SI No. 2157 Nurses, Midwives and Health Visitors (Professional Conduct) Rules 1987, Approval Order 1987, Rule 10 (3) (d)], the appeal case centred on and questioned use of this rule. Rules current at the time of writing still contain the facility for rebuttal, although it is rarely used.

55 A leading article in the *Nursing Times*, suggested that the outcome was 'a muddle', *Nursing Times*, 8 March, 85(10), 1989, p. 23. The matter was further discussed in Flint, C., 'A matter of judgement', *Nursing Times*, 22 March, 85(12), 1989, p. 19 and in Davies, C., 'Free speech! Caring practice must be safe practice', *Midwives Chronicle and Nursing Notes*, 102, No. 1216, 1987, p. 159. This latter article provoked some further correspondence and debate.

56 Prior to the Rosser case, there had been seven appeals and four judicial reviews (for details of the distinction between the two, see Appendix 3). Four of the appeals were dismissed. A rehearing was ordered in two cases, and one had led to a change in the Rules after the senior judge had ruled that the respondent's representative was not equipped to deal with prejudicial evidence concerning the history. The first judicial review was brought by the UKCC itself requesting an interpretation of two statutory rules. The others were dismissed, although an appeal against one was upheld on a matter of law. CC/89/C17, Annex 4.

57 This case was later subject of an article in the academic nursing press questioning the judgement of the UKCC. See Long, T. 'To protect the public and ensure justice is done: An examination of the Philip Donnelly case', *Journal of Advanced Nursing*, 17(1), 1992, pp. 5–9.

58 See UKCC, M4.7.2, Contentious Decisions.

59 See UKCC, M4.7.2, Contentious Decisions.

60 The Jhugroo case is important, however, in the matters of powers to suspend and of interpretations of the concept of suspension. Neither of the suspension powers the UKCC had sought under the 1992 Act involved the intent to remove for a specified period after which registration would be restored. The UKCC conceded that it had power to remove for a specified period and from this point routinely considered this penalty in its procedures. It has never applied it, however. Council's view is that suspension for a specified period, that is, with automatic restoration, is inappropriate because it operates as a punishment rather than as a mechanism of public protection. This makes an interesting contrast with the GMC.

61 Even though the 1992 Act had enabled Council to include non-Council members on its disciplinary and fitness to practise committees, neither the primary nor the secondary legislation specifically required lay representation. This was in contrast to the situation of GMC. (See also Chapter 8.)

62 *Nursing Times*, 9 June, 89(23), 1993, p. 5.

63 Ibid. The matter did not end here. The son of the patient who had died applied for a judicial review of the restoration decision. The case was dismissed at a hearing in May 1994.

64 In contrast to the swift decision to appoint a consumer panel, members of the Third Council decided to wait and see whether the expanded Council membership eased the situation. This reticence at using the new power to co-opt non-Council practitioners onto the PCC finally ended in 1996. The reasons given for the change were those of necessity in the face of heavy caseloads. See Minute 22/96(3), and CC/96/18.

65 In relation to the Bundhun case, the UKCC received correspondence from eleven registered practitioners and eleven others, including the daughter of the victim, a branch secretary of, and the Head of Health at UNISON.

66 Cited in *Sunday Times*, 25 June 1995.

67 See Cassidy, J., 'Registering outrage', *Nursing Times*, 20 September, 91(38), 1995, pp. 14–15, and for the reply, Hussain, T., 'In defence of UKCC conduct cases', *Nursing Times*, 11 October, 91(41), 1995, p. 24.

68 A vote of 98.2 per cent was recorded. See *Nursing Standard*, 1 May, 10(32), 1996, p. 7.

69 At the seminar on 5 September, Council paper CC/95/58, 'Guidelines for members considering applications for restoration' was discussed.

70 The list of possible questions was contained in Annexe 1 to CC/95/58. These included the nature of the applicant's employment since removal; why the applicant considers himself/herself ready to re-enter the profession; what lessons had been learnt; which area of the profession the applicant would wish to re-enter; what steps had been taken to keep up with developments and whether some professional up-dating would be appropriate before starting back at work; how applicants could assure the committee that they could now be safely restored.

71 CC/96/32; Minute 37/96(3).

72 CC/96/32, p. 4.

73 Minute 37/96(3).

74 Minute 37/96 (3.5); CC/96/32, paras 22–3.

75 Though not a restoration case, the level of controversy suggested the value of a review.

76 In a letter the UKCC's Director of Professional Conduct, Mandie Lavin, noted that since the inception of the consumer panel in 1994 there had been a consumer member in 86 per cent of professional conduct cases, a figure which she hoped would increase once the consumer panel numbers doubled. Letter from Mandie Lavin to John Dorling, Department of Health, 5 December 1996.

77 Letter from Sue Norman to Yvonne Moores, 6 December 1996.

78 Minute 8/97(6).

79 CC/97/09, 'Professional conduct – protecting the public: issues arising from high-profile cases', p. 3. Some members regarded the issue of life bans as a red herring, arguing that Council could effectively bar certain practitioners for life through repeated refusal at restoration hearings – a strategy buttressed by a change in policy, by keeping records of hearings for life instead of for five years (see note 60). No equivalent regulatory body has the power to issue life bans.

80 Minute 8/97(6).

81 Ibid. PCCs had not used the power to remove for a specified period (a power contained in Section 12 of the 1979 Act) even though the judgement in the Jhugroo case had made clear that this power was available to them. In linking specified period removal with the additional requirement for a restoration hearing, Council was affirming its disapproval of specified period suspension *per se* (see note 60).

82 Minute 27/97(4), September 1997. Council also agreed that records of removals and restorations should be kept for the life of the practitioner bringing Council policy in line with that of other regulatory bodies. Also, by the last Council meeting of the term, draft guidance for members on this issue was produced. Minutes of Council meeting 4 March 1998; CC/98/10.

83 UKCC, *Professional Conduct – Occasional Report on Standards of Nursing in Nursing Homes*, 1994.
84 UKCC, *Annual Report 1995/96*, p. 11
85 UKCC, *The Council's Proposed Standards for Incorporation into Contracts for Hospital and Community Health Care Services*, 1995.
86 UKCC, *Issues Arising from Professional Conduct Complaints*, 1996.
87 Mention of this issue had been made in the Annual Report for 1988/9. Members noted that 'practitioners who have made a mistake due to pressure of work (often in administering medicines) and have been open and honest about it are often disciplined by their managers' – a practice, which it was felt, was in danger of encouraging 'dishonesty to the potential detriment of patients'. UKCC, *Annual Report 1988/89*, p. 6. The issue had been addressed earlier in the UKCC advisory document *Administration of Medicines*, 1986.
88 Statistical analyses of cases coming before the PCC are compiled annually, showing not only the number of cases and their disposal but also the field of practice of respondents and the nature of the allegations made against them. The classifications are not altogether easy to interpret, however, and the document has attracted little interest. See *Statistical Analysis of the UKCC's Professional Register*, (various years).
89 See Appendix 3, Table A3.2.
90 From 1995 onwards, Annual Reports had noted the very great discrepancy between percentage of men on the register and percentage of male respondents.
91 UKCC, *Annual Report 1997/98*, p. 4. In September 1998, the first year of the Fourth Council, a proposal came forward for the first time for research based on the work of the Health Committee, CC/98/C31.
92 SEC MIN 5/94(5); SEC MIN 24/94(1); SEC MIN 35/94(1); SEC MIN 05/95(1).
93 See CC97/07.
94 See, for example, UKCC, *Annual Report 1990/91*, p. 7.
95 For a contrary view, see Pyne, *Professional Discipline* (third edn), pp. 100–1.
96 As this book went to press a consultation document on medical performance procedures was issued *Supporting doctors, protecting patients: A consultation paper on preventing, recognising and dealing with poor clinical performance in the NHS in England*, London, Department of Health, 1999.
97 UKCC, *The Future of Professional Regulation,* 1997.
98 The three lay Council members were already involved in PPC. This proposal, taken together with an agreement, bring a 'due regard' practitioner from the practitioner panel and to split the PPC into two groups of seven to cope with the growing workload, meant each case would first be seen by four Council members, two consumers and one practitioner from a relevant field. CC/98/09.
99 JM Consulting, *The Regulation of Nurses, Midwives and Health Visitors: Report of a review of the Nurses, Midwives and Health Visitors Act 1997*, Bristol, JM Consulting, 1998.

6 Standards of professional practice
PREPP and after

Once its strategy for the reform of pre-registration education was accepted 'in principle' by the government, the UKCC's attention focused on the need for explicit Council standards for post-registration education and practice, a body of work that from August 1989 came to be known as PREPP.[1] The issue was particularly pressing, in view of the wide array of courses of different lengths and standards that had grown up, and the plethora of new job titles, roles and responsibilities that were beginning to emerge with changes in the NHS. There was also a strong desire to develop the concept of registration to ensure that every person who gained entry to the Council's register remained competent to practise, and enhanced their personal professional development, in the years that followed. This notion of using the register as a positive tool to maintain professional standards beyond the point of entry had surfaced early in the lifetime of the UKCC, being a key component of the discussions of Working Group 2 during the shadow period (see Chapter 2), but progress during the First Council had been limited by a combination of practical difficulties and the prominence of the review of pre-registration education.

Early forays into this field[2] had suggested that there was a wide array of challenges. Among them were the sheer size of any updating or professional development requirement for over half a million registrants; the problems of rationalising a highly complex structure of post-basic qualifications that was still growing as a result of the activities of the National Boards and academic departments; the hopes in the professions of a clear system of clinical career progression; the fears of practising nurses, midwives and health visitors about requirements which affected their registration status and hence livelihood and the wariness of midwives and community nurses who feared that new arrangements might not properly reflect their specialist areas of practice. Nor was the matter solely an internal one. Employers had a strong vested interest in keeping flexibility in the grading and deployment of staff, and feared that the statutory bodies' activities in this field might compromise their freedom to act. For all these reasons, PREPP proved to be a long-running project. By the time it came to the end of its formal life, however, the concept of standards was also being taken forward in other ways. Specialist professional officers were in post, and greater dialogue with people working in particular practice areas was evident. The idea of standards in practice, alongside standards of education and conduct, was beginning to take shape.

The first phase of PREPP, 1988–90

At their first meeting, in November 1988, members of the Second Council agreed that a comprehensive review of post-registration education and practice issues was urgently required.[3] EPAC held a two-day meeting at the Chequers Hotel in Newbury the following April and agreed that the review, which was to last no more than twelve months, should cover three interconnected areas. First, it needed to find a way of describing the different levels or spheres of professional practice that could incorporate existing specialisms and allow for the further development of clinical fields and expertise. Second, it had to address the closely related issue of the educational preparation for the different roles identified. Third, and regardless of the particular sphere of practice, there was the need to establish just what the requirements for maintaining competence in practice would be and how they would be monitored.[4]

Work was to proceed through working groups comprising EPAC members, representatives of the National Boards, and others co-opted as and when required, and a Steering Group, chaired by Professor Margaret Green, was established to provide guidance. Two existing UKCC officers, Heather Williams and Maggy Wallace, were appointed to act as Project Director and Deputy Director respectively, and were asked to devote 50 per cent of their time to this work. They were joined by an administrator and a research assistant. Over the summer, informal contact was made with the National Boards in the hope of avoiding confusion and the duplication of activities, and it was agreed that communication with the wider professions should follow the pattern developed during Project 2000. Consideration was also given as to how UKCC staff could be kept informed of the project: an opportunity, it was felt, that had been missed during Project 2000. It was agreed that a '"drop in" for tea and buns' would be held on the first Monday of each month so that everyone whose work was affected by the project could have the chance to share ideas and see what progress had been made. PREPP was formally launched in August 1989.[5]

Early discussions and initial reactions

From August until the end of the year, the project team reflected on the key issues and their relationship to wider health care needs, and, informed by a seminar attended by the professors of nursing in the UK, drafted an initial discussion document.[6] A complex and wide-ranging agenda was outlined. Professional practice, it was suggested, encompassed three spheres – practice following initial registration, specialist practice and advanced practice. Definitions of each, however, remained loose. Project discussions had already indicated that members held varying views on the distinctions between specialist and advanced practice, and all wished to avoid, at least at this early stage, too close a linkage with NHS grades and career structures. Effective and relevant educational frameworks were required for the different spheres. These, it was argued, might attract academic accreditation as well as professional approval and be linked with outside developments such

as credit accumulation and transfer. On the third issue, of maintaining competence, the main suggestion was for the introduction of system of review, possibly
linked to periodic re-registration with the Council. Looking back on the UKCC's
previous consultations on periodic refreshment, the paper acknowledged the
professions' concerns over the cost and manpower implications of such reforms,
as well as the potential inconsistency between a system of mandatory periodic
refreshment and the Council's Code of Professional Conduct which clearly stated
that the responsibility to maintain and improve professional knowledge and
competence remained with the individual practitioner. It was hoped that the
project group's new proposal for a 'personal professional profile' would ease some
of these concerns.

The discussion document was circulated in January 1990 to the National
Boards, professional organisations and health authorities, and to any individuals
who requested it. Its main arguments and suggestions were also published in
Register, the UKCC's bulletin for registrants, along with a prepaid questionnaire.
Commentaries on the project soon began to appear in the professional press.
During the spring, the profession was able to question members of the project
group directly at twenty PREPP roadshows held around the UK. The level of
involvement during this initial discussion phase was substantial. Nearly 30,000
replies were received (compared to the 2,500 written responses received during
the Project 2000 consultation). Overall, it was estimated that well over 400,000
people contributed to the debate.[7] This surprisingly large figure, however, was
only achieved by including the total membership in cases where a membership
organisation submitted a response.

This informal, preparatory round of discussions with the professions swiftly
flagged up areas of particular interest and concern. Responses confirmed that the
special needs of the newly registered practitioner were widely regarded as an
important target for action. On the other hand, feedback on the proposals for
maintaining competence revealed widespread concerns over the implications of a
mandatory scheme. As a *Nursing Standard* editorial noted, a 'cloud of uncertainty
about when and how mandatory refreshment would be implemented' coloured
the professions' reaction to the discussion paper.[8] For example, who would oversee an individual's 'personal professional profile'? Would the proposed profile be
linked to management initiatives? If so, was there a danger that it could become a
punitive rather than a positive instrument for practitioners? Concerns were also
expressed over possible reactions of employers. Would they be prepared to support
professional updating? Who, indeed, would meet the cost?[9]

In addition, while the professions seemed to support the idea of continuous
learning to support standards of practice, severe doubts existed over the model of
levels or spheres of professional practice at the heart of the PREPP discussion
document. Concerns over the definitions of 'specialist' and 'advanced' practice
were widespread, especially among the existing 'specialist' groups of midwives,
health visitors and district nurses. The three terms also appeared to have fuelled
fears of 'elitism and an over-emphasis on academia' created in the context of
Project 2000, and exacerbated the concerns of those the *Nursing Standard* called
'practice-based nurses' already worried about their future in the profession.[10]

Over the summer of 1990, the project group analysed responses and reviewed its position in preparation for the publication of a full consultation document in the autumn.[11] Members agreed that proposals for professional updating and maintaining competence should also explore the desirability of including a period of statutory study leave. It was also agreed that the personal professional profile should be separate from any management systems of individual performance review. Next, it was clear that proposals on the model of professional practice would need to explain more clearly that the majority of practitioners would not become 'specialist' or 'advanced' practitioners but would develop their practice within the initial sphere. Indeed, the terminology used to describe the three spheres of practice needed to be rethought, given the lack of consensus on what constituted 'specialist' practice and its relationship to existing specialisms, such as midwifery, health visiting and district nursing. This whole area, the chairman of the project group admitted, was proving to be 'a minefield'. The complex situation facing community practitioners persuaded Council to recommend the establishment of a separate but parallel Community Education and Practice Project (CEPP) (see p. 127).[12] The project team also identified the need for a costs and benefits analysis of the PREPP proposals, and for a range of developmental activities that included an exploration of how the proposed profiling system might be delivered and verified, implications for recordable qualifications, the establishment of a logical and comprehensive framework for credit accumulation, the development of standards for the teachers of nurses and midwives,[13] and much else besides. A new Steering Group was set up at the end of October 1990 to monitor the further work arising out of PREPP, to provide expert advice to staff and to the consultants undertaking the costs and benefits analysis, to identify additional areas of work and to provide progress reports to Council.[14]

A formal consultation

The PREPP consultation document was published at the end of October 1990.[15] The following January an extended summary, *PREPP and You*, and a question-naire card was mailed to every nurse, midwife and health visitor with an effective registration. There were nine major recommendations. For newly registered practitioners it was recommended that a period of support or 'preceptorship' (lasting between three and six months) should be introduced. This, it was hoped, would help consolidate the competencies achieved at registration and enhance the confidence of new practitioners. Support was to be provided by an experienced colleague ('preceptor') with some preparation for the role. These were not to be new statutory requirements, but instead statements of good practice which were to be introduced by employers no later than January 1993.

Five recommendations addressed the issue of maintaining competence and developing professional knowledge. All nurses, midwives and health visitors were to demonstrate that they had 'maintained and developed their professional knowledge and competence' by completing a 'personal professional profile' and taking a minimum of five days statutory study leave every three years. Practitioners wishing to return to practice after a break of five years or more would have to complete a 'return to practice' programme. Registration was to embrace a new concept of 'eligibility to practise' with three components: submission of a notification of practice form every three years; evidence of successful completion of the personal professional profile or 'return to practice' programme; and the payment of the periodic registration fee. Those wishing to return to practise after a break of less than five years were to submit a notification of practice and, within the following calendar year, provide verification of the satisfactory completion of a personal professional profile.

When it came to the difficult issue of the model of professional practice, two recommendations were offered. 'Initial', 'specialist' and 'advanced' had been replaced by the terms 'primary', 'advanced' and 'consultant'. Those wishing to practise as 'advanced' practitioners were to have a Council-approved recordable qualification. This was not simply a change of label but reflected the fundamental problem of how to define a level of practice skill and expertise that could both incorporate existing 'specialists' and allow for the continued development of roles. By removing the term 'specialist' from the model of practice, it was hoped that the objections of practitioners with existing post-registration qualifications would lessen. Until these issues were clarified, no progress could be made on the detail of the educational preparation required for advanced practice.

At the report's launch, Dame Audrey Emerton, the Chairman of the Council, said that the proposals provided 'a realistic blueprint for improvement and development' and that Council looked forward to 'discussing these exciting proposals with the professions, the health services and, very importantly, consumer organisations during the six-month consultation period'.[16] This was the first time consumer organisations had been formally included within a UKCC consultation exercise. The first phase of PREPP had covered a great deal of ground. Yet it was already clear that a number of extremely complex and sensitive issues needed to be broached. Practitioners, not surprisingly, were worried about the new goalposts represented by mandatory refreshment and renewal of registration. Moreover, while efforts had been made to define a model of practice that was inclusive and non-hierarchical, those who regarded themselves as specialists were understandably anxious about the new framework. The extent of these anxieties would be confirmed during the consultation. All this was complex enough – further down the line, however, would be the reactions of employers, government and consumer organisations.

Phase two: developing the proposals, 1991–2

The results of the consultation

Responses to the PREPP consultation document were collated during the spring and summer of 1991, and considered by the Council in closed session in July.[17] Once again, the magnitude of the exercise was striking: a total of 35,999 documents were received during the six months' consultation period, the vast majority of which were responses to the questionnaire issued in *Register*.[18] It was not possible to quantify the exact number of people contributing to the debate, as individuals could have responded in more than one way; but it was clear that the PREPP proposals had been well noticed by the profession and wider afield. The nursing press, in particular, devoted a considerable amount of space to the issues involved, acting as a conduit for the exchange of information and opinions.

The consultation revealed undoubted support for Council's efforts. The RCN praised the proposals for striking the 'right balance between a statutory frame-work to ensure that the programmes of education are implemented in practice, and the individual practitioner's own personal responsibility to develop them-selves professionally'.[19] No significant differences had emerged at this stage between professional groups. Yet, there was clearly a range of doubts and questions. The funding implications of the PREPP proposals continued to dampen enthusiasm. The *Nursing Standard* commented that 'nobody could pretend that making sure more than a half-million nurses receive regular, continuing education is going to be cheap', and a later article by the *Nursing Times* confirmed a belief that nurses would be obliged to pay for PREPP out of their own pockets.[20] The formal responses of the trade unions echoed these concerns. NUPE Assistant General Secretary, Roger Poole, for instance, was quoted as saying that while the report had elements which the union was keen to support, the issuing of proposals 'without considering who will fund it is like putting the cart before the horse'.[21] COHSE, too, was particularly worried about the cost implications of maintaining eligibility and, though supportive of the broad principles of PREPP, felt unable to endorse the PREPP package in the absence of proper funding.[22]

While the principle of professional updating was broadly supported, doubts persisted over methods. The *Nursing Times* greeted the proposals as 'interesting, progressive and hold[ing] great potential' but drew attention to concerns over the system of verification and the need for national guidelines.[23] The arrangements for study leave were also questioned, with some respondents expressing the view that the recommended 'five days every three years' would soon come to be seen as the maximum rather than as a minimum requirement.[24] On the mechanisms of main-taining eligibility, a large majority of midwife respondents expressed their wish to retain an annual, rather than a three-yearly notification of intention to practise, a view endorsed by the Council's Midwifery Committee.[25]

Most worryingly for Council, the revised definitions of the spheres of practice as 'primary', 'advanced' and 'consultant' did not erase concerns and, arguably, added to the confusion of a profession increasingly exposed to the growing array of post-registration and continuing education opportunities offered by higher education institutions and the RCN. Two further factors added to the complexity. Both the Welsh National Board (WNB) and the ENB had indicated their own plans for continuing education for nurses, midwives and health visitors around the same time as the PREPP consultation document.[26] Health service managers, too, received the report at a particularly 'frenetic' time. In the lead-up to imple-mentation of the NHS reforms, and with senior nurses already absorbed with the minutiae of Project 2000 and Working Paper 10, PREPP found itself competing for attention. It was, to say the least, a less than perfect environment in which to reflect upon Council's proposals.

After the July 1991 Council meeting, a press statement was released outlining, in broad terms, the current position on PREPP. Three key decisions had been made. The PREPP recommendations on support and preceptorship, and maintaining eligibility to practise, were to be implemented. Preparations for the drafting of rules and guidance material could now begin. Work on definition of 'primary', 'advanced' and 'consultant' practice, however, would continue alongside a detailed examination of the educational preparation required for those wishing to practise in an 'advanced' role.[27] Thirdly, work on costs and benefits and on the nature of community education and practice, along with other more detailed issues, was to continue during the remainder of 1991.

Costs and benefits analysis

Work on the costs and benefits of Council's proposals, once again led by Price Waterhouse, had begun in early 1991 while the PREPP report was out for consultation. The task was not an easy one. The proposals were not yet sufficiently specific or detailed for precise costing. Moreover, while the potential benefits of PREPP were felt to be significant, they were extremely difficult to measure quantitatively. Outside factors further complicated the situation. It was, as the management consultants themselves noted, a very difficult time to be collecting quantitative information from the health service, with the various NHS reforms impacting upon health authorities' ability to respond to requests for figures. The costs and benefits analysis, it was decided, would have to 'tease out' the likely resource requirements, assisted by an expert panel and reinforced by a series of field trips to health authorities who were known to have undertaken costing of existing post-registration activities.[28]

Initial findings were presented to Council in March 1991. Four months later the PREPP Steering Group issued a report summarising the conclusions reached in the light of the management consultants' analysis.[29] The proposals were not costed or evaluated individually, but presented as a comprehensive package. Precise values of likely benefits were extremely difficult to achieve, particularly as the full extent of the changes would take a decade or more to realise. The initial costs of implementation, spread over the first four years, were estimated to be in the range of £25–50 per practitioner, (equivalent to £15–30 million), while continuing costs were likely to fall in the range of £129–169 per year for each practitioner (£50–100 million per year) or between 0.75 and 1.5 per cent of the cost of employment. Further study and perhaps even trials in sample areas, it was noted, could narrow the range of these estimates, but the costs and benefits sub-group felt confident that they were sufficiently precise to demonstrate that the PREPP proposals were both 'highly beneficial and financially feasible'.[30] If just a 1 per cent improvement in the average effectiveness of all practitioners, and a higher percentage for those categorised as 'isolated practitioners', could be achieved, it was suggested, this would seem enough to justify the level of investment required for implementation.[31] Council, therefore, was able to satisfy itself that the costs of introducing PREPP were a reasonable management investment; but it still had to persuade others, especially government and employers, this was the case.

By the summer of 1991, Council had travelled a considerable distance with two elements of the PREPP package – preceptorship and maintaining eligibility. As preceptorship was not to be a statutory requirement, Council was able to produce guidance material for the profession and employers fairly quickly. This was issued in January 1993 along with a promise to review the experiences of newly registered practitioners and their preceptors after a year or so. Policies for maintaining eligibility to practise and for professional updating had also progressed. In July 1991, Council agreed that self-verification of the personal professional profile offered the most 'effective method of confirming that an individual has maintained and developed their professional knowledge and competence'.[32] However, further consideration was required on the nature of the profile's content and systems of audit.[33]

Bringing in areas of specialist practice

It was clear that a number of challenges still faced the project, and that these would have to be explored in the context of a fast-moving world in both the health service and in the educational sector. One of these challenges was how to identify and accommodate the post-registration education needs of different community-based practitioners whose practice environment was undergoing rapid and major change.[34] At the beginning of 1991, following a high-level 'summit meeting' with the representatives from the National Boards, professional associations and the health departments, and a series of internal workshop sessions, Council had agreed to approach this issue by establishing a separate but parallel project.[35] The aims of CEPP were to develop what came to be called 'community health care nursing', to identify the knowledge and skills required for effective practice in the community and to specify how these requirements link with PREPP's concepts of 'primary', 'advanced' and 'consultant' practice. The CEPP sub-group was also asked to specify the links between the competencies required of P2000 registrants and the qualifications of existing community nurses and health visitors.[36]

A consultation document was drafted over the summer of 1991 and published in October. Unlike the main PREPP report, no specific recommendations were offered. Instead, the document laid out several points for discussion. Community health care nursing was identified as a unified discipline, albeit one encompassing a range of specific areas of expertise – such as health visiting, district nursing, occupational health nursing, school nursing, community psychiatric nursing and community mental handicap nursing. Preparation for these linked but distinctive roles, it was suggested, should include a core programme as well as specialist modules. One of the most difficult issues was the need to devise an educational framework that could accommodate traditionally trained practitioners (a substantial proportion of whom already had additional registerable or recordable qualifications and considerable experience) as well as newly registered P2000 nurses.[37] Consultation on PREPP had already demonstrated that this was an area fraught with difficulties and considerable care was taken in the CEP document not to exacerbate these tensions. It was proposed that existing practitioners with registered or recordable qualifications in areas of community practice would automatically be considered as qualified community health care nurses, but those wishing to acquire an advanced practice qualification would need to take additional modules in appropriate areas. Responses, however, indicated continuing worries over the recognition of identities and existing expertise. Many thought Council intended to introduce a generic community health care nurse (something, indeed, that held particular attractions for employers). Fears that existing qualifications and experience would not receive due recognition were widespread. Those practising in the community without recordable qualifications – including many of the growing band of practice nurses – were also worried about their future position. The decision to approach the issue of post-registration education and practice in the community in a separate report had not been able to stem anxieties. Council still had to contend with considerable confusion and many doubts and anxieties.

By this time the main project group had returned to the notion of 'specialist' practice, and now set about testing its application to the various disciplines within the fields of nursing and midwifery. A Council seminar in January 1992 provided members with the opportunity to share their views. The principle of 'special preparation' for those engaged in 'specialist practice' was widely favoured by the nursing members of Council.[38] It was immediately clear, however, that the notion of 'specialist' practice did not find favour among the midwives. Midwifery, it was argued, was already a specialised sphere of practice that neither could nor should be further subdivided. Nevertheless, some support was given to the idea of 'enhanced' practice which, it was felt, could describe a 'depth and breadth of additional knowledge and skill' without narrowing the focus of midwifery practice. In February 1992, Council agreed to describe post-registration practice as consisting of primary, specialist (nursing) or enhanced (midwifery) and advanced spheres, and established broad definitions of each. All recognised, however, that this was just the first step: the complicated matter of determining the educational preparation for the higher spheres still had to be broached.[39]

Thus, by the beginning of 1992 the UKCC had reached an important stage in the PREPP project. The responses to the PREPP report had been assimilated, material relating to the costs and benefits of the proposals had been assembled and analysed and an additional consultation exercise on community education and practice had been undertaken. Council had agreed policies on support for the newly registered practitioner, and on maintaining and developing professional knowledge and competence and eligibility to practise, and arrangements for the implementation of these aspects of PREPP were being made. However, making a reality of the key elements of the project remained a long way off. First, it was clear that more 'robust' estimates of the costs and benefits of change would have to be attained before firm proposals for the implementation of PREPP could be laid before the government.[40] July 1992 brought a decision by the government – delivered to the Council in person by Baroness Cumberlege, the Parliamentary Secretary at the Department of Health – that it would undertake this supplementary work itself. While the government indicated its support for preceptorship and the provision of return to practice courses, it was concerned by the potential cost of Council's proposal for five days mandatory study leave over three years.[41] The government's decision to develop its own costings was regarded with disappointment and concern by the Council, while an already cautious professional press began to wonder whether PREPP would be a 'toothless tiger'.[42] Council's control of the next stage of the process, therefore, was significantly weakened. Equally concerning was the fact, that despite enormous efforts and consultation, Council had been unable to generate a firm consensus around the notions of primary, specialist/enhanced and advanced practice. This was to make Council's next consultation exercise – on the nature and standard of the educational preparation for specialist and advanced practice – extremely difficult.

Phase three: establishing standards, 1992–8

Council now focused its attention on how the register might be used to denote higher levels of post-registration education and experience. Between 1992 and 1993, the PREPP team, now led by a new Steering Group,[43] worked towards clarifying the definitions of specialist and advanced practice, setting standards for preparation for these roles and for nurse, midwife and health visitor teachers, and establishing new criteria for recording post-registration qualifications on the register. Problems with the definitions of 'primary', 'specialist'/'enhanced' and 'advanced' continued to surface. The notion of 'specialist' practice, in particular, was repeatedly scrutinised and questioned. Its definition was complicated not only by the position of existing practitioners with post-basic qualifications and specialist experience, but also by the increased range of roles in the clinical environment and the growing array of courses and qualifications offered by universities, the RCN and the National Boards. The pressure to move forward, however, was intense, and when in February 1993 the government confirmed that it was not prepared to take a final decision on the introduction of mandatory study leave until it had received all of the PREPP proposals, it was decided that a consultation paper on the kind of educational preparation required of those wishing to practise as specialist practitioners should be agreed at the March Council meeting – the final session of the Second Council.[44]

Consultation on Council standards for post-registration education

The consultation paper on Council's proposed standards for post-registration education was issued at the beginning of the Third Council term in May 1993.[45] It outlined Council's latest definitions of primary, specialist/enhanced and advanced practice, the educational preparation required of those wishing to practice as specialist and advanced practitioners in both community and institutional settings,[46] the position of existing practitioners with post-basic qualifications[47] and the standards required for teachers.[48]

The results of this second (or third, if the separate Community Education and Practice consultation is included) formal consultation again proved mixed.[49] It appeared that general support existed for using the register to indicate higher levels of skill and experience. Consensus on the detail, however, remained elusive. Established practitioners already in possession of post-basic qualifications continued to wonder what the streamlined 'standards' framework proposed in the document would mean to them. Midwives remained doubtful of the appropriateness of the notion of 'enhanced' practice. Many respondents expressed the view that Council's framework was too hierarchical and rigid to accommodate the growing range of practitioner roles and career development opportunities. The definition of advanced practice, in particular, was deemed overly prescriptive. Concerns were raised over the employment and grading implications of the proposed framework, the budgetary and human resource implications and the timescale for implementation. Above all, it was clear that the matter could not be tied up at this stage. In October 1993, Council members agreed to revisit the description of 'specialist' nursing practice and the outcomes identified for community health care nursing, reconsider the applicability of the notion of 'enhanced' midwifery practice and rethink the notion of advanced practice. It was a large agenda.[50]

March 1994 was a landmark date in Council's efforts to realise PREPP, as members agreed what was hoped would be the final report on standards of education and practice. The resulting document, *The Future of Professional Practice. Council's Standards for Education and Practice following Registration* clarified the definition of specialist practice and attempted a more explicit articulation of the links between the possession of a specialist qualification, the Council's new standards and the register. There was, it reiterated, 'a clear difference between practising within a specialty and being a nursing specialist'. Nurses at this latter level, it stated, were expected to 'demonstrate higher levels of clinical decision-making and will be able to monitor and improve standards of care through supervision of clinical practice, clinical audit, developing and leading practice, contributing to research, teaching and supporting professional colleagues'. The document suggested that a strict delineation of the number and type of specialist qualifications was not appropriate at this stage: programmes and specific roles, it argued, should be allowed to evolve in response to service need. Eight separate areas of specialist community health care nursing, however, were identified. These included the well-established practice areas of health visiting, district nursing, occupational health nursing, school nursing, community mental health nursing and community mental handicap nursing. Defined standards were also outlined, for the first time, for general practice nursing. Programmes of education for these specialist areas were to be of equal length and standard, and structured around a common core with appropriate specialist modules for each of the different areas. Midwifery's uncertainty over the term 'enhanced' practice was acknowledged and replaced by a general statement on the continuing nature of post-registration midwifery education, which was not to be linked to the acquisition of specific qualifications for additional roles. A more flexible approach to advanced practice was also advocated, and formal preparation or qualification linked to Council's register was not proposed for advanced practitioners at this stage. In addition, the term 'primary practice' was replaced by 'professional practice' to remove the potential for confusion between this and primary health care nursing, and to emphasise the fact that most nurses and midwives would spend the majority of their careers in this sphere of practice. Council also announced that its new policies on re-registration would come into effect on 1 April 1995.

Formal discussions on the implementation of PREPP with the four government Health Departments began immediately, and in May the government announced that it would support the project. Work on the implementation of Council's standards for maintaining registration could now begin in earnest. Information for registrants and their employers on the PREP changes was produced,[51] and Council's officers and solicitor worked on new Rules for the implementation of the new standards for maintaining registration. These came into force on April 1 1995 as SI 1995 No. 967, The Nurses, Midwives and Health Visitors (Periodic Registration) Amendment Rules Approval Order. Council also reviewed its position on preceptorship – a position which had been made public, as a statement of good practice in January 1993[52] – and began to prepare additional guidance to clear up a number of misunderstandings that had arisen and to ensure that the policy was implemented in a flexible and facilitative manner.[53]

Further reconsideration in the face of change

By April 1995, therefore, all of the UKCC's standards for post-registration education and practice were formally in place. This achievement, however, was somewhat overshadowed by ongoing difficulties with Council's standards for specialist and advanced practice. The recommended standards for the teachers of nurses and midwives were also coming under considerable criticism.[54] In the period of these debates, changes in the health services and in nursing practice in particular had made the UKCC's task of issuing clear, workable and responsive statements more difficult. Traditional boundaries between the health professions were becoming more fluid in response to a range of practice developments, local needs and national policy objectives (such as the first stage in the reduction of junior doctors' hours as a result of the New Deal). The flexible approach to the development of nursing and midwifery roles contained in the UKCC's *The Scope of Professional Practice* (see Chapter 3, p. 55) had also played an important part.[55] In addition to increasing the skills and decision-making responsibilities of all practitioners, these changes were leading to a further proliferation of new roles and titles within and around nursing. The growth in the numbers of clinical nurse specialists and nurse practitioners was particularly striking. There was, moreover, a distinct lack of consistency about these roles and titles.[56] Was it a moment for a complete rethink about this particular aspect of PREP?

Aware of the enormous implications of these changes and, more particularly, of the absence of a common understanding or definition for either advanced or specialist nursing practice, the UKCC decided for its standards framework to revisit its articulation of advanced and specialist practice, to see if a more definitive position could be agreed. Throughout 1995, examples of what might be construed as advanced nursing roles were examined, but it became increasingly apparent that progress on standard setting could not be made until Council had developed a more comprehensive understanding of the nature of practice at this level. In January 1996, UKCC officers, supported by an outside consultant, began a series of research and evaluation activities in the hope that these would aid Council to refine its position. A review of the existing research literature was undertaken in conjunction with a 'listening exercise' with Council members, outside experts and other 'stakeholders' in the health services. In October 1996 a consultative conference was held, with around one hundred invited participants, to test out the views generated during the previous nine months.[57] The overriding theme was the widespread confusion which existed around the roles, titles and responsibilities of practitioners who might be seen as practising in 'advanced' spheres. Other concerns expressed included the need to avoid a 'checklist' definition of advanced practice that might inhibit its dynamic and autonomous nature. The weight of opinion was that detailed standards should not be set for advanced practice, though support was given to the retention of the concept. It was felt that detailed consideration should now be given to whether the notion of specialist practice could be orientated less towards roles or functions in a specialty *area* and used more as a description of the standards required for a *level* of practice – a standard that would be applicable regardless of the environment or specialty in which a practitioner worked.[58]

From March 1997 these issues were taken up by a 'specialist practice' task group.[59] Contributors agreed that PREP was 'an innovative and far sighted policy' but its definition of specialist practice had not kept pace with the fast-moving developments in the field and had become entangled with various definitions of specialism and specialty. This was a serious problem, confusing practitioners, employers and consumers of health services alike. The need for a set of standards regulating specialist practice was not discounted by those involved in the review: indeed, a number of the written submissions to the task group had indicated that the current situation in relation to clinical nurse specialists and nurse practitioners was 'perceived to be potentially unsafe, inequitable and [as offering] insufficient public protection'. Nevertheless, the task group's review had indicated a lack of certainty among all interested parties about the role of the UKCC in setting standards for post-registration education and practice.

In December 1997, as Council's third term drew towards its close, members agreed that the UKCC needed to take a new and stronger lead in bringing greater clarity to this vexed topic. Policy on the shape of the new NHS was at this point emerging from the new Labour government. This indicated that the scope of practice of nurses, midwives and health visitors and the clinical and educational opportunities available to them would be extending still further in years to come.[60] Rather than try to build a complex set of standards around existing and projected roles and educational programmes, it was agreed that the UKCC needed to take a step back and establish a simpler framework based on an unambiguous currency of safe 'threshold standards' across all health care settings.[61] The work of the specialist practice task group had shown particular concern over the ambiguities around nurse practitioners and clinical nurse specialists. Some practitioners in these roles met the standards for the recording of specialist practitioner qualifications. Others did not. Public protection demanded a 'more robust system of regulation, associated with fitness to practise, or competence rather than the possession of an academic award'.[62] As the fourth Council term began, this fresh attempt to move forward had crystallised into the notion of regulating a *higher level of practice* rather than particular roles and spheres.[63]

An evolving concept of practice standards

While all this was going on, energies had also started to be channelled into other areas of thinking about standards. The influx of new kinds of member with the elections of 1992 and, after 1996, the arrival of new staff and the creation of new ways of working, both facilitated this. The production, in the summer of 1992, of the revised *Code of Conduct* and of *The Scope of Professional Practice* was an acknowledgement of rapidly changing roles that put the onus on the practitioner to take responsibility for assessing competence and patient safety when extended roles were proposed (see Chapter 4). The UKCC role was starting to be more that of supporting decision-making than that of laying down in detail what should be done in the increasingly complex and diverse settings of health care.

And yet the idea of standards in practice settings was starting to emerge alongside standards of education and conduct as the Second Council's objectives had made clear. There was a continuing thread of concern over the adequacy of what the Code called 'the environment of care' and questioning of how the UKCC could intervene here. It was a delicate path – the legislation gave no route to single out practice as separate from education and conduct, or to set standards that would trespass on employer prerogative. However, those in the Third Council, many of whom did not have a statutory background, pressed for the UKCC to act. They wanted to insist, for example, on minimum levels of resources and staffing and to require (in a context where middle levels of nurse management had been removed in new Trusts) that registrants should have access to clinical supervision to support them in their work. The growing involvement of non-Council members in the work of committees and, especially after the 1995 organisational review, a way of working that included much direct consultation with the professions and others, pointed in the same direction.

Starting in 1995, UKCC publications took a noticeably new turn. In September, Council revised and re-issued a list of ten proposed standards for inclusion in purchaser/provider contracts. The response to an earlier version, designed to support practitioners in their attempts to give good and safe care, had been disappointing.[64] The document was now given more publicity. It argued that purchasers should require providers to confirm the current registration status of their employees and should monitor this. They should require assurances that the provider was complying with the code as a condition of the contract, and ensure that staff had opportunities for professional development and access to clinical supervision, and that policies were in place to allow staff to express concern about standards. This represented an uncompromising position on standards for good practice, albeit that the title of the documents was 'proposed standards'. The line was softened when work on clinical supervision emerged the following spring. A position statement made clear the UKCC's support for the concept of clinical supervision for nurses and health visitors.[65] The UKCC was prepared, however, only to 'commend' it as 'an important part of strategies to promote high standards' leaving detail to be agreed locally. On professional conduct matters, Council was in some ways on stronger ground. The Nursing Homes Report of summer 1994 had demonstrated that. November 1996 brought the most uncompromising statement yet on policies that the UKCC believed were needed for the effective management of services and support and supervision of staff.[66]

By now, new organisational arrangements had begun to settle down and a number of additional staff were in post. New projects got under way and old ones were brought to fruition in the context of a revised business plan, with an explicit objective to review standards across the board, and of newly formed directorates. The Standards Promotion Directorate, with new professional officer posts in specialised areas of practice, began to support the Midwifery Committee and the Nursing and Community Health Care Nursing Committee in reviewing existing standards, and started also to explore professional conduct cases to see how more proactive support could be provided. The bringing to fruition of *Guidelines for Professional Practice* (July 1996) was one early result. This was followed by *Guidelines for Mental Health and Learning Disability* (April 1998). While the latter document followed the outlines of the former, it was notable for the ways in which, following extensive consultations, it was able to link the Code very directly to issues arising in the field. This was clear in the way it tackled consent, for example, and the sensitive matter of personal relationships and boundaries. It also made direct links with current thinking on risk management and evidence-based practice.

People had begun to talk of a policy cycle in which research and information coming into the UKCC from a variety of sources including consultation and commissioned research, would inform standards. These would be monitored and evaluated, resulting in the further development of the standards. Certainly there was much more activity towards the end of the Third Council in terms both of research and of consultation. A document on the continuing care of older people (November 1997) showed the value of substantial consultation. It directly addressed factors which could enable nurses to make an effective contribution – an appropriate educational culture and a committed management, for example. It posed questions to help registrants examine their practice and teased out examples of good practice. It was not a standards document as such, but it was not difficult to imagine how it might serve as the precursor to one.

Looking at all this from the outside, however, it was not easy to grasp just what the directions of the work were. Twin tracks seemed to be emerging. On the one hand, there was work focused on helping registrants to use the Code to think through issues in their own fields of practice. On the other hand, there was work that was edging towards naming standards that those providing a service must meet if nurses, midwives and health visitors were to use their skills safely and effectively.

Late in 1997, the UKCC, in its submission to the legislative review then under way, had pointed out that the rapid developments in the field of education had 'tended to divert the work of the UKCC and the National Boards towards standards in education . . . at the expense of standards in practice'. It went on to argue that the regulatory processes 'now need to be re-focused' to balance the two.[67] The implication was that this strategic change was under way though not as yet complete. The reviewers, however, took an uncompromisingly critical view of this aspect of regulation. They were clear that Council should have the power to make rules in all three areas – practice, education and conduct. However, while the UKCC had set standards in all three areas:

> This has been done piecemeal and not presented in a way that is accessible to those not closely involved. Anyone asking what the standards are will find, as we have, a confusing mix of strategic standards (such as Rule 18(A) for education outcomes, or the Scope of Professional Practice) and other much more detailed documents – of which the Midwives Rules are just one example. They will also find that the National Boards have added to or interpreted the educational standards to varying degrees in each country.[68]

Whatever the achievements, including what many regarded as a landmark achievement of setting standards for continuing eligibility for practice through validated professional development, the reviewers felt that it was time for a fresh start. The government agreed.

Conclusion

The story of post-registration standards is a complex one whose outlines are only just beginning to emerge with any clarity. PREPP, launched in 1989, was in fact three projects in one. The first, and most straightforward, concerned the value of establishing a system of support for the newly registered. The second was about using the mechanisms of registration to help maintain and improve standards of competence. The third – and by far the most difficult – attempted to define the nature of professional practice beyond the point of registration and to set a framework of post-registration educational standards. Determination to involve the profession and to honour in full its legislative requirement to consult with interested parties meant a series of consultations – with the profession, with employers and also, for the first time, with consumers. Much of the feedback about what Council was trying to achieve was positive, yet the framework it was seeking to establish remained elusive; and anxieties were not allayed by what appeared from the outside to be an immensely protracted process and a steady stream of confusing documents. Council grappled with all this at a time of very great change in education and in practice. New roles and relationships in employment, new courses in higher education, new frameworks of continuing education at National Board level, and debate about vocational and occupational standards, all served to make the picture even more complex. The UKCC had undoubtedly moved a very considerable distance since 1979. With the PREP conditions for continuing eligibility to practise and re-registration in place, an entry on the register meant much more than it did in the past in terms of protecting the public. The question was whether there was still more to do to ensure public protection, and whether the UKCC in its current form was the body to do it.

Notes

1 The term PREPP was used until March 1994, when the Council agreed its standards for post-registration education and practice. After that date the 'project' was formally complete and Council's work in this area became known as PREP.

2 These included a consultative document in 1982 proposing an 'effective' register which would indicate current eligibility to practise (see Chapter 2), a set of 'good practice' guidelines on re-entry programmes for nurses and health visitors in 1986 and a consultative document in 1987 on periodic refreshment. See EPAC MIN 84/24; EPAC MIN 84/28; EPAC MIN 85/04; UKCC, PS&D/86/06, 'Guidelines of good practice, return to practice programmes for nurses and health visitors', May 1986; CC/88/16. See also UKCC, K4.1, K4.2 and K8.1.

3 MIN 113/88(a), November 1988; CC/88/75.

4 See minutes of EPAC meeting, 13–14 April 1989, at Chequers Hotel, Newbury, Berkshire. The project terms of reference were agreed at the May 1989 Council meeting.

5 UKCC press release, 'A major new project', 16 August 1989.

6 UKCC, PREPP/89/02, 'Methods of working'; UKCC, PREPP/89/03, 'The development of the project', September 1989; CC/89/88 Annex 1; UKCC, K4.4 (A3), 'Discussion paper on post-registration education and practice', January 1990.

7 UKCC, PREPP/90/11, 'Analysis of responses to discussion document, article in "Register" and roadshows' (n.d.).

8 *Nursing Standard*, 12 February, 4(22), 1990, p. 3.

9 See, for example, *Nursing Standard*, 1 November, 4(6), 1989, p. 3; *Nursing Standard*, 14 March, 4(25), 1990, p. 16.

10 *Nursing Standard*, 12 February, 4(22), 1990, p. 3.

11 A report on the situation was introduced to Council members at a private seminar on 19 July. Council formally received the report in closed session the following day. The report was also sent in confidence to the National Boards. See C MIN 53/90, July 1990; CC/90/C40.

12 MIN 47/90(e), July 1990; MIN 58/90(d), September 1990. See also CC/90/68.

13 For a history of the debates and decisions in relation to preparation of nurse and midwife teachers see Wallace, M., *Lifelong Learning. PREP in action*, Edinburgh, Churchill Livingstone, 1999.

14 The Steering Group was chaired once again by Professor Green. It comprised seven members, with representatives from each of the four home nations and the major professional groups. The whole of the UKCC professional unit were also members, and additional members could be co-opted if required. UKCC, K4.(A7), letter to members of PREPP Steering Group, 26 October 1990; SG/PREPP/2, 'Steering Group Post-Registration Education and Practice: terms of reference and details of further

work'. See also UKCC, K4.4 (A7), PREPP Steering Group, notes of meeting held 15 November 1990 and C MIN 73/90, November 1990.

15 UKCC, *Report of the Post-Registration Education and Practice Project*, October 1990.

16 UKCC press statement, 'The Report of the Post-Registration Education and Practice Project – the UKCC consults on major proposals', 30 October 1990.

17 CC/91/C16. A preliminary analysis of the consultation response was completed for the May Council meeting. The full report on the response to the consultation was produced in June 1991 and submitted to Council in July 1991.

18 The report to Council gave a considerable amount of attention to the methodology used in the analysis. The responses were analysed in two ways: firstly, by analysing group responses and, secondly, by analysing responses to each of the recommendations.

19 The RCN's view was stated by Christine Hancock and quoted, together with a range of other views in O'Byrne, J., 'Linking study, education and practice', *Nursing Standard*, 7 November, 7(5), 1990, pp. 16–17.

20 *Nursing Standard*, 7 November, 5(7), 1990, p. 19. See also Millar, B., 'Investing in the future', *Nursing Times*, 20 February, 87(8), 1991, pp. 29–30.

21 *Nursing Standard*, 7 November, 5(7), 1990, p. 19.

22 Representatives of the Council met with representatives of COHSE to discuss their response to the consultation document. MIN 44/91, July 1991.

23 *Nursing Times*, 7 November, 86(45), 1990, p. 3.

24 CC/91/C16, p. 18.

25 The major purpose of the midwives' annual notification of intention to practise is to enable the local supervisor of midwives to know which practitioners are to be supervised in any given year. Because of this, the form is processed through the supervisory network. The new system proposed in PREPP would involve the practitioner dealing directly with Council. Both systems, it was agreed, could operate concurrently.

26 In February 1989, the WNB had published its *Framework for Continuing Education: the Development of Professional Practice*, Cardiff, WNB, 1989. This was amended in January 1990 and replaced in March 1991 with a circular WNB 91/3 under the same title. It continued to be reviewed and amended after this point. In early 1991, the ENB published *Framework for Continuing Professional Education and the Higher Award*, London, ENB, 1991.

27 UKCC press statement, 'Post-registration education and practice (PREPP) – the next steps', 30 July 1991.

28 For more information on the discussions of the Panel and the Price Waterhouse team, see UKCC K4.4(A5), Vol. 1, section 7.

29 CC/91/C15, July 1991.

30 Annexe to CC/91/C15, pp. 2–4.

31 A statement based on the summary report was issued as an annexe to the PREPP press statement of 30 July 1991.

32 UKCC press statement, 'Post-registration education and practice (PREPP) – the next steps', 30 July 1991.

33 CC/91/71, November 1991. See also PREPP/SG/91/15 for details of a three-part 'eligibility form', with sections for notification of practice, notification of satisfactory completion of a personal professional profile and payment of periodic fee.

34 The NHS and Community Care Act 1990, the Children Act 1989, and the implementation of Project 2000 were all beginning, or about to impact on those practising in the community.

35 MIN 59/90(d), September 1990; Council seminar paper, 'Community practice and education: paper for informal meeting on 15 November 1990; ChGp/C/1, 'Draft paper for chairman's initiative to address community practice and education issues', September 1990; Summit paper 10, 'Summit meeting on community education and practice: chairman's brief for session 1'; CC/91/C01; C MIN 8/91, January 1991.

36 C MIN 8/91, November 1991; CC/91/C01.

37 CC/91/C12, Annexe 1.

38 CC/92/C08.

39 C MIN 15/92(2), February 1992. Additional work on the accumulation and transfer of credit obtained for post-registration education was also needed, but progress was limited until firm policies had been agreed on the standard of professional and academic learning for specialist and/or advanced practice. Standards for the preparation of teachers also needed to be explored and agreed.

40 CC/92/14, Annexe 1, letter from Dame Audrey Emerton to Mrs Virginia Bottomley, Minister of State for Health, 21 February 1992; CC/92/14, Annexe 2, letter from Mrs Virginia Bottomley to Dame Audrey Emerton, (n.d.); PSG/92/08, Annexe 2, letter from Mr Robin Orton, NHS Management Executive, Department of Health, to Mr Colin Ralph, Registrar, UKCC, 7 April 1992.

41 Letter from Ms S. Norman, Principal Nursing Officer, Department of Health to Mr Colin Ralph, 22 July 1992. Department of Health press release, 16 October 1992, 'Baroness Cumberlege announces survey of nurses', midwives' and health visitors' study leave'. A government survey of practitioners' current experience of study leave and a survey of nursing and midwifery colleges to elicit the average cost of providing a 'study day' duly took place during the autumn and winter of 1992/93.

42 Naish, J., 'A toothless tiger?' *Nursing Standard*, 29 July, 6(45), 1992, p. 2. See also pp. 1 and 5, and *Nursing Standard*, 22 July, 6(44), 1992, pp. 3 and 5, and Minute 47/92(4), July 1992.

43 The Steering Group comprised the chairman of the Council and the chairmen of the Midwifery Committee, HVJC and DNJC. It had the power to co-opt additional members as and when necessary. It was once again chaired by Professor Margaret Green. Maggy Wallace was appointed as director of this phase of the project.

44 Minute 13/93, February 1993; CC/93/12.

45 UKCC, *The Council's Proposed Standards for Post-Registration Education*, May 1993; Registrar's Letter 8/1993, 21 May 1993. See also article on PREPP in UKCC's *Register*, Spring 1993, no. 12, p. 10.

46 Programmes leading to specialist nursing or enhanced midwifery qualifications, it was recommended, should be modular and of no less than six months' study at degree level. Programmes leading to the advanced practitioner qualification were to be available only to those in receipt of a specialist qualification of no less than three months' duration and at the level of higher degree. Both qualifications were to be recorded on the Council's register.

47 Transitional arrangements to ensure that existing practitioners were recognised within the new proposals were under consideration at the time the consultation document was issued. It was envisaged that those already in possession of a recordable qualification (from a course lasting six months or more) who have undertaken practice in the appropriate area would 'automatically' be recognised as specialist practitioners, and that mechanisms would be put in place for other practitioners who wished to gain access to a specialist, enhanced or advanced programme.

48 Teachers of nursing and midwifery were to be graduates with an advanced qualification recorded on the Council's register (when, in March 1994, Council agreed that no advanced qualifications were to be recorded on the register, the requirement was changed to holding a specialist qualification), and had to possess an appropriate teaching qualification at either graduate or post-graduate level.

49 The consultation lasted for five months. 437 responses were received.

50 Minute 55/93/7(3), October 1993.

51 Factsheets on PREPP were prepared, a PREPP helpline was introduced and a series of joint UKCC/National Board conferences were held at various locations throughout the UK. See also Wallace, *Lifelong Learning*.

52 Registrar's Letter 1/1993, 'The Council's position concerning a period of support and preceptorship ; implementation of the PREPP proposals', 4 January 1993.

53 A questionnaire survey was used to evaluate the implementation and interpretation of the policy in 1994. New guidance was issued, Registrar's Letter 3/1995, 'The Council's position concerning a period of support and preceptorship', 25 January 1995.

54 Particular concerns were expressed by community practice teachers, many of whom feared a dilution of standards under the new arrangements. Further consideration of this issue was undertaken by a Teachers Task Group and, in the summer of 1996 an external consultant, Ruth Champion, led a new consultation exercise. In June 1997, Council approved a standards framework for the preparation of teachers of nursing, midwifery and health visiting, and detailed implementation work began. For further information see CC/97/21, CC/97/47 and Wallace, *Lifelong Learning*.

55 One view being expressed at the time, however, was that the formal requirements of PREPP did not fit well with the UKCC's *Code of Professional Conduct* and its *Scope of Professional Practice* document – both of which stressed the responsibility of individual practitioners to ensure that they practised with due competence and according to their knowledge and skill.

56 The professional literature revealed the extent of these changes. See for example, Hopkins, A., *et al*, 'Shifting boundaries in professional care', *Journal of the Royal Society of Medicine*, 89, 1996, pp. 364–71; Brown, R., 'The politics of specialist/advanced practice: conflict or confusion?', *British Journal of Specialist Nursing*, 1(3), 1995, pp. 944–8; Burke-Masters, B., 'The nurse practitioner's surgery', *Self-Health*, March 22–3, 1988; Buchan, J., *Grade Expectations: clinical grading and nurse mobility*, Brighton, Institute of Manpower Studies, University of Sussex, 1989; Casselden, D., 'The role of the neo-natal nurse practitioner', *Nursing Times*, 4 October, 91(40), 1995, pp. 42–3; Mackie, C., 'Nurse-practitioners managing anti-coagulation clinics', *Nursing Times*, 3 January, 92(1), 1996, pp. 25–6.

57 The project was led by an outside consultant, Abi Masterton, lecturer at the School for Policy Studies, University of Bristol. Minute 6/97(6), March 1997. See CC/96/46 for more details of the project group's work.

58 CC/97/06, p. 4; Minute 6/97(6), March 1997. See also Roques, A., 'A floor not a ceiling', *Nursing Standard*, 19 March, 11(26), 1997, p. 16.

59 The task group initially comprised Council members and officers. Later, a group of external experts was added. Also, whilst acknowledging the decision of midwifery to stand outside the specialist practice standards, the group invited a member of the Midwifery Committee to participate. Abi Masterton was the project manager. See CC/97/46.

60 Department of Health, *The New NHS, Modern – Dependable*, London, The Stationery Office, 1997. These themes were further explored in NHS Wales, Welsh Office, *Putting Patients First*, London, The Stationery Office, 1998; DHSS, Northern Ireland Office, *Fit for the Future: A New Approach: The Government's Proposals For The Future Of The Health And Personal Social Services In Northern Ireland*, Belfast, DHSS, 1998; Scottish Office, Department of Health, *Designed to Care: renewing the NHS in Scotland*, Cm 3811, Edinburgh, The Stationery Office, 1997. See also CC/98/41, Annexe 1, 1998.

61 CC/98/19, p. 3. The work was taken forward by a Steering Group comprising Council members, officers, and external experts (a number of whom had been members of the previous task group on specialist practice).

62 CC/97/46.

63 CC/98/19. As the Fourth Council got under way, a new Steering Group was set up, chaired by Professor George Castledine, Vice-President of Council. A consultation carried out between August and October 1998 showed considerable support, but how all this was to fit in the government's agenda was an open question (see Chapter 10).

64 UKCC, Registrar's Letter 37/1992, 'Standards for Incorporation into Contracts for Hospital and Community Health Care Services', 14 December 1992.
65 For more on midwifery's distinctive position on supervision, see Chapter 7, pp. 149–150.
66 UKCC, *Issues arising from professional conduct complaints*.
67 UKCC, *The Future of Professional Regulation*, para. 2.4.
68 JM Consulting, *The Regulation of Nurses, Midwives and Health Visitors*. Report on a review of the Nurses, Midwives & Health Visitors Act 1997, Bristol, JM Consulting, 1999, para. 72.

Part III

Stakeholders and standards

7 Holding the professions together

The complex negotiations leading up to the passage of the 1979 Act resulted in a number of provisions to safeguard the position of 'minority' interests. Three distinct groups – nurses, midwives and health visitors – were named in the title of the Act and subsequently in the titles of the new statutory bodies. Section 2(6) of the Act stated that 'in the discharge of its functions the Council shall have proper regard for the interests of all groups within the professions, including those with minority representation'. A similar requirement was placed upon the National Boards in Section 6(2). Protection for minority interests was further enshrined in certain distinctive organisational structures at both Council and National Board level.

Midwives won a number of significant legislative safeguards. Key elements of extant midwifery legislation, such as provisions restricting who may attend a woman in childbirth, were carried over into the 1979 Act, and the regulation of midwifery practice through statutory rules was maintained.[1] The primary legislation also required the establishment of statutory standing Midwifery Committees at both UKCC and National Board levels. Composed of a majority of practising midwives, these were to be consulted on 'all matters relating to midwifery'. This was a strongly worded statement, buttressed, in the case of midwifery practice rules, by two further clauses;[2] but, as this chapter will indicate, the absence of a precise definition of what constituted a 'midwifery matter' left room for the development of conflicting interpretations and tensions. Health visitors gained a distinct, if less powerful, presence in the primary legislation. Not only was the profession to be identified in the title of the Act, but health visitors were to be represented through a standing committee, including a majority of practising health visitors. Unlike the arrangements for midwifery, however, this was to be a joint committee of the Central Council and the National Boards, a situation that, as we shall see, brought its own complications.[3]

What, then, of the much larger and more diffuse body of nurses? Although, as we have already seen in chapter 1, the framers of the 1979 Act were anxious to avoid a proliferation of specialist committees at UK level, the primary legislation did not close off this option completely. It allowed further joint committees – a power that was utilised in the shadow period to form the District Nursing Joint Committee,[4] and gave the new Central Council discretionary powers to establish further standing committees. During the 'shadow' period, however, members decided against the creation of more specialist committees, preferring to represent mental nurses, mental handicap nurses, occupational health nurses, school nurses, children's nurses and the growing number of nurses with post-basic training in clinical specialties through a single Educational Policy Advisory Committee. The National Boards, by contrast, established a range of specialist committees to assist them, for example, in approving institutions and courses of training.

When statutory responsibilities were handed over to the new regulatory bodies in July 1983, the professional committee structure of the Central Council was thus composed of a statutory standing Midwifery Committee, two standing Joint Committees for Health Visiting and for District Nursing, and EPAC.[5] The standing orders of this last committee stated that its membership should include representatives engaged in the practice of children's nursing, mental illness nursing, mental handicap nursing and occupational health nursing, as well as allocating a specific place to a member of the Midwifery Committee and the Health Visiting and District Nursing Joint Committees.[6] This, in conjunction with the committee arrangements of the four National Boards, provided the basic professional committee structure of the statutory bodies for around ten years. When the time came for an external review, elements of this structure were criticised as cumbersome and born of political expedience – a judgement that we will review in the course of this chapter.

Amending legislation in 1992 redefined the National Boards as smaller executive bodies and, in line with this, repealed provisions for the establishment of joint committees and of the standing midwifery committees at Board level. The statutory Midwifery Committee of the Central Council was retained but no other professional committees were explicitly required by the amended primary legislation. Following the assembly of the Third Council, a second 'practice' standing committee, the Nursing and Community Health Care Nursing Committee, was created to give representation to the other professional groups regulated by the Act. This, it was hoped, would enable all the nursing specialties to contribute to strategic debates about practice standards. Both 'practice' committees were to be joined by an Education Committee, with a membership that included representatives of adult nursing, children's nursing, midwifery, health visiting, mental health nursing, mental handicap nursing and occupational health nursing.[7] This new structure, and other changes brought about as a result of the 1992 Act, altered the ways minority groups could articulate their particular needs.

The principal aim of this chapter is to provide an exploration of what was achieved, and the difficulties that were experienced, by the various professional groups within these regulatory structures. It is not possible, in the compass of a single chapter, to consider in detail the perspective of every specialist group under the UKCC umbrella. Some of the tensions experienced by specialist groups have already been noted in other chapters. This chapter will build on these references, paying particular attention to the structural forms that were available and the scope they have given for the articulation of special needs and interests.

Midwifery: a 'special' place within a common regulatory structure[8]

Midwives brought to the new statutory structure a long and distinctive history of professional regulation.[9] This was a powerful yet ambiguous legacy. On the one hand, the processes of midwifery regulation, based on legislation passed during the first years of the twentieth century, bore the stamp of the profession's relatively humble beginnings.[10] The dominant presence of medical men on the CMB for England and Wales,[11] the use of detailed practice rules outlining the limits of the midwife's responsibilities, the development of local authority supervisory arrangements and the funding of the Board through the receipts of local taxation,[12] could all be interpreted in this light.

On the other hand, midwives were extremely proud of the extent to which it had been possible to develop positive interpretations of processes that, to others, could appear restrictive or controlling. Whereas nurses might regard the midwives' practice rules as evidence of the low trust accorded them by the medical profession, to midwives they were a symbol of their statutory right to be autonomous practitioners, and a statement of their profession's awareness of the primacy of public protection. Similarly positive interpretations were given to statutory supervision of midwifery practice and arrangements for the annual notification of intention to practice. This section will suggest that these conflicting interpretations – nowhere explicitly put into words – fed tension and misunderstanding between nurses and midwives, and help explain the conflicts which arose as the two groups tried to work together in a new, and somewhat cumbersome, framework of shared regulation.

Midwives' hopes and expectations of the new statutory body were high. Since the mid-1970s there had been concern that the direction of NHS policy was weakening the distinctiveness of midwifery. Over a decade of medical emphasis upon the safety of hospital deliveries, strong moves towards making a pregnant woman's first point of contact the GP and not the midwife and increasing specialisation of the work of hospital midwives were all interpreted as curtailing the midwife's freedom to use clinical judgement, turning them into maternity nurses.[13] It would not be long before the more vocal among them sought concrete evidence that the new arrangements were capable of maintaining the distinctiveness of the midwifery profession.

Mixed experiences of shared regulation

Meeting on average five times a year, the UKCC Midwifery Committee quickly established a full and wide-ranging agenda. While informal arrangements had existed between the former statutory bodies for midwifery to enable them to share information, the new regulatory framework focused attention on the need to devise and agree a set of midwives rules and a code of practice that were applicable for the United Kingdom as a whole.[14] In January 1984, a working group comprising the four practising midwife members of the Council (one from each

National Board) and a further member of the Midwifery Committee, was established to take this work forward.[15] The new statutory structure required consultation, and in May 1984 a paper was ready for distribution. This was the first time that practising midwives were asked to share their views on the rules governing their education and practice with the statutory body and Council members were encouraged by the interest shown.[16]

Midwifery had both training and practice rules enshrined in secondary legislation.[17] First designed at the turn of the century for an occupational group that included a large proportion of poorly educated women, over the intervening years practice rules had become a tool of public protection, in a way that had no comparison within nursing.[18] To the midwife, practice rules were a public declaration of professional skill and a way of signalling, perhaps even securing, the midwife's space as an independent practitioner. This distinctive part of the regulation of midwifery, midwife members of the new statutory bodies agreed, needed to continue. Yet the form and tone of the practice rules was felt to be in need of updating.[19] Members of the Midwifery Committee spoke of the desirability of a 'fresh approach', allowing for a variety of local circumstances, and for professional development and change.

The complement to this revision was the further development of the *Midwife's Code of Practice*, a companion document to the practice rules that had been devised earlier by the CMB (England and Wales). It was felt that if advice designed to 'guide the midwife in her own performance review and in the establishment and maintenance of optimum standards of practice' could be issued to practitioners through the Code, then only the most fundamental issues would need to be contained within the secondary legislation.[20] Not only would this have practical value in enabling the UKCC to amend its guidance to midwives without recourse to Parliament, it could signify and, in turn, foster a changing regulatory culture – one that clearly placed the professional judgement of the individual practitioner at its heart.

The new editions of the Rules and the Code of Practice, published in May 1986,[21] exemplified the new approach in two ways. First, delineation of the professional relationship between a midwife and a medical practitioner when working together was moved from the statutory Rules to the Code of Practice.[22] Second, the Code was the preferred place for outlining the duties of a midwife when attending a woman requesting a home birth when the circumstances were unsuitable.[23] Both changes put the onus of decision-making on the midwife herself and represented a clear move away from a narrow and constraining interpretation of the concept of practice rules. This stance was in line with the UKCC's general desire to build a flexible framework for professional practice: a theme that was explored during Project 2000, and which would find further articulation during the lifetime of the Second Council, both in the next edition of the Midwives' Code and Rules and in the nursing profession's development of the *Scope of Professional Practice*. At this point, however, the underlying issues were not brought out into the open in a way that engaged the different constituent elements of the UKCC.

With these new documents in place, the Midwifery Committee continued to focus on how regulatory processes long familiar to, and trusted by, midwives should be taken forward. In 1985 and 1986 new administrative arrangements for the notification of intention to practise were prepared and reviewed. In 1987, a review of the policies and approval mechanisms related to mandatory updating and return to practice courses was undertaken, and it was agreed that the current rules and arrangements should continue, at least for the time being.[24] Although nurses and health visitors were also interested in these issues from the very first years of the new statutory body, it did not prove possible to develop arrangements appropriate to their professions at this point. Instead developments proceeded in parallel.

Parallel development, however, could not be a solution when it came to a new system of pre-registration education (see Chapter 4). The stated aim of the new regulatory body was to develop a rationalised and integrated scheme. The distinctiveness of midwives and nurses would need to be confronted. Midwife members of Council were strongly of the view that the deficiencies of current midwifery programmes were different from those affecting nursing, and that the training needs of midwives differed substantially from those of nurses. The difficulty lay in getting this point across in a constructive manner in the short time available.[25] As Project 2000 progressed, the inclusion of midwifery within the two-year Common Foundation Programme and a one-year branch model of professional preparation became a problematic issue. At this point, midwifery training normally consisted of an eighteen-month course taken following registration as a nurse. Midwives felt that a one-year midwifery programme was insufficient preparation for the highly specialised and autonomous practice of the midwife,[26] and while the Project Report's endorsement of midwifery as 'a profession different from but complementary to nursing' was warmly welcomed, many midwives remained unconvinced that Project 2000 would fit their particular needs.[27] As the UKCC prepared its submission to the government, midwives within the Council reiterated their unhappiness with the Project's recommendation for experimental one-year branch programmes in midwifery. In October 1986, Council accepted that experimentation with the CFP/branch model should not proceed in midwifery at this stage and agreed that an increase in the number of three-year direct-entry midwifery programmes should be recommended to the government alongside plans to continue the eighteen-month post-registration preparation.

The episode had been revealing. In spite of strong commonalities, midwives and nurses did not share a truly common language, and the structure adopted under the 1979 Act in some ways perpetuated differences. Business in the Midwifery Committee was taken forward rapidly and tended to be recalled in a positive light by those involved. Project Group meetings and those of Council itself, however, were clearly more tense. Until 1993 there were just four midwife members of Council, each of whom was also a member of a National Board. If midwifery was to have a voice at all levels and in all arenas, this meant an extremely demanding schedule for the individuals concerned. Close contact between midwives at Council and Boards was a consequence of the structure, but it also perhaps encouraged the perception of midwives as a group apart.[28]

How did midwifery appear through external eyes? The departmental review in 1989 concentrated on the relationship between the national and the UK components of the statutory framework. Much less attention was given to the experiences of the different professional groups. The reviewers accepted what the professions themselves styled as the 'tribalism' in their culture, arguing that it would need more than legislative change to overcome, without really exploring whether the structures developed under the primary legislation actually exacerbated unresolved tensions. Given this important omission, it was not surprising that the debate within the midwifery profession about the appropriateness of shared regulation intensified during the late 1980s and early 1990s.

Working with new legislation

The passage of the 1992 Act was closely watched by midwives.[29] The new constitution of the Council, with its membership of sixty, brought an increase in the number of midwife members from four to eight. This went some way to ease the extremely heavy workloads of individual midwife members. In the parliamentary debates on the Bill, the Secretary of State for Health, Virginia Bottomley, had underlined that midwifery's 'special' position within the common regulatory structure would 'continue to be recognised by that structure, as it has been since 1902'.[30] The powers and functions of the UKCC Midwifery Committee were to remain the same. Under the new Act, indeed, the Midwifery Committee was to be the only named committee (apart from the statutory Finance Committee) required by primary legislation. The new standing orders brought an increased membership of between fourteen and eighteen members. The majority were to be persons who worked or had worked in the professional field of midwifery, including eight elected UKCC midwives. Other members were to include two medical practitioners appointed after consultation with the appropriate professional bodies and, for the first time, two representatives from consumer organisations with a special interest in midwifery and maternity services.[31] The legislation also shifted responsibility for the setting of standards for midwifery supervision from the National Boards to the UKCC – a move that was widely welcomed as logical and positive. Not only did it provide the means to achieve a greater measure of consistency in the development of standards, but it also secured the involvement of the elected profession in an important practice-related activity. By requiring the Boards to provide the local supervising authorities with advice and guidance consistent with the Council's rules and requirements, moreover, the Act ensured that a national focus for this important aspect of midwifery regulation was retained.[32]

Nevertheless, there were elements of concern. First, with the removal of the requirement that statutory Standing Midwifery Committees be established at Board level, a key forum for debate close to the point of service delivery had gone and, without named places among the Boards' membership, midwifery representation there was not guaranteed. Of even greater concern, though, was the 1992 Act's failure to address what many representatives of the midwifery profession, including the Council of the RCM, felt to be the weakest aspect of the extant legislation – the lack of definition of 'matters relating to midwifery' on which the Committee was to be consulted. A particularly tense debate had already surfaced around this matter in 1989 when first the ENB, and then the WNB, decided to give its education officers generalist instead of specialist responsibilities. The RCM was also disappointed that a clause requiring the Council not to 'unreasonably reject any recommendation' of the Midwifery Committee was not included in the amended legislation. The question of just what constituted a 'midwifery matter' would return to forefront of debate during the lifetime of the Third Council.

The legislative changes required the UKCC to amend and make additions to the midwives' Practice Rules and to redraft the Midwife's Code of Practice. This opportunity to explore and enhance key aspects of midwifery regulation was well taken by midwives within the UKCC.[33] Their efforts to encourage a positive perception of the Practice Rules and the Code can be regarded as an extension of earlier work. The discussion of requirements relating to post-natal visiting provides a good illustration of this aim. During the early 1990s, concerns were beginning to surface about the implications of recent changes and cutbacks in the health services. A significant number of practitioners contacted the UKCC to express their concern that managers were beginning to restrict the level of their visiting of mothers in the post-natal period. In response the UKCC indicated how the midwives' Rules could be used against attempts to interfere with professional activities. Employers could be reminded that the Rules defined the post-natal period as not less than ten days and not more than twenty-eight days after the birth and, in conjunction with the Code, clearly stated that the midwife retained professional responsibility for mother and baby during this period.[34]

The UKCC's new role in setting standards for the supervision of midwives also gave the Midwifery Committee the opportunity to review the existing situation and to plan for the development of more uniform standards. An analysis of current supervisor-to-midwife ratios, undertaken during the first year of the new Council using the UKCC's registration statistics, indicated that sharp variations existed between different parts of the UK. For the statutory body charged with developing standards for the supervision of midwifery, this was an important finding. Nevertheless, as the numbers of supervisors of midwives employed by the Local Supervising Authority (LSA) was essentially a staffing issue, it would have been extremely difficult for the statutory body to set an optimum ratio in its secondary legislation. Rather than attempt this, Council decided instead that the new edition of the Midwife's Code of Practice should include a recommendation that each supervisor should supervise no more than forty practising midwives. It was also agreed that, while it was 'for each LSA to determine its organisational arrangements', the Code should clearly state Council's view that the LSA function should be assigned to a 'practising midwife who is professionally experienced in the supervision of midwives'.[35] Publication in the Code, it was felt, would give these important issues authority and a high profile. More generally, the language of the new edition of the Code was carefully chosen to re-emphasise the enabling nature of the midwives' Practice Rules, and to indicate the 'broader context of professional responsibility and accountability within midwifery practice'.[36] This, of course, was not a completely new departure: it consolidated a process begun in 1986,[37] and complemented other elements of the UKCC's work, such as the publication of the *Scope of Professional Practice* and the series of guidance documents on important practice issues.

The Council's ongoing work on PREPP carried the potential for tensions to develop between the two professions. As Chapter 6 has shown, the formation of detailed policy on a standards framework for specialist and advanced practice did not make sense in midwifery terms.[38] Clinical supervision provided another case in point. While professional opinion on its current effectiveness and, indeed, its relevance to autonomous and responsible practitioners varied considerably, statutory supervision had become an emblem of midwifery's distinctiveness.[39] As Karlene Davies, then deputy general secretary of the RCM, put it, midwives needed to consider the possibility that the rising interest in a non-mandatory system of clinical supervision might challenge midwifery's 'statutory basis for supervision' and lead to the incorporation of midwives 'within the new nursing peer review model'.[40] Within the UKCC, there was an element of disappointment that midwifery's long history of supervision and, indeed, the Midwifery Committee's on-going work on setting standards for supervision did not receive more attention from their nursing and health visiting colleagues.[41] Nevertheless, it was accepted that each needed to explore the notion of professional supervision on their own terms. The Midwifery Committee therefore continued to explore the development of standards of statutory midwifery supervision in parallel to the Council's work on clinical supervision.[42]

The 1995 internal organisational review refocused the attention of some midwives, within the Council as well as outside it, on the suitability of the current system of shared regulation. Concerns that had surfaced during the legislative review returned. There was anger that no midwife was elected specifically to represent midwives on the Organisational Review Steering Group,[43] and a proposal to bring all education matters under the remit of a Joint Education Committee was rejected by the Midwifery Committee. Its view that the Midwifery Committee itself should be able to commission its own work on educational matters was reconsidered and accepted by Council in September 1995.[44] Concern was also expressed that the new senior management structure, organised on functional lines, would disadvantage midwives.[45] In March 1996 the chairman of the Midwifery Committee resigned from Council over these issues.[46] The episode also reopened a debate in the professional press about the possibility of separate legislation for midwives. At one point, indeed, the RCM began a campaign to take over midwifery regulation itself.[47] This aim, however, was relatively short-lived, and not all the press took up the issue. More recently, the RCM has asserted its desire to see a Midwifery Directorate established at the UKCC 'to ensure that midwifery's position as a separate and distinct profession is recognised'.[48]

During 1996, stability returned to the Midwifery Committee. Together with the Nursing and Community Health Care Nursing Committee (NCHCNC) it agreed a position statement on the role of practice nurses in the delivery of antenatal care.[49] The Committee continued to work, alongside the Education Committee and the NCHCNC, on the development of standards for the preparation of teachers of midwifery and nursing. A number of issues directly related to clinical midwifery practice were also considered, such as the question of midwives being unable to administer intravenous fluids in the community when they can do so in a hospital setting.[50]

The government's review of legislation would inevitably reopen the question of how shared regulation between midwifery and nursing was working. JM Consulting's report, released in February 1999, acknowledged midwives' dissatisfaction. Recommendations for a Nursing and Midwifery Council with equal numbers from the two professions, and for the inclusion of a Director of Midwifery Regulation among the executive staff of the new body,[51] went a long way to mollify midwives' concerns. But the government's response, accepting that health visitors also should be named and have representation, clouded the issue in midwives' eyes and left them once again in what they felt was a compromised position.[52] The fundamental question of how far their distinctiveness was recognised was back on the table. As Chapter 9 will show, they remained profoundly doubtful and lobbied strongly for amendments in the run-up to the 1998 Health Act.

In all, the relation between midwifery and nursing had remained uneasy throughout the period of the three Councils. While midwifery developed its regulatory policy and practice in new ways in the unified structure that was put in place with the 1979 Act, tensions continued to surface and reached an acute state on more than one occasion. The histories and practices of midwives and nurses were sufficiently dissimilar to require different structures and approaches, yet sufficiently similar to cause confusion. JM Consulting had concluded early on that midwifery's detailed regulation of practice was simply an outdated legacy from the past that needed to be swept away,[53] yet had gone on to acknowledge that midwives deserved distinct regulation. And the government's response compounded rather than clarified the situation. The nettle of shared regulation remained to be grasped.

Changing structures for health visiting and community health care nursing

At the end of the 1970s, health visitors and district nurses viewed the efforts to establish a shared regulatory structure with some concern (see Chapter 1). To many community-based practitioners, Briggs had reflected the continued domination of hospital nursing interests. District nurses were particularly disappointed that their hopes for a mandatory training requirement had been dashed. The absence of a statutory committee to replace the Panel of Assessors for District Nurse Training, just when its work in securing new standards for district nurse training was beginning, also caused concern. Many health visitors too remained unconvinced of the need to reorganise. Like the Panel, the CETHV was a relatively young body, having been created under legislation passed in 1962; and as UK-wide it was not seen to suffer from some of the problems faced by the regulatory bodies for nursing and midwifery.[54] The passage of legislation for a new regulatory structure, moreover, came at the end of a challenging decade for community-based practitioners. Health visiting practice in England, for instance, had been fundamentally affected by the reorganisation of the health and social services under the Local Authorities Social Services Act of 1970 and the 1974 NHS (Reorganisation) Act, raising concerns about the future security of the profession's special role in health promotion. With health visitors now working as part of a large nursing service dominated, numerically, by nursing colleagues engaged in curative work in hospital, the specificity of the profession needed, more than ever, to be clearly understood.[55] In 1977, the CETHV had published a statement on the principles of health visiting practice.[56] This was quickly seized on by the profession as a timely statement of who they were. Would the new shared regulatory structure be able to maintain the momentum, and safeguard the special identity of the health visitor? This section will mainly focus on health visitors, as a named profession under the Act, but it will look also at the experiences of district nurses, since both groups had similar committee arrangements during the statutory bodies' first two terms of office.

Working through joint committees

The primary legislation required each National Board to include a health visitor among the members nominated to serve on the Central Council. No similar specifications were made for district nursing or, indeed, any of the other 'minority' nursing groups, although in practice the Boards tended to include a district nurse among their nominees. The 1979 Act also required the establishment of a joint committee of the UKCC and National Boards for health visiting, and opened the way for the establishment of a similar arrangement for district nursing. Governed by similar terms of reference, both joint committees were to act as expert resources to the Council and the Boards, and to initiate the consideration of matters related to the development of education and the promotion of improved standards of practice. Both committees were to consist of between eighteen and twenty-seven members, the majority of whom were to be health visitors and district nurses respectively. The membership of the joint committees was also to include two registered medical practitioners, four persons qualified to advise on matters of professional education, one person with experience in health service management and one with experience in local government. Committee meetings were to occur at least five times a year and in each of the four countries.[57] This entailed a considerable amount of work and travel for the members and officers.

These structural arrangements were not ideal. First, as joint committees of the National Boards and the Central Council, both the Health Visiting Joint Committee and the DNJC had an executive role as well as an advisory one.

Consequently, they were delegated a number of executive functions from the National Boards, such as approval of institutions, courses and examinations. This brought a considerable amount of operational detail to the agendas of the committees and, arguably, detracted from their ability to act in a strategic manner. Much of the first year or so was spent assisting the Boards in the development of approval procedures. After that, a considerable amount of agenda time was spent on considering applications for new courses.

Second, a considerable amount of effort needed to be given to the development of effective communication links between the joint committees and their parent bodies, and also between the two joint committees themselves.[58] This task was complicated by the different meeting arrangements of each National Board. In practice there was no month when all five bodies had formally arranged meetings, making a uniform system of communication impossible. It was agreed that circulation of agreed joint committee minutes to the UKCC and the National Boards would take place. It was also hoped that closer links would arise from the cross-membership of the several bodies and from the input of the professional staff who would meet prior to each joint committee meeting. In practice, however, cross-membership was a mixed blessing. Both the HVJC and the DNJC were closely affected by the initial uneasy relationship between the UKCC and the National Boards, particularly the ENB (see Chapter 3). It should also be remembered that as the National Boards were free to establish their own internal structures, a number of operational differences emerged. The National Board for Nursing, Midwifery and Health Visiting for Northern Ireland (NBNI), for instance, did not delegate approvals to the joint committee, but executed these through its Education Committee. The NBS, moreover, established a Primary Care Committee which, in practice, considered a similar range of issues to the two joint committees.

In addition to these operational difficulties the committees, particularly the DNJC, began life under something of a cloud. The establishment of a DNJC had not been universally approved by members of the Shadow Council, some of whom felt that a combined Primary Health Care Committee would be a less divisive and more effective structure. The Shadow Council's decision to represent the different nursing fields through EPAC rather than through a wide range of standing committees also weakened district nursing's case for special treatment. The DNJC, therefore, started life with the proviso that the structure would be reviewed within the lifetime of the First Council.[59]

The members, however, were keen to get on with the business in hand and to make the best of their arrangements. Aware that their involvement in operational detail could detract from their ability to act strategically, members of the HVJC agreed to develop a strategic plan and to delegate some of the routine work to officers.[60] From the summer of 1984, the Committee experimented with dividing into sub-groups for parts of its work.[61] After a year, the system was reviewed. The facility to discuss course submissions in the Approvals Sub-Group had worked well, enabling the Committee to engage in a fuller discussion of matters of policy. Greater flexibility however was needed for the sub-groups. Group agendas needed to be able to accommodate issues referred to the HVJC by Council or the Boards, and members needed to be able to move between groups if their expertise was needed. Recognition also needed to be given to that fact that, on occasions, the full committee would want to participate in discussions. A less structured arrangement of *ad hoc* sub-groups, convened as and when the work demanded it, was consequently adopted.[62]

Efforts were also made to share professional issues with other groups within the statutory structure. In 1985, for instance, the HVJC held a meeting with the UKCC Midwifery Committee to discuss issues relating to obstetric preparation for health visitors. The following year a series of meetings was held between the HVJC and the ENB's Midwifery Committee to examine the particular difficulties experienced by health visitors in England in gaining access to obstetric experience.[63] More generally, health visitor members often found it useful to work with other members from 'minority' groups, building a range of shifting alliances on different issues.

Especially important were the efforts of members of the two joint committees to work closely together. An early indication of this was the committees' decision to co-operate over course approvals where health visiting and district nursing courses were sited in the same institution.[64] In 1986, the relationship between the committees was taken a stage further when representatives of the HVJC and DNJC met informally to discuss issues of common interest and the following year a joint meeting was held between the full committees. During the First Council's term of office both committees acknowledged the value of sharing discussions on a range of issues. In October 1985, for instance, a joint meeting was held between the two committees and the team working on the Cumberlege review of community nursing. Close co-operation between the two committees also occurred during the development of recommendations for Project 2000, particularly over the needs of the specialist practitioner.

As the first term of office drew to a close in the summer of 1988, the joint committees reviewed their efforts at improving their working arrangements. Both memberships agreed that 'it was natural that both committees had to establish themselves before being ready to explore how certain activities could be shared'. It was also agreed that considerable benefit could now be expected from increased joint activities.[65] Under the second term of office, indeed, joint meetings between the HVJC and DNJC were to become a regular feature.

During the first five years, therefore, the joint committees found ways to pool their resources and to create space within their agendas for the discussion of wider policy issues. As standing committees of the statutory bodies, the joint committees were able to present reports to Council thus ensuring that issues of concern to health visitors and district nurses would regularly be heard by their colleagues from other areas of nursing and from midwifery, and that views and any decisions would be minuted. However, a degree of tension did exist, particularly during the early days, over the role of the committees and the need to achieve a balance between business referred from the Council or the Boards, and agenda items raised from committee members themselves. While valuable initiatives to help

secure a more strategic role for the committees were undertaken, their fundamental orientation towards routine executive matters remained.

A changing environment: 1989–93

During the late 1980s and early 1990s two important developments affecting the
work of the statutory body occurred close together: the restructuring of health
care delivery through the NHS and Community Care Act and the departmental
review of the provisions of the 1979 Act.[66] The NHS and Community Care Act
presaged major changes to the context of health visiting and district nurse practice, and raised considerable anxiety among community-based practitioners. The
introduction of the new arrangements for GP contracting, were of special
concern. Health visitors were particularly fearful that fundholding GPs would
choose not to purchase health visiting services but instead rely on the increasing
number of directly employed practice nurses. A mass lobby of parliament in 1989,
supported by the HVA, publicised their concerns.[67]

Alongside this uncertainty and professional anxiety, the recommendations of
the Peat Marwick McLintock legislative review carried profound implications for
the health visitor and district nurse members.[68] While the report welcomed the
efforts of the HVJC and DNJC to improve their working arrangements, it
suggested that a single primary care committee of the UKCC would be a more
logical and efficient structure. Many of the members of the joint committee
sympathised with this analysis: now that each National Board had clear policies
for approvals in place, there was less reason to persist with the rather awkward
joint structure. Also, a broad-based primary health care committee would better
reflect the diversity of community-based practice at a crucial period of change in
the health services. A firm decision on the future committee arrangements for
health visitors and community nurses was not felt to be appropriate until the
government had made clear its position on the future shape of the statutory
bodies.[69]

Minority representation received considerable attention during the parliamentary debates on the amending legislation. Speaking for the opposition during
the committee stage in the House of Lords, Lord Carter noted the 'anxiety
expressed by the Health Visitors' Association'. The profession, he suggested, 'was
experiencing an alarming and unprecedented change on the education and
practice side and a profound change in the management and delivery of care in the
community as a result of the implementation of the community care plans . . .' The
loss of the HVJC, and the statutory guarantee of health visitor membership on the
National Boards, had created the feeling that health visitor representation was
being 'eroded'.[70] Similar concerns were raised in the Commons.[71] In response, the
government made the assurance that in practice the membership of each Board
would include, either as an executive or a non-executive member, a registered
health visitor (and a registered nurse and a practising midwife).[72] Future provisions for the representation of district nurses and mental health and mental
handicap nurses were also strongly debated. Yet, while the concerns of health

visitors and other practitioners were acknowledged in both Houses of Parliament, the legislative framework did not give clear guidance as to the form any replacement structures should take. Questions of how 'due regard' for the interests of minority groups could be secured were again on the table for the UKCC.[73]

A more inclusive structure after 1993?

By the time the new Council assembled in the spring of 1993 it was decided that Council's business could best be transacted if all areas of nursing practice were represented together in a combined NCHCNC.[74] At its first meeting, held in May 1993, the UKCC Registrar stated that the new committee 'had a major responsibility for assisting the Council in establishing and improving standards of nursing and community health care nursing across the breadth of nursing'.[75] The reconstituted Council would be asking its members to adopt a broad strategic role in their committee work; one that would take them beyond their own particular area of professional interest. This model was not without its critics. During the debate on the standing orders of the new committee, an alternative proposal was put forward for the establishment of two new committees, one for nursing and one for community nursing.[76] While the combined approach won through, a refinement of the proposed standing orders was accepted, so that exactly half of the nursing membership of the committee would be people engaged in some kind of community practice.[77] Also, the committee's terms of reference included a specific requirement of the committee to 'consider all relevant matters relating to community health care' as well as to nursing more generally.[78]

A brief look at the agendas of the NCHCNC during the first couple of years confirms that a considerable number of primary health care issues were addressed. These spanned a wide range of topics, and included discussion of the impact of government primary health care policies as well as practice-focused issues, such as the administration of oral vitamin K to young babies by health visitors. Nevertheless, the professional press indicates that considerable anxieties were held by both groups, and especially by health visitors, during this period of transition. Further developments in government policy created a backdrop of anxiety. The introduction of direct management of health visitors by fundholding practices, for instance, heightened fears about health visiting's future as a separate profession.[79] Concerns were also growing about how the value of public health services, particularly health visiting, could be quantified and marketed.[80] At times the profession felt that the UKCC did not always appear to appreciate their distinctive position. PREPP was a case in point (see Chapter 6). Particular concerns were expressed over the identification of community health care nursing as a unified discipline, though one that encompassed different areas of expertise. This, it was felt, might be seen by purchasers as a green light to push for a generic community nurse.[81] Other worries included the alignment of school nursing with paediatric nursing instead of linking it to health promotion and public health and, more broadly, the impact of the UKCC's decision not to give all groups of community health care nurses separate registration status.[82]

An altogether bigger challenge to health visiting as a discrete profession for the purposes of regulation, however, came from the management consultants conducting the second fundamental review. JM Consulting found little to suggest the need for the continuation of separate health visitor registration. In its view, separate registration for health visitors was an 'historical anomaly' and a reflection of the 'tendency to tribalism within the nursing profession'.[83] The profession's response was ambivalent and uncertain. While some expressed their concern at the possibility of health visiting losing its separate registration, others acknowledged the validity of a simplification of regulatory processes.[84] In the event, all this was overtaken by a government keen on giving health visitors an extended role as part of its public health agenda, and for this reason willing to listen to those who wanted to keep health visitors named in legislation.[85] As we have seen earlier, this upset the applecart as far as a model of shared regulation between nurses and midwives was concerned. It also did little to address the concerns of those who felt that the key issue for public protection was to think about primary care more broadly and to ensure that all those working in the isolation of community practice should be in possession of mandatory qualifications.

The nursing specialties: building diversity and flexibility in a unified structure

What of the other occupational groups within nursing? Mental health, mental handicap and paediatric nurses undoubtedly saw themselves as having a distinctive identity within the family of nursing, shaped by their history of separate training and registration.[86] The creation of the new statutory bodies, moreover, came after a decade or so of anxiety about the future of the supplementary registers, fuelled by poor levels of recruitment into specialist training and the development of psychiatric units in general hospitals.[87] For mental handicap nurses, the future appeared especially uncertain. As established occupational boundaries weakened in the shift to community-based care, the emergence of a new caring profession linked more to social work than to nursing seemed a real possibility.[88] Worries about the still growing range of clinical nursing specialties after the demise of the JBCNS also surfaced at this time.

The 1979 Act did not contain any specific requirements with regard to the representation of specialist nursing groups, beyond the general clause that 'due regard' be paid to their interests.[89] Concerns about the implications of this omission surfaced during the drafting of legislation and continued beyond the parliamentary debates into the 'shadow' period of the new statutory bodies. Two issues occasioned particular comment: the decision not to allocate specific 'seats' to specialist nursing groups in the election scheme for the National Boards, and the Shadow Council's decision to represent the interests of specialist nursing groups through a single EPAC. With nursing activities diversifying, and the range of clinical specialities proliferating, it would have been extremely difficult to have done otherwise. A similar constraint inevitably affected the organisation of the small professional staff at the UKCC. While there were Professional Officers for the three named professions, specific posts for the various nursing specialities were not created. The Professional Officer for Nursing, however, brought professional qualifications and experience as a registered mental nurse.

The views of specialist nurses on these matters are less visible in the organisation's records than those of midwives, health visitors and district nurses. Issues relating to nursing practice in specific fields or disciplines were undoubtedly raised by groups or individual Council members, either through the agendas of Council, its committees or through other, more informal channels. For instance, in 1984, Council agreed to the establishment of a five-member working group to prepare draft comments on an EEC Consultation paper on psychiatric nursing,[90] and in 1987 a similar strategy was deployed for the consideration of a report on paediatric nursing training in the EEC.[91] In 1986, Council members from the mental handicap field expressed their concerns about the high proportion of mental handicap nurses working in large hospitals coming before the PCC of Council. This led to a meeting with the Minister of Health, Tony Newton, on the UKCC's concerns about the run-down of the large mental handicap and psychiatric hospitals.[92] Earlier, in 1984, the UKCC was asked to submit written evidence to the House of Commons Social Services Committee inquiry into community care and the adult mentally ill and mentally handicapped,[93] and in 1989 and 1990 members with a background in mental handicap and mental health nursing were included on the Council's own working group on the government's community care policies and on the Community Education and Practice sub-group.[94] It might be argued, however, that without a practice-focused committee, either for mental health/mental handicap or nursing in general, there was not a regular forum for the discussion of these and similar issues. The value of a practice-focused forum for nursing was not strongly articulated at this time. Unlike midwifery, nursing did not have statutory Practice Rules to provide a ready-made focus for discussions on standards of practice, and it was not until the UKCC began to work on post-registration issues that standards of nursing practice in specialised areas became more clearly articulated.

Meetings with the statutory bodies, and the lobbying of MPs before and during the parliamentary debates on the Nurses, Midwives and Health Visitors Bill, once again raised the issue of specific standing committees for specialist nursing interests. During the committee stage in the House of Commons, for instance, an amendment requiring the establishment of UKCC standing committees for mental health, mental handicap and also for enrolled nursing was put forward by the Labour MP Sylvia Heal. The lack of reference to these groups in the recent UKCC consultation document on the CEPP, she suggested, had raised concerns.[95] Of the thirty-one people involved in the work of the CEPP sub-group, only two held a Registered Mental Nurse (RMN) qualification, and one a Registered Nurse Mental Handicap (RNMH) qualification. None had qualifications in community nursing. 'Examples like that', Heal argued, 'are symptomatic of the alienation that minority groups presently feel at Board and Council level'.[96] Concerns were also being expressed about the lack of progress on the development of European Union (EU) sectoral directives to recognise the specialties of mental health and mental handicap nursing, and the drop in the number of students entering those two branches of pre-registration training. A legislative requirement for standing committees for key minority groups, she suggested, would go some way to protect their identity, advance initiatives in these fields and ensure that their special needs received due recognition within the statutory bodies. The amendment was defeated.[97]

New ways of working

Following the 1992 Act, the nursing press continued to debate the representation of minority nursing interests on the statutory bodies, focusing in particular on the new electoral scheme of the Central Council.[98] Letters complaining about the inadequate representation of minority nursing groups on the Council indicated a strong professional view that the UKCC should be more representative of diverse professional interests. The UKCC responded by pointing out that its role was to create and maintain the professional register, control admission to it and, where necessary in the public interest, remove practitioners from it. It was acknowledged that in order to fulfil these public duties appropriately, the Council needed the contribution of 'practitioners in all aspects of professional practice' – a matter aided through legislative powers to involve non-Council members in the work the UKCC's committees – but this did not equate with formal representation.[99] Such tensions between public protection and professional representation were to persist and, indeed, to remain a key element in the ongoing debate about the future shape of the regulatory bodies.

The NCHCNC, which operated from April 1993, included practising nurses from the fields of adult nursing, children's nursing, mental handicap nursing, mental health nursing and occupational health nursing, as well two health visitors, two medical practitioners and two consumer representatives.[100] The minutes of this Committee indicate that many items required outcomes to be considered in a general way. The Committee, moreover, was keen to explore the impact on nursing of broad policy changes, such as the new arrangements for the health and social care of people in the community and the implications for nursing of the New Deal on junior doctors' hours.[101] On the other hand, a range of specialist nursing matters were given space within the Committee's agenda. Two of the first issues mentioned in the Committee's business plan, for instance, concerned 'minority' nursing groups. As the Department of Health was about to launch a review of mental health nursing, on which the UKCC was to be represented, the Committee stressed the need to progress work in this area. Consideration of the future of mental handicap nursing was felt to be required, especially given the recent significant changes to the purchasing and provision of services for clients with special needs, and the growing concern among practitioners about their future role and training.[102] In April, the Council agreed that a small task group of members be convened to consider issues associated with mental handicap nursing.[103] Strong support for this initiative came from the UKCC's professional staff which at this time included the Assistant Registrar for Professional Conduct,

Tariq Hussain, a former Council member with a background in the mental handicap field. To help collate sufficient information to make an informed strategic
statement, meetings were held with outside experts. Considerable work was
also undertaken on mental health nursing, with the UKCC hosting a special
consultative conference in January 1995 for mental health nursing practitioners,
managers of mental health services, educationalists, representatives of consumer
organisations, professional organisations and trades unions and the specialist
officers of the government health departments.[104] One of the issues raised during
this conference, interestingly, was whether the recognition of the value of mental
health nursing accorded by the statutory bodies needed to be reflected in the
elected membership of the Council. It was suggested, indeed, that when Council
considered its election scheme in May 1995, attention should be given to the
possibility of allocating seats to mental health practitioners from each of the four
UK countries.[105]

Already, however, Council was changing its way of working, extending its
interaction with those outside its membership, facilitating dialogue with people
directly involved in particular practice areas and putting itself in a stronger
position to develop practice standards. Further changes came in 1996 following
the acceptance of a recommendation by the steering group of the internal
organisation review that future work on the development of standards should be
undertaken by a wide range of task groups commissioned by the Council or its
committees and comprising Council members, officers and, significantly, external
experts also.[106]

The move towards a more generic committee structure was also counter-
balanced by the development of a greater number of field-specific Professional
Officer posts. Professional advisors with specific expertise in children's nursing
and mental health had been appointed at the UKCC since the early 1990s but,
following the organisational review, three new Professional Officer posts were
created for Mental Health/Learning Disability, Paediatrics, and Adult/General
Nursing, adding to the existing posts for Midwifery and Health Visiting/
Community Nursing, and Professional Conduct and Research. Given the role of
the professional staff in helping the Council to identify issues of interest to the
UKCC, and their ability to help steer matters onto the agenda of Council, its
committees and their task groups, this expansion of the range of professional
expertise at officer level was extremely significant.

By the end of the Third Council, therefore, 'due regard' was beginning to be
expressed in a new, less formal and more flexible way, with greater input from
officers and from outside. A landmark document, the *Guidelines for Mental Health
and Learning Disabilities Nursing*[107] was the first area-specific document on
practice issues to be produced by the Council apart, of course, from its work on
the standards of midwifery practice. This new way of working, however, brings its
own questions. Whereas before, the UKCC may have appeared bureaucratic and
rigid, this apparently more open structure raises new questions about governance
and accountability, such as whose view should be represented on individual task
groups and how 'representatives' should be selected.

Conclusion

It was clear at the outset that the question of how 'due regard' might be paid to the interests of 'minority' groups would be a problematic matter. The lengthy title of the Act, and the form that the new statutory bodies took, testify to the intensive lobbying undertaken by the different professional groups to try to ensure that their position would not be eroded. The complicated structure that emerged was unlikely to prove durable – it was perhaps both inevitable and inevitably short-lived. Council's Midwifery Committee remained broadly the same during the lifetime of the shared regulatory framework. However, as we have seen, shared regulation proved to be a particularly challenging matter for midwives, and doubts periodically surfaced over the viability of the special structural arrangements within a statutory body dominated in numerical terms by nurses.

It is too easy, perhaps, to accuse the nursing and midwifery professions of 'tribalism' – as both groups of management consultants who have reviewed the work and organisation of the statutory bodies have tended to do. The challenges of shared regulation are complex ones and, given the variety of practice areas encompassed by the UKCC, solutions for one group were always going to create problems for another. By the middle of the Third Council's term of office, the structural arrangements for 'due regard' were very different from those initially adopted. They were now focused on the two 'practice' committees, closely linked with a broad-based education committee, and balanced by an expanded range of professional officer expertise and the facility to establish special 'task groups' comprising both insiders and outside experts. At the close of the Third Council in March 1998, it was too early to say with certainty whether the solution was a better one: while some of the shortcomings of the initial approach had been resolved, the new arrangements were generating some problems of their own. What initially seemed an internal issues of how different occupational groups related to each other has now become part of a larger debate about the role of lay representatives in the regulatory processes and structures and, indeed, about how protecting the public and representing interests can best be aligned.

Notes

1 Nurses, Midwives and Health Visitors Act, 1979, Sections 15 and 17.
2 Clause 4(3) of the Act stated that 'any matter involving a proposal to make, amend or revoke rules relating to midwifery practice' was to be assigned by the UKCC to its Midwifery Committee. This was buttressed by the late inclusion of a clause [Section 4(4)] stating that the Secretary of State 'shall not approve rules relating to midwifery practice unless satisfied that they are framed in accordance with recommendations of the Council's Midwifery Committee'.
3 The parent bodies were required to consult the Health Visiting Joint Committee on 'all matters relating to health visiting' and were not to act on 'on any such matters before receiving a recommendation of the Joint Committee' within a specified period of time.
4 Nurses, Midwives and Health Visitors Act, 1979, Section 8(4) and (5).
5 For a time, the Council was also supported by a Research Committee, and from 1989 by a Standards and Ethics Committee.
6 CC/84/7.

7 This was replaced after the internal organisational review of 1995 by a Joint Education Committee with a membership drawn equally from the two practice committees – Midwifery, and Nursing and Community Health Care Nursing. Both of these education committees also included members from the general education field and consumer and medical organisations. Student representation was likewise included. See Chapter 8 for an exploration of the involvement of 'lay' members and external experts in the work of the UKCC.

8 The reference is to a speech by the Secretary of State for Health, Virginia Bottomley made during the passage of 1992 Act on 4 March 1992 Act quoted in Minute 20/92, see p. 148.

9 State registration of midwives, and a legal definition of midwifery practice, were achieved in England and Wales in 1902. Primary legislation for Scotland followed in 1915, and in 1918 for Ireland. After the partition of Ireland in 1922, the Republic of Ireland continued with this body until 1951 when An Bord Altranais was established for the regulation of both nursing and midwifery. In Northern Ireland, the Joint Nurses and Midwives Council (Northern Ireland) Act 1922 set up a new regulatory body for nurses and midwives. In 1970 a new act established the Northern Ireland Council for Nurses and Midwives, which had wider powers for midwifery and nursing education.

10 Though additional primary legislation and statutory instruments had been achieved during the 1920s and 1930s, and a consolidating Act passed in 1951, the legislative basis for the regulation of midwifery education and practice remained the original 1902 Midwives Act. See Donnison, J., *Midwives and Medical Men. A History of Inter-professional Rivalries and Women's Rights*, London, Heinemann Educational, 1977.

11 Initially, there were no midwives on the CMB (England and Wales) at all. In contrast with other regulated professions, they were precluded from holding the majority of places on their statutory body. It was not until 1973 that a midwife was elected by the CMB (England and Wales) as its Chairman. For a comment on the ways in which the legislation put midwives in a 'uniquely disadvantaged position' among the professions, see Donnison, *Midwives*, p.174.

12 When the first Midwives Act was passed in 1902, the relatively low income of midwives led to the requirement that the expenses of the CMB, with the exception of examination fees, should be met by the local authorities. This arrangement, which continued until the reorganisation of the National Health Service in 1974, laid the duties of county councils on the new area health authorities and made midwives the only professional group whose regulation was subsidised by ratepayers. One of the most serious consequences of this system of funding was the Board's tendency to restrict its expenditure on educational developments, conscious of the unwillingness of local authorities to increase their subventions.

13 See the RCM, *Evidence to the Royal Commission on the NHS*, London, RCM, 1977; CMB for Scotland, Northern Ireland Council for Nurses and Midwives, An Bord Altranais, *The Role of the Midwife*, Edinburgh, The Board, 1983; and the House of Commons Social Services Committee's *Perinatal and Neo-Natal Mortality Report* (Short Report), London, HMSO, 1980 – all of which mentioned concern at the continued underuse of midwives' skills. See also Sandall, J., 'Continuity of midwifery care in England: a new professional project?', *Gender, Work and Organisation*, 3(4), 1996, pp. 218–19.

14 MIN 7/83; MIN 32/83; CC/83/19.

15 MIN 69/83; CC/83/50; MC MIN 58/83; MIN 26/84; CC/84/23.

16 Section 22(3) of the 1979 Act required Council to consult the representatives of any group of persons who appeared likely to be affected by the proposed Midwives Practice Rules. Around 200 responses were received by the close of the consultation in September 1984, and a further 100 or so submissions after that date. Respondents included LSAs, health authorities, professional organisations and trade unions,

midwifery colleges, individual midwives and groups of midwives. MIN 62/84(ii); UKCC, *New Midwives Rules and Code of Practice: A Consultation Paper*, 1984. MC/84/23, p. 5; MC MIN/44/84(b). Also see also Chapter 8, page 175 for discussion of the Committee's decision not to include consumer groups within the consultation process.

17 Like the Practice Rules, the Midwives' Education and Training Rules also needed to be harmonised. Certain rules, too, needed to be removed as they were felt to be more appropriately included in the regulations or guidance issued by the National Boards.

18 Donnison, *Midwives*, pp. 179–82.

19 See MC/84/23, p. 11.

20 MC/85/08.

21 Nurses, Midwives and Health Visitors Act 1979 (Midwives Amendment) Rules Approval Order, SI 1986 No. 786; UKCC, *The Midwife's Code of Practice*, 1986.

22 Extant rule 58 had stated that when both a medical practitioner and a midwife were present at a case, the midwife had to follow the doctor's instructions. The UKCC's decision to remove this rule was not welcomed by all medical practitioners. In September 1985, the Chairman of the Midwifery Committee, the Professional Officer for Midwifery and a further midwife member of Council met with the President of the GMC and Professor Sir John Dewhurst to discuss the issue. The GMC suggested that the UKCC might wish to consider whether the Rules and the Code made it sufficiently clear 'where the ultimate responsibility lies' in cases attended by both a doctor and a midwife. The Midwifery Committee felt that the issue was clear, but it agreed to keep the matter under review. See MC MIN/34/85, October 1985.

23 The extant rules in Northern Ireland had contained a provision of this nature. Rather than incorporate this into the new UK-wide practice rules, it was decided that this was a matter more appropriately contained in the Midwife's Code of Practice. A similar change was the decision of the Midwifery Committee and the Council not to specify in rules the duties of a midwife when a woman or her partner refused the advice to call in a registered medical practitioner.

24 For brief summaries of these issues see the section on midwifery in the UKCC's *Annual Reports*. Consideration was also given to a number of practice issues, such as the use of new equipment for the relief of pain in labour.

25 There was only one midwife member on the EPAC/P2000 Project Group. The Professional Officer for Midwifery, however, provided an additional source of midwifery expertise.

26 It was also pointed out that a training model of this kind would not comply with the European midwifery directives.

27 UKCC, *Project 2000. A New Preparation for Practice*, 1986, p. 50, para. 6.33.

28 A second midwifery Professional Officer post was created during the mid-1990s following an internal organisational audit, conducted in January and February 1993, which recommended the allocation of extra staffing resources to midwifery.

29 In April 1991 a top-level meeting was held between the Chairmen and senior staff of the statutory bodies and the RCM Council to examine the implications for midwifery of the proposed changes to the constitution and functions of the Council and National Boards. The RCM also kept a close eye on the passage of the Bill through Parliament. See UKCC, 1/8/3, Review of the UKCC and National Boards, 1988–1991.

30 *Parliamentary Debates* [Commons], 205, 4 March 1992, col. 394.

31 MIN 35/93(3); CC/93/30 Annexe 3.

32 A new clause was added to Section 16 of the 1979 Act which empowered the UKCC to make rules prescribing the advice and guidance that is given by the National Boards to LSAs.

33 Work began on this issue in 1991. See minutes of Midwifery Committee, 6 June 1991, MC/91/22; minutes of Midwifery Committee, 3 October 1991. Changes were agreed by Council in November 1992 and the necessary statutory instrument to bring the rules into effect was passed in September 1993. A task group to begin the revision of

the Code of Practice was set up in 1993. Council approved the Midwifery Committee's recommendations for amendments in January 1994.

34 Registrar's Letter 11/1992, 'Community post-natal visiting by midwives', 18 May 1992.

35 UKCC, *The Midwife's Code of Practice*, 1994, paras 45–48.

36 MC Minute 28/93.

37 See Winship, J., 'The UKCC Perspective: the statutory basis for the supervision of midwives today' in Kirkham, M. (ed.), *Supervision of Midwives*, Hale, Books for Midwives, 1996, pp. 38–57.

38 Rejecting the notion of specialist midwifery practice completely, however, raised the possibility that midwives would be disadvantaged in terms of pay and conditions and, indeed, in job opportunities in such fields as neo-natal care, family planning clinics, etc. When the legislation for PREP was drafted, therefore, midwives within the statutory bodies fought to leave the possibility for a specialist tier to be introduced in midwifery, if it became appropriate in the future.

39 For some idea of the different views on supervision held within the midwifery profession see Kirkham (ed.) *Supervision of Midwives*, especially chapters by Demilew, J., 'Independent midwives' views of supervision', pp. 183–201, and Winship, 'The UKCC perspective'.

40 Davies, K., 'Is statutory supervision central to our professional identity?', *British Journal of Midwifery*, 2(7), July 1994, p. 304.

41 MC Minute 38/94.

42 In September 1995, for instance, a joint research project on the supervision of midwives was launched with the ENB; UKCC, *Annual Report 1995/96*, p. 4.

43 The chairman of the Midwifery Committee, Sarah Roch, was co-opted onto the Steering Group following Council's discussion of this issue on 31 May 1995. She resigned from this position in July.

44 C Minute 51/95(2).

45 Minute 57/95(2). While there was nothing to prevent midwives from applying for and receiving any of the new Directorate posts, it was felt to be unlikely that a top-level practising midwife would apply since, under the terms of Rules 27(a) of the Midwives' Rules, she would lose her 'practising' status if she took up a post which did not explicitly require a midwifery qualification.

46 Minute 6/96. See also Roch, S., 'Midwives must determine midwifery matters', *Modern Midwife*, 5(10), October 1995, p. 7; Roch, S., 'Midwifery: pride and prejudice?', *British Journal of Midwifery*, 3(11), November 1995, p. 573; Roch, S., 'Equal opportunities for midwives – too much to ask?', *Modern Midwife*, 6(3), March 1996, pp. 4–5.

47 RCM, *Midwifery Legislation: the Issues and the Options*. Position Paper No. 14, London, RCM, 1996. An alternative view, exploring the potential dangers of the RCM's pressure for a separate regulatory body for midwifery can be found in an article by Reg Pyne, 'A cautionary tale for midwives', *British Journal of Nursing*, 10 August, 4(15), 1995, pp. 853–4. This was reprinted in the *British Journal of Midwifery*, 3(9), 1995, pp. 463–4.

48 *Nursing Standard*, 14 January, 12(17), 1998, p. 6; 'Look to the future', *Nursing Times*, 21 January, 94(3), 1998, p. 14. This was at the point where JM Consulting were requesting feedback on their interim report on the Nurses, Midwives and Health Visitors Act (see Chapter 9).

49 MC Minute 05/96(5); MC/96/02.

50 In June 1996, the Council agreed to apply for the inclusion of intravenous fluids in the list of medicines which midwives can carry in the community. Minute 35/96 (1.8).

51 JM Consulting, *Report on the Review of the Nurses, Midwives and Health Visitors Act 1997*, 1999, pp. 3–6, 8 and 10.

52 This response, deeply influenced by the government's wish to expand the public health role of health visitors, was to reject the view that health visitors were a specialist group

of nurses and did not need to be named in the title of the Council or recognised on the register. It hence overturned the careful two-profession balance that JM Consulting had devised. See NHS, HSC 1999/030, p. 6.

53 JM Consulting, *The Regulation of Nurses, Midwives and Health Visitors. Invitation to comment on issues raised by a review of the Nurses, Midwives and Health Visitors Act 1997*, 1998, p. 16.

54 Health Visiting and Social Work (Training) Act, 1962. On the CETHV see Wilkie, E., *A Singular Anomaly: A Case Study of the CETHV, 1962–1974*, London, RCN, 1984. Though responsible for the award of the statutorily required health visiting certificate, and respected for its work in raising educational standards, the CETHV did not keep a register of health visitors and had no disciplinary role.

55 The 1970 Local Authorities Social Services Act followed the recommendations of the Seebohm Report of 1968, establishing local authority social service departments and ending the links between the two training councils for health visiting and social work. After the 1974 health service reorganisation an increasing number of health visitors became 'attached' to individual GP practices. See Office of Population Censuses and Surveys, *Nurses Working in the Community: a survey carried out on behalf of the DHSS in England and Wales in 1980*, London, HMSO, 1982. For the concerns expressed by health visitors see Dingwall, R., *The Social Organisation of Health Visitor Training*, London, Croom Helm, 1977, p. 143; Clode, D., 'Of primary concern', *Health and Social Services Journal*, 12 May, 88, 1978, p. 538.

56 CETHV, *An Investigation into the Principles of Health Visiting*, London, CETHV, 1977. The statement identified four basic principles of heath visiting practice: the search for health needs; the stimulation of awareness of health needs; the influence on policies affecting health; and the facilitation of health-enhancing activities. See also the CETHV's follow-up pamphlet, *The Investigation Debate*, London, CETHV, 1980.

57 DNJC/84/7.

58 See, for example, HVJC MIN 18/83, and HVJC MIN 18/83 and 19/83; HVJC/83/ 11. For the issue of communications between the two joint committees, see HVJC MIN 23/94.

59 See CC/84/98; CC/86/C8; C MIN/28/87; CC/87/C12.

60 HVJC MIN 89/83; HVJC/83/60, p. 5.

61 Three 'policy' sub-groups were established on inter-professional learning, the application of technology in health visiting training and the development of criteria for professional conduct, and a fourth sub-group – for approvals – was also set up.

62 HVJC MIN 62/85; HVJC/85/92.

63 HVJC/85/8. In 1989, the rule requiring prospective health visitor students to have either specific midwifery or obstetric experience was annulled.

64 HVJC MIN 16/84 (a); HVJC/84/23.

65 The Joint Committees proposed that they should normally meet on the same day and have both a shared agenda and specialist agendas. They also wished to see a measure of shared membership. However, this last recommendation was not endorsed by the Council and the Boards. See minutes of joint meeting between HVJC and DNJC, MIN 88/28.

66 The UKCC established a special working group to consider the emerging policy on community care. Its membership included representatives from the HVJC and DNJC and other Council members, particularly those with a background in community mental health and mental handicap nursing. A second working group was established on the NHS and Community Care Bill.

67 See, for example, 'Facing the challenge of GP contracts', *Health Visitor*, 62(12) 1989, pp. 363–4 and Jackson, C., 'Pulling the plug on the NHS', *Health Visitor*, 63(2), 1989, pp. 43–5.

68 Peat Marwick McLintock, *Review of the United Kingdom Central Council and the Four National Boards for Nursing, Midwifery and Health Visiting*, 1989, ii–v.

69 A questionnaire on meeting arrangements was issued to members of the joint committees in November 1990, and in December a proposal from the WNB that serious consideration be given to the establishment of a single Primary Health Care Committee was received by the joint committees. Members felt that the implications of setting up such a committee would need to be carefully explored once the government had made clear its position on the Peat Marwick McLintock Report and Council's own activities on PREPP were further advanced. This view was reiterated by Council in January 1991.

70 *Parliamentary Debates* [Lords], 532, 26 November 1991, col. 1286.

71 *Parliamentary Debates* [Commons], 201, 13 January 1992, cols 702–3.

72 *Parliamentary Debates* [Lords], 532, 26 November 1991, col. 1287.

73 The 1992 Act did leave the way open for the establishment of new standing committees of Council under Section 2(3), explicitly linking this power with Council's duty to have regard to the interests of minority groups. No groups, however, were specifically named in this context. See also Registrar's Letter 17/1991, 'Statement of the Council's position and intent regarding the Nurses, Midwives and Health Visitors Bill', 12 November 1991.

74 HVJC Minute 93/11.

75 NCHCNC Minute 1/93(4).

76 Seventeen of the newly assembled Council members voted in favour of this alternative, twenty-seven were against and three members abstained.

77 Minute 35/93(3); CC/93/30, Annexe 4.

78 NC/93/01.

79 National Health Service Management Executive Task Force, *New World, New Opportunities. Nursing in Primary Health Care*, London, NHS Management Executive, 1993; Department of Health, *Choice and Opportunity. Primary Care: the Future*, London, HMSO, 1996. See also 'Back to bondage', *Health Visitor*, 66(6), 1993, p. 187; Symonds, A., 'Health visiting and the new public health', *Health Visitor*, 66(6), 1993, pp. 204–61.

80 See for instance, HVA, *Weights and Measures: Outcomes and Evaluation in Health Visiting*, London, HVA, 1995.

81 Concerns were also raised about the length of the proposed six-month preparation for community health care nurses. See, for example, Appleby, F. and Robotham, A., 'Less means less', *Health Visitor*, 66(9), 1993, p. 332; 'UKCC u-turn on training', *Health Visitor*, 66(12), 1993, p. 428.

82 For the concerns of school nurses see 'School nurses rebuff UKCC plans', *Health Visitor*, 66(7), 1993, p. 237.

83 JM Consulting, *The Regulation of Nurses, Midwives and Health Visitors*, p. 6.

84 See for instance, 'Caught in the Act', *Health Visitor*, 71(2), 1998, pp. 40, 41, 46.

85 NHS, HSC 1999/030, p. 6.

86 In the early days of nurse registration, the so-called specialists tended to be 'disparaged as semi-educated and unduly susceptible to medical domination' by those trained in a general hospital setting. See Dingwall *et al.*, *An Introduction to the Social History of Nursing*, London, Routledge, 1988, p. 91; pp. 132–3.

87 Bendall, E. and Raybould, E., *A History of the General Nursing Council for England and Wales, 1919–1969*, London, H. K. Lewis and Co. Ltd., 1969, pp. 211–2.

88 The development of a new professional group to provide care for people with learning disabilities was mentioned in the Briggs Report and further explored by the Jay Committee on Mental Handicap Nursing and Care. This latter committee reported in 1979 just as the new statutory framework for nursing was being created. The proposal aroused considerable resistance within the various nursing organisations, which quickly set about reshaping the education and role of mental handicap nurses. A new training curriculum was issued by the GNC in 1981. See *Report of the Committee on Nursing*, (Briggs Report) Cmnd 5115, London, HMSO, 1972, paras 557–65, and recommendation 75. See also Dingwall *et al.*, *An Introduction to the Social History of Nursing*, pp. 140–2.

89 The 1949 Nurses Act had required the GNC to establish a Mental Nurses Committee. Sick children's nursing did not have its own standing or statutory committee under the GNC. See Bendall and Raybould, *A History of the GNC*, p. 155–6. The Briggs Co-ordinating Committee had debated whether similar provisions should be required of the new statutory bodies, but it was felt that detailed specifications of this kind would work against the Act's overall aim of integration.

90 MIN 67/84 (2). This matter was initially raised through EPAC.

91 MIN 94/87(e); CC/87/75.

92 MIN 13/86 (b); MIN 29/86 (b); MIN 43/86 (b); MIN 65/86 (f). In November a meeting was held between the Minister of State for Health, the Chairman of Council and three Council members, Mr Hussain, Mr Jackson and Miss Oxlade. See MIN 85/86.

93 See UKCC B4.14, 'Evidence to the House of Commons Social Services Committee Inquiry into Community Care, with special reference to the adult mentally ill and mentally handicapped', 1984.

94 See UKCC, Papers of the Working Group on Community Care, 1989–90 and CC/91/20.

95 Sylvia Heal's sister, Ann Keen is a prominent figure within community nursing, serving as director of the Community and District Nurses Association (CDNA). Keen herself became a Labour MP in 1997, and was later appointed as Parliamentary Private Secretary to Frank Dobson, the Secretary of State for Health.

96 *Parliamentary Debates*, House of Commons Standing Committee, 28 January 1992, col. 16.

97 Ibid.

98 See, for example, 'Hard work ahead', *Nursing Times*, 31 March, 89(13), 1993, p. 3; 'UKCC leave us out in the cold', letter to *Nursing Times*, 24 March, 89(12), 1993, p. 12.

99 'UKCC answers election charges', *Nursing Times*, 14 April, 89(14), 1993, pp. 12–3.

100 The membership requirements specified the inclusion of two persons specifically qualified to advise the Committee on matters of general education, two members of the Midwifery Committee, two registered medical practitioners (one of whom to be actively engaged in medical education), two students on programmes leading to registration with the Council, and one member from a consumer organisation. Specific representation for the main nursing groups was also guaranteed for the new Education Committee, with adult nursing, children's nursing, mental health nursing, mental handicap nursing and occupational health nursing each to have at least one representative among the committee's membership.

101 NC/93/05; NCHCNC Minute 17/93.

102 Minute 12/93. The debate included the issue of whether mental handicap nursing should remain a branch of Project 2000 or be replaced by a post-registration programme. See, for example, *Nursing Standard*, 30 June, 7(4), 1993, p. 10, three articles on learning disability nursing in *Nursing Times*, 30 June, 89(26), 1993, pp. 47–9.

103 Minute 32/93; CC/93/24; Minute 42/93; CC/93/35.

104 CC/95/23.

105 Ibid.

106 The revised Joint Education Committee was also to be able to explore the development of profession-specific education standards through appropriately constituted, project-managed task groups. This was important since the membership of the committee did not specify places for the specialist nursing groups. UKCC, *Organisational Review, Report of the Steering Group*, p. 19; CC/95/C09, p. 5.

107 UKCC, *Guidelines for mental health and learning disabilities nursing*, 1998.

8 Widening involvement in the work of regulation

Until recent times, it has been taken as axiomatic that statutory regulation of the professions is properly a matter for the professions themselves. Today, this no longer goes unquestioned. There are increasing demands that regulatory systems should be more open, accountable and responsive, and a greater questioning of how others – allied professionals, non-professionals, employers, service users – might become more fully involved in regulation. This chapter traces the growing involvement both of representatives of 'consumers' and of representatives from 'ordinary' practitioners in the UKCC's efforts to establish standards of education, conduct and practice. Viewed from the inside, the pattern is without doubt one of considerable development in thinking and practice and of adjustment to a changing external environment. Judgements from the outside, however, have often been that the UKCC is remote and inaccessible. And, while more people and more diverse people have been involved in the work of regulation, it has still proved difficult to convey to the different stakeholders just what the role of a regulatory body is and should be.

Elections and appointments: legacies of representation before 1979

Historically, the statutory bodies established for the regulation of the health professions have been composed of varying proportions of elected and appointed members. The original constitution of the GMC, in 1858, envisaged a body composed in great measure of the leaders of the profession. The majority (eighteen) would take their places as nominees from the royal colleges, the universities and the existing licensing bodies. They would be joined by another six appointed by the monarch on advice from the Privy Council. It was not until almost a hundred years later, in 1950, that statutory provision was made for including three lay members among the Crown appointments on the GMC.[1] By this time, however, practice had already begun to change. From 1926, the King had included one lay person among those whom he nominated, as a way, it seems, of ensuring that the public maintained some measure of direct vigilance over the Council, especially in matters of discipline.[2] The idea of a small number of directly elected representatives had also taken hold. The overall pattern, however, was one of continuing reliance on the most senior members of the profession, establishment figures who were possessors of honours and titles, who were known in government circles and part of a ruling elite.[3]

The first CMB, in 1902, reflecting the caution of the medical profession and the parlous state of training for midwives at the turn of the century, also called on the elite of medicine. All members were nominated, but at least four of the nine were to be medical practitioners and there was no place at this point specifically reserved for a midwife.[4] The 1919 Nurses Registration Act again provided for an all-appointed Council, this time of twenty-five. Sixteen members who were or had been nurses were to be appointed by the newly formed Ministry of Health after consultation with nursing bodies. Five more were to be appointed after consultation with people knowledgeable about nursing education and the range of general and specialist work. Two were to be nominated by the Board of Education and a further two were to be included who were 'not doctors, not nurses, not employers'. After the initial period, there was provision for the sixteen nurses to be directly elected. A cursory glance at the names and backgrounds of the members of the GNC at this time suggests that those elected were leaders rather than the rank and file. They were persons who had already risen to prominence as heads of nursing, for example, in some of the major teaching hospitals. The people who filled the small number of lay positions were also socially prominent individuals, well known in government circles for their commitment to public service.[5] All rules and all major decisions were to be approved by the Ministry of Health. The Ministry took a particularly interventionist line both with nursing and with midwifery, whose line of accountability transferred in 1919 from the Privy Council.[6]

A key concern of Ministers in making appointments in the case of nursing has always been to seek a balance between the different groups and areas of work within the field. The 1919 Nurse Registration Act, for example, instructed that Ministers must 'have regard to the desirability of including in the Council persons having experience in the various forms of nursing'.[7] By 1949, the legislation was delineating in great detail the people who were to be elected and appointed to the reconstituted GNC for England and Wales. Seventeen were to be elected, drawn by a complex process from and elected by those on different parts of the register and in different parts of the country. Three were to be appointed by the Minister of Education; two were to be appointed by the Privy Council (at least one of whom was to be a university representative). Of the twelve members appointed by the Minister of Health, two were to be registered nurses employed in local authority health services; two teachers of nurses; one a male nurse; and one a ward sister in an approved general training school. There were to be three persons experienced in hospital management, in addition to three unspecified members.[8] Less attention seems to have been paid to the qualities required for those who were not nurses. Once educationalists had been appointed and doctors had been given a place, the places that remained were few. Both here and in the case of midwifery,[9] however, governments, as noted above, had the added fallback that there was little action that the statutory bodies could take without approval by the minister.

An opportunity for review of the custom and practice of appointments and elections to regulatory bodies came in the mid-1970s. The GMC, in financial difficulties, had proposed to activate a retention fee to be paid annually by all doctors, which would be a condition of remaining on the register. This generated considerable unrest. Some doctors had objected on the grounds that they had paid for life and should therefore not be asked for more money; others, however put the point that, if they paid, they should be directly represented and thus have a say in the running of the GMC. Non-payment looked likely. But if the GMC removed names from the register for non-payment, how was the NHS to function? The Merrison Committee was set up to examine the issue. It took the opportunity to review just what professional regulation meant and who should be involved.[10]

Merrison was convinced that a regulatory body had to be a professional regulatory body. A register, essential for public protection, could only be maintained, the committee felt, by those with knowledge of the issues involved. To maintain standards, furthermore, a regulatory body needed to be thoroughly independent of government and of employers (although the public interest dictated that parliament should have the power to intervene if the profession was not doing its job). Merrison's model involved a large Council, of ninety-eight members in all. There should be fifty-four directly elected members, whose experience in practice would be particularly important in decisions about fitness to practice. The universities and royal colleges should play a significant part in the major business of the Council: that is, the setting of educational standards. They should have direct nominees, thirty-four in all. There should also be ten lay members.

Merrison's thinking on lay representation had a number of facets. First, a lay contribution was acknowledged as valuable. Lay members, the committee argued, would prevent discussions becoming too narrow and could be expected to 'focus attention on matters likely to worry ordinary members of the public'.[11] This argument could not be taken far, however, since

> It is the essence of a professional skill that it deals with matters unfamiliar to the layman, and it follows that only those in the profession are in a position to judge many of the matters of standards of professional competence and conduct which will be involved.[12]

Second, 'lay' was defined in a deliberately broad and encompassing way. Although it was conceded that lay members are 'in some sense the public's voice on the GMC',[13] a lay person – to Merrison, and to the framers of the 1978 Medical Act which followed it – meant anyone not in possession of a registrable medical qualification. 'Lay' therefore, included nurses and others working in the health field. Those who could be called the 'truly lay' – those, in other words, whose only relationship with medicine was as a patient[14] – were not separately identified. In naming lay members, the Privy Council, Merrison felt, should consult widely with government departments and NHS authorities, since these were involved with the public. It was a model that called for 'the great and the good': prominent public figures, who had already undertaken public duties chairing health authorities or sitting in membership of local and regional committees.

Merrison's proposals represented what was perhaps the last moment when so confident a statement of the superiority of the professions, their right to control their own affairs and their ability to act in the public interest could be made.[15] The recommendations widened involvement by conceding a much greater place for the rank-and-file practitioner, while at the same time preserving and strengthening the place of the elite educational establishment in decision-making. The inclusion of as many as ten places for lay members was also significant. Probably unintentionally, it paved the way for the strong user voices that were to be raised over the next decade. Delicate negotiations, however, were necessary to translate the report into reality. Significantly, the government was prepared to sit back and wait until a consensus within the medical profession was reached. This perhaps, more than anything else, indicated that it was an era in which regulation of the professions by the professions was not in question.

The Nurses, Midwives and Health Visitors Act came one year after the new Medical Act was on the statute book. The Briggs Committee, in its brief treatment of these matters some years earlier, had insisted that the regulatory body needed independence from the service. It emphasised leadership, arguing that the profession, speaking through a single central council, should 'play the major part in identifying . . . needs and in making sure they are adequately met'.[16] National Boards would give voice to national level considerations, while inspecting and approving colleges and administering the details of policy. Briggs had also envisaged a tier below the Boards, where local initiative and experiment could be fostered. The report suggested six or eight colleges coming together to co-operate with the service on matters such as organising placements and deciding on numbers to be trained. Briggs saw an elected element to the central council, arguing that it gave the opportunity for involvement of nurses and midwives at all levels. The report, however, went into no detail on lay members, simply stating that 'non-nurse members should include among others doctors, people with knowledge in the field of general education, health service administrators and financial experts'.[17] There was no mention of an explicit consumer or patient perspective.

There was little further debate on these matters of composition and representation as the 1979 Nurses, Midwives and Health Visitors Bill passed through parliament. The Secretary of State's appointments to the Central Council were to be drawn from within the professions, to attempt to ensure the representation of particular groups and to create a balance between the different parts of the UK. They were also to come from registered medical practitioners as well as from those people deemed to be 'of value to Council in the performance of its functions'.[18] In practice, this was interpreted as providing for the Briggs trio of experts in education, management and finance. It was decided that, while the UKCC would set up and meet the cost of an electoral scheme and run elections, these elections would better take place within countries and be to the National Boards. The Boards then had the possibility of nominating either elected or appointed members for Council.[19]

The government of the day firmly believed that professional regulation was something requiring only the lightest oversight by Parliament. The debate, where there was one, largely concerned questions of balancing the representation of internal groups. Much was made in the Act of the need to consult groups within the professions before substantive decisions were made. Parliament, however, still retained the right to approve rules through the mechanism of statutory instruments.[20]

The first ten years

Participants

In the shadow period, members of both Council and National Boards were appointed by the Secretary of State for Social Services in consultation with the Secretaries of State for Scotland, Wales and Northern Ireland. Some of the twenty-seven Council members were active in the main in professional associations, others had direct experience of the former statutory bodies. For the most part, they were senior figures, high in the hierarchies of management or education. The remaining six appointees included two from the medical profession, two with expertise in general education and two from a management/finance background. Both sets of appointments followed the established pattern. There was clear concern to secure balance, to have 'due regard' for the interests of all groups within nursing, midwifery and health visiting. Matters of balance also shaped discussions of the internal committee structure (see Chapter 2). There was far less overt discussion of the role or contribution expected of lay members – apart from an appreciation of what they offered in the areas of finance and general education.[21]

The position did not change dramatically with the first full Council. Those who had been successful in the first elections to the National Boards tended to be those already active in professional structures of their respective countries. It was far less easy for ordinary practitioners, with a limited public profile, to establish themselves as potential candidates. After the elections to the National Boards had taken place, and the Boards had decided which members to send to Council,[22] the Secretary of State announced the names of those who would be appointed to complete the Council membership. Balance was the order of the day. Among the appointees were five male nurses, all with qualifications in mental health, a children's nurse and an occupational health nurse.[23] Two particularly well-known figures from nursing – Catherine Hall, the General Secretary of the RCN and Chairman of the Shadow Council, and Zena Oxlade, a regional nursing officer who was the last Chairman of the outgoing GNC for England and Wales, were also appointed. As for the lay element, there were three medical practitioners (a general practitioner, an obstetrician and a surgeon), three people with a background in finance and two general educationalists.[24] In all, both the Shadow Council and the First Council comprised an established elite – senior professionals used to serving their colleagues on national or regional bodies, well versed in committee protocol and the demands of public service. They were both prepared and able to put in the long hours, since most no longer had direct clinical commitments within the health services.[25] The only members with current clinical posts were two enrolled nurses.[26]

The potential for further participation

How far did the internal structures of Council during the first ten years invite or enable the participation of lay members and practitioners in the work of regulation? What formal arrangements were in place to generate and channel contributions from registrants and those outside the statutory bodies? What other avenues of communication were deployed?

Co-option of outside people, both lay and professional, could be made to all of Council's committees with the exception of the PCC and Health Committees, so long as they constituted no more than one-third. Also, while primary legislation laid down certain aspects of the committee structure of Council – such as the requirement that the Midwifery Committee contain a majority of practising midwives – much was left for the Council to decide. Lay members of Council were deployed throughout the range of Council's activities, with the notable exception of the Health Committee and its panel of screeners. A particularly strong lay presence, together with use of co-option, was to be found on the Finance Committee. Six out of its thirteen members, including the Chairman, Roger Holland, were from outside the professions regulated and three of these lay members were drawn from outside Council membership.[27] The HVJC and DNJC each included five people (co-optees as well as Council members) to advise on matters of general professional education; there were also two co-opted medical practitioners; one co-optee from health service management and one from local government on each joint committee. EPAC also included two non-Council educationalists. The Midwifery Committee, as already noted, had a strong professional slant. As well as the primary legislative requirement for a majority of practising midwives, Council's standing orders required the membership to include four practising midwives from among the Council membership nominated by the National Boards, and two medical practitioners. During the first term, the committee also contained seven co-opted members, who included midwives in clinical practice, teaching and service administration, a paediatrician and a lay member, the Hon. Mrs L Price.[28]

The legislative requirement upon Council to undertake consultations before setting its policies in rules was a further way of increasing the influence of those outside the Council. Apart from the requirement to consult National Boards, the Act left considerable scope for Council to determine who should be approached. The practice of consultation could draw in the rank and file, and there were comments from the professional press commending the new Council for opening up previously hidden issues of regulation to the ordinary practitioner. The publication in May 1984 of a consultation paper on new UK-wide Midwives' Rules and Code of Practice, for instance, gave practising midwives the chance to share their views on the rules governing their education and practice with the statutory body, for the first time in the profession's history.[29] While the response was considerable,[30] the episode also reveals the limits of the First Council's approach to outside consultation. The Act required Council to consult the representatives of any group of persons who appeared likely to be affected by the proposed Midwives Practice Rules. This was not taken to include consumer organisations on the grounds that the matter was one of 'professional practice and not the delivery of the service'.[31] The consultation document was not circulated to consumer organisations, but Council nevertheless did receive a number of responses from community health councils and other consumer groups. Project 2000, of course, was a major opportunity to engage with those delivering a nursing service on a wider scale. Not everyone was convinced that this was the right way to go (see Chapter 4), and some might argue that this was 'managed consultation', more information-giving than actually listening and responding. Furthermore, with over half a million names on the register, efforts at consultation within the professions could only reach the tip of the iceberg. There was much to learn about how to prompt comment inside and outside the professions as well as how to analyse and interpret responses to a consultation.

Other efforts to gain direct contact with and influence ordinary practitioners were also afoot. The new Code of Professional Conduct was widely circulated and sent to every new registrant and there was a commitment to review the first edition after a year. Council also actively encouraged practitioners to attend professional conduct hearings held around the UK, and members and officers would routinely speak to observers at the end of hearings, asking if they had understood the proceedings and had found the experience of interest and value. Attendance at Council meetings was and is another possibility. Space, however, remains limited, and in this period the early stages of debate on substantial policy issues tended to be channelled into the closed agenda. Later this division was to come into question, and much more business was conducted in open session.[32]

As well as this communication outward, however, there was growing communication inward. Prompted perhaps by the Code and by the efforts being made to make the work of the UKCC known, and challenged by changes in their daily work, ordinary practitioners and nurse managers began to make direct contact with the Council for advice. In 1985, a new grade of Professional Adviser was added to the staff, to handle the increasing number of telephone and written enquiries on education, conduct and practice issues. As the first term of office was drawing to a close, plans were made to recruit a new Administrative Officer to develop the Council's communications and public relations work. One significant development on this front was already in train. The creation of the live register made it possible to produce a UKCC newsletter for registrants. *Register* was launched in summer 1987 – though at the beginning it was little more than a digest of Council's main activities and policy decisions, rather formal and bland.

By the end of the first term of office, it was clear that Council had begun to experiment with ways of opening up issues of regulation to a wider constituency. The main focus of communication remained the nursing, midwifery and health visiting professions. As yet there was little appreciation that contact and, indeed, accountability might need to be extended to users of nursing, midwifery and health visiting services.

More two-way traffic: 1989–92

In setting its objectives for the second term, Council put on paper for the first time an overt statement that its regulatory work in improving standards in the professions was being carried out *in order to* protect the public. Once put in this way, it became important to ask how such a commitment could be delivered and assessed. Specific new activities associated with this included, for the first time, the establishment of closer links with consumer bodies and a more systematic monitoring of their views on Council policies through opinion-sampling and consultation. This commitment was given practical demonstration in October 1990, with the inclusion of a range of consumer organisations in the consultation on the PREPP.

A further step was taken at the start of 1991, when a preliminary meeting was held between the Chairman and senior officers of the UKCC and the representatives of a small number of consumer organisations, including the Association of Community Health Councils for England and Wales, the Patients' Association, the Consumers' Association and the Association for Improvements in Maternity Services. The intention was to make a 'modest first step' towards the creation of a 'network of contacts' between Council and user groups.[33] It was a revealing first meeting. One of the main issues to emerge was the lack of consumer representation on the Council. Attendees were informed that the 1979 Act did not provide for specific consumer appointments (though, of course, it did not preclude it), and that the matter could change once the government acted upon the findings of the recent departmental review of the Council and National Boards. In this and in other ways, the meeting demonstrated how little was known about the detail of the Council's work or, indeed, its powers in legislation. The consumer representatives, for instance, were eager to press the Council on matters of workforce planning and staffing ratios – both issues that some of those with long service in the Council felt fell outside the UKCC's statutory remit.[34] The meeting, however, resulted in the establishment of a regular Annual Standing Conference with consumer bodies – the first of which took place in October 1991.[35]

Both Council and consumer representatives had a chance to shape the agendas of the consumer conferences. The 1992 conference, for instance, began with an explanation of the legislative changes to be introduced under the 1992 Act, the revised edition of the Code of Conduct and the introduction of the UKCC's new policy document *Scope of Professional Practice*, and progress on PREP. This was followed by discussion of a number of issues of direct concern to consumer bodies. These included the impact of recent changes in community care and the implications for users of health services of the NHS draft guidance document on 'freedom of speech' for NHS staff, then out for consultation. By the end of the second term, and partly prompted by the new consumer conferences, contact had been made with a number of voluntary bodies, and the circulation list for UKCC publications had expanded and become more diverse. Further developments were to come during the third term, as reflected in the stronger public-interest strategic objective of the new Council (see Chapter 3).

Working with a new kind of committee

In early 1988, prompted in part by the kinds of issue that were emerging in professional conduct cases, the outgoing First Council considered its mechanisms for debating and developing policies on ethical and practice issues. The existing strategy of using *ad hoc* groups, for instance to develop the Code of Professional Conduct and its supplementary documents, was felt to have served well but did not help systematically to identify issues and process them speedily. In July 1988, therefore, Council agreed to establish a Standards and Ethics Committee – a decision carried through by the incoming Second Council.[36] The new committee included four co-optees among its initial membership of twelve. The importance of having a specific consumer voice amongst the membership was also stressed. For the first time, four large consumer organisations (the Patients' Association, the Association of Community Health Councils for England and Wales, the Association of Local Health Councils in Scotland and the Association of District Committees in Northern Ireland) were asked to nominate suitable candidates. Jean Robinson, the nominee of the Association of Community Health Councils for England and Wales and a lay member of the GMC, was selected. She was joined by a lay academic, Dr Ruth Chadwick, then lecturer in philosophy at the University of Wales, Cardiff, together with a further nurse and a midwife.

The Committee became a key forum for debating ethical and standards-related issues, both those brought to the UKCC from outside bodies, and those generated from within. It became the principal site for the discussion of consultation papers sent from government departments and other organisations. During its first full year of operation (1989–90), for instance, the Standards and Ethics Committee considered: draft guidelines for local research ethics committees produced by the Department of Health; the implications of a new Committee on the Ethics of Gene Therapy established by the health ministers in England, Wales and Scotland; the report of the voluntary licensing authority for *in-vitro* fertilisation; the Human Embryology Bill; the concerns of a number of community health councils over the increasing number of senior health authority staff with financial or other interests in private health care facilities, especially registered nursing homes and the report of a Department of Health advisory group on nurse prescribing. This kind of activity continued into the Third Council. In 1993, the Committee helped prepare evidence to the House of Lords Select Committee on Medical Ethics, which was set up to consider a range of 'end of life' issues. This issue remained on the agenda of the Standards and Ethics Committee and formed the basis of a joint UKCC and GMC meeting on the matter. The following year, the Committee considered, amongst other issues, the findings of the independent Committee of Inquiry into the deaths and injuries on the children's ward at

Grantham and Kesteven General Hospital between February and April 1991 (Allitt inquiry); a Department of Health paper on the regulation of nursing homes and the executive summary of the Greenhalgh Report on the interface between junior doctors and nurses.[37] With these high-profile, politically sensitive issues of concern to practitioners and public on the agenda, the UKCC was starting to appear more outward-looking and responsive.

The Standards and Ethics Committee also became a more direct focus for the Council's efforts to improve its responsiveness to ordinary practitioners. During 1989, for instance, confusion over the role of nurses in residential care homes led the Committee to arrange a special consultative meeting with representatives of the Registered Nursing Homes Association, the Social Services Inspectorate and the chief nursing officers of the government health departments. In 1990, the Committee explored the increase in requests for advice from or regarding practice nurses and a working group was convened to consider what steps Council could or should take in this area. Later in 1990, members agreed that, while it should continue to provide the main forum for issues raised by outside bodies, greater emphasis should be given to issues identified by ordinary practitioners and members of the public.[38]

At the heart of all this lay a new monitoring and analysis system with two principal elements. The first involved a more systematic logging of items of interest from the national, regional and professional press, the broadcasting media, parliamentary debates and select committees, government statistics, the reports of the Health Service Commissioner and from the cases and evidence heard by the UKCC's PCC. The second element was the identification of issues of concern to practitioners and the public raised through telephone calls to, and correspondence with, the UKCC's professional staff and advisory service – a process that became known as 'contacts analysis'. One issue identified in this way was the standard of documentation and record-keeping – a matter that was followed up by the Standards and Ethics Committee and by the UKCC's professional staff in a new Council publication.[39]

It was at this time too, that the UKCC began to make closer and more systematic contact with other regulatory bodies in the health sector. A particular effort was made to maintain regular contact with the GMC. In early 1989 the two bodies agreed to establish a Joint UKCC and GMC Liaison Committee, to act as a forum for the consideration of issues of mutual interest and concern. Starting in March 1990, there were biannual meetings.[40] Early agendas addressed such issues as the extending role of the nurse, the report of the government Advisory Group on Nurse Prescribing, the proposed reduction in junior doctors' hours, the impact of the new GP contract on practice nurses, the UKCC's work on maintaining registration and professional competence beyond registration and the GMC's consideration of the feasibility of a performance review procedure for doctors.[41] Links with nursing bodies overseas were also developed – another new objective of the Second Council. Specific targets included seminars on international matters for Council members and the establishment of an international network between regulatory bodies for nursing and midwifery.

An uneasy legislative repositioning

The health departments' first review of the working of the Council and National Boards got under way as the Second Council started its term of office. In the short time available, there was no way that management consultants Peat Marwick McClintock could take on the developments in involving the professions and the public that have been discussed here. Their review, furthermore, had strict limits – it was to confine itself to the efficiency and effectiveness of the structures. As we have seen in Chapter 3, they felt that the whole structure was much too cumbersome. They recommended a clearer line of division between a directly elected, standard-setting Central Council and National Boards who put standards into practice, negotiating with education and service. Boards should be accountable to the Department of Health. Council, they felt, should be altogether more accountable to the practitioners who paid for it through fees.

This was a position that had distinct echoes of the Merrison report's confident view that the profession, given its expertise, could and should carry out the work of regulation in the interests of the public at large. Had Peat Marwick McClintock come to their review a little later, when the work of the panel of consumer representatives was in full swing, or had their remit been to consider the nature of regulation more directly, their conclusions might have been different. The question of whether those whose purpose was to keep a register to protect the public could also be accountable to the profession was to come to the fore more urgently later in the decade, when another firm of management consultants took a different view. As it was, the package of recommendations was largely accepted and enshrined in legislation. It endorsed *self*-regulation and put profession above public in a way that would not remain unquestioned for long. Nothing was said about lay appointments or about the involvement of lay people in the work of the Council.

In one respect, and given the review that was to come at the end of the Third Council, the Peat Marwick McLintock model was particularly prescient. It recommended a smaller Council, with a panel of practitioners who could be called upon to sit on conduct committees. This would not only add to efficiency but would be a further way of encouraging more direct participation of practitioners in the work of Council. Lobbying by the UKCC, convinced that what was needed to carry out the heavy load of professional conduct work was a larger council not a smaller one, was successful.[42] The recommendation was turned on its head.

The government was willing to give legislative time only for non-controversial changes (see Chapter 5). The role of 'lay' or consumer participants in the regulatory process did get raised, however. Roger Sims MP asked the government for clarification about the lack of a specific allocation for consumer members among the Secretary of State appointees. The Minister of State for Health, Virginia Bottomley, replied that the government would certainly expect lay representation to play an important part in these appointments; but she did not choose to expand on this or, indeed, to reflect upon the specific contribution of consumer representatives.[43] The issue returned during the committee stage and at the third reading. This time Mrs Bottomley stated that the government accepted that the wider public interest in the regulation of the professions should be adequately reflected in the appointed membership, and assured parliament and the professions that she 'would wish to take account of the need to reflect the interests of health service consumers and would take wide soundings about the appropriate individuals who could make that special contribution to the council'.[44]

The years between 1989 and 1993 had been interesting times for those who had seen at first hand the work of the earlier Council. Both the Standards and Ethics Committee and the consumer conferences had brought new people and new topics into the ambit of regulation. In all the controversy that was to come – the high-profile debates about professional conduct, the events leading to the organisational review – the pattern of increasing consumer involvement was not as well acknowledged as it might have been. It continued, however, to gather pace.

Multiple challenges and an influx of new ideas

Under the revised primary legislation, the Third Council in 1993 was a larger body, with forty members directly elected by the professions and twenty appointed by the Secretary of State. Of the twenty government appointments, eleven were lay members. Once again, these latter appointees included medical practitioners, people with financial expertise and experience in health service management, educationalists and academics. As had been suggested on the floor of the House, however, the appointments now included two people who were very specifically identified as bringing a consumer voice to the Council.[45] Once again there was an opportunity to bring in non-Council members, both professional and lay, through the process of co-option, and the amended primary legislation now allowed the UKCC to include non-Council members (lay or otherwise) on all of its Committees.[46]

In October 1993 the Council took the decision to open up the membership of the PCC to non-Council members by agreeing to the establishment of a panel of consumer representatives – a decision partly influenced by the growing public unease at some of the recent decisions of the Committee.[47] Consumer members of Council were also invited to join the Chairman and Deputy Chairmen of the PCC on an *ad hoc* committee to look at the issues raised in PCC hearings. It was decided, however, that the consumer panel should not be involved in the work of the closed PPC – a position that was changed at the final meeting of the third term. Interestingly, Council also decided not to use the increased flexibility of the 1992 Act at this time to establish a panel of practitioners for professional conduct, preferring to wait and see if the expanded Council membership eased workload difficulties. This policy was reversed in March 1996.[48]

Lay members of Council now sat on all Council committees. The Education Committee (established as a replacement for EPAC) included a lay educationalist and a consumer representative. This committee now also, for the first time, included students among its membership.[49] The Midwifery Committee now included four non-midwife or health visitor members among its nineteen members. Two of these were medical practitioners, while the other two represented the consumer perspective.[50] The NCHCNC had four non-nurse/midwife/health visitor members, though this time out of a larger membership of twenty-four. The Standards and Ethics Committee once again had a strong lay membership – eight out of twenty-two members. These, however, were still largely a group of 'experts' – two medical practitioners and three academics as well as three consumer members of Council.[51]

The start of the first elected Council was a particularly turbulent and uncertain time as far as understanding of the work of the UKCC and patterns of involvement in it were concerned. The electoral process had encouraged candidates to discuss their aims for the Council in the professional press, and both UNISON and RCN members were prominent in this. One individual, Graham Pink, became very high-profile in his campaign that the UKCC should stand up for the ordinary nurse and be less secretive about its decisions. He appeared on the front cover of the *Nursing Times*; letters in support of him were published and he gained a large share of votes.[52] When it came to the business of setting objectives, it was clear that members were confused and frustrated about the limits of their legislative remit, and how far they could act to promote the interests of practitioners (Chapter 3). The RCN congress in June showed just how much outside dissatisfaction was mounting. An account of the congress in the nursing press reported that Council was 'taking a battering in debate after debate'. The story opened with words that must have been hard for the new Council to hear: 'What has the UKCC got in common with a jellyfish? In the opinion of one delegate . . . it's spineless, toothless, useless and stings you every three years'.[53]

Press questioning of just what the UKCC was doing and how it was doing it was to reach a climax the following year, as the investigation into the Chief Executive continued to run. The UKCC 'should be made to justify the decisions it makes', said an editorial in the *Nursing Times* – public voting, demystifying disciplinary committees and fewer closed discussions should be put in place. A *Nursing Standard* leader the week before had called for a complete culture change to shift the perception of the UKCC as 'an establishment rolling slowly forward on a set agenda'.[54] At this low ebb, the UKCC took the decision to carry out its own review to reposition itself and gain a new sense of its identity and role. It provided the fresh start many were waiting for.

1995 – a watershed

The organisational review, aided by the Office of Public Management, gave the UKCC a new way of looking at itself and a new language for expressing its role. Armed with this it was able to reframe its objectives and put into words and into practice ways of working – some of which were already in hand – that were more open and responsive. The key recommendations have already been discussed.[55] They included creation of a Management Board, reorganisation of standards work and upgrading of communications. In a document presenting these changes to a wider audience, the President, Mary Uprichard, echoed Council's continuing commitment to discharge its statutory responsibilities in the public interest. She added: 'In a health system that is rapidly changing, it is important that the UKCC is able to respond to the changes and, *in collaboration with consumers and providers of health services*, to shape the future [emphasis added].'[56]

One controversial aspect of the structural change, however, was the loss of the Standards and Ethics Committee, with standards and ethical issues instead becoming the responsibility of the two practice committees – working in conjunction with specially convened task groups. Members feared that the move would be perceived 'as a lowering of the status of the consideration of ethical issues by the Council'. Concern was also expressed that the relocation of standards-related questions to the practice committees would lessen the current level of input from non-Council members.[57] It was accepted that a compromise position needed to be found. In November 1995, Council agreed that the practice committees should be assisted in the area of ethics by a standing task group, the Ethics Advisory Panel, a series of annual ethics conferences or seminars and a designated Professional Officer with responsibility for ethical issues.[58] These measures were introduced from April 1996. Problems persisted, however. Members of the new Panel were disappointed that its terms of reference did not allow it to set its own agenda; there were a number of early resignations and the August 1997 meeting had to be cancelled owing to lack of business. A review of the working of the Panel followed but no definite plans were made by the end of the Third Council term.[59]

The work of the Council during this period, however, certainly saw important fruits of the collaborative perspective that Mary Uprichard had emphasised following the organisational review. The communications unit, directly accountable to the Chief Executive, focused on more active management of media and public relations, the co-ordination of publications, conferences and other external events designed to promote the work of the UKCC. Regular 'Meet the UKCC' days were now part of this. New efforts were made to ensure that the public was aware of the UKCC and its role in protecting the public's interests; the decision was taken to publish an explanatory information leaflet and to distribute it via community health councils and Citizen's Advice Bureaux.[60] Members were given guidelines on their corporate role and on expectations of them both in respect of specific Council business and as 'ambassadors' of the UKCC. A database of members' skills was set up to help ensure that the UKCC made better use of its members.

Particularly notable was the way in which the direct participation of the professions in the standard-setting work of the Council gained momentum; and the style and content of publications changed. Chapter 3 referred to the use of consultative conferences, on mental health nursing, on nursing homes and on clinical supervision; it noted how *Guidelines for Professional Practice* set out to respond to practitioner concerns. The Council's *Proposed Standards for Incorporation into Contracts for Hospital and Community Health Care Services*, published in September 1995, also had the benefit of consultative conferences prior to its publication. It prompted a leading article very different from the ones in 1994.

The UKCC was now described as 'audacious'. Could it, the editor of *Nursing Management* asked with clear relish, become 'the SAS of statutory bodies?' More detailed work on standards in particular clinical areas – carried out by task groups supported by the new specialist Professional Officers – sent a signal to the profession that that the UKCC was engaging collaboratively with issues of specific clinical concern. The Fourth Council was to see the importance of engaging with students of nursing and midwifery being reiterated by the Joint Education Committee, and a proposal for the establishment of an annual delegates conference for students.[61] In all these instances, it was being more clearly acknowledged that Council needed to encourage participation if it were to demonstrate to its many audiences how standards were developed, and what it was doing to promote them.

Research was commissioned to find out how the UKCC was viewed by registrants (see Chapter 3, pages 65–6). As the fourth term got under way, there was also a survey of 500 employers of nurses, midwives and health visitors – in the private sector as well as the NHS – addressing such issues as the registration confirmations service, the telephone system, the professional advice service, the ordering of publications, the handling of professional conduct cases and of complaints. On the one hand, the results were encouraging, suggesting that the UKCC was being seen in a better light by significant proportions of its stakeholders. On the other hand, criticisms of remoteness and bureaucracy had not altogether gone away. Election turnouts also remained very low.[62]

Consumers were sometimes able to bring new perspectives to issues of regulation.[63] In September 1996, Council reviewed its policies for including consumer representatives on the PCC, and agreed to add further members to the panel of consumer representatives.[64] The method of selection – appointment following nomination by specific organisations – remained the same. The alternative of seeking nominations through advertisements in the national press was not taken up at this time. In June 1996, Council agreed that in future two consumer representatives would sit on every restoration case. At the final meeting of the Third Council, members also agreed to involve non-Council members (lay and practitioners) in the work of the PPC, and in April 1998 both consumer panel and practitioner panel members joined the Committee.[65] A report back confirmed that the development was regarded as a success, and that the involvement of consumer and practitioner panellists had enriched the discussion and decision-making of the Committee.[66] In September 1998, the Fourth Council considered the possibility of extending the scope of the consumer panel still further, to include involvement in work of the Health Committee and its panel of screeners. It was a change that would require the amendment of Council's Professional Conduct Rules, and Council agreed to consult on this.[67] A year into the fourth term, results demonstrated 'overwhelming support' for this action and, in the light of Council's commitment to continue to expand the involvement of consumers in its work in serving the public interest,[68] members agreed to seek the necessary legislative change.[69]

By the final year of the third term, the UKCC was beginning to frame and organise the annual standing consumer conference, its principal method of monitoring the views of consumer bodies in different ways. The list of organisations invited to send representatives had been greatly expanded with the help of the consumer members of Council. In 1996, sixty-eight bodies were approached, in comparison to thirty-five the previous year. The number of attendees had risen. During the first few years of the annual standing conference, an average of twelve representatives of consumer bodies attended. By 1996, this had increased to twenty-five, rising to thirty-seven in 1997. Discussions with consumer representatives in preparation for the sixth conference, moreover, had suggested the value of combining the annual conference with consultation exercises on current UKCC policies and projects. While it was not the only issue on the table at the 1996 conference, delegates were given the opportunity to express their views on the UKCC's project on the nursing and health visiting contribution to the continuing care of older people during an early stage of its development.[70] This approach was repeated the following year, with the afternoon session of the seventh consumer conference set aside for consultation on specialist practice.[71] Feedback from this event pointed the way for further change. Increased use of smaller working groups of consumers on subject-specific topics, more consultation with consumers during the early stages of publication of Council documents, a greater use of outreach work with service users, as well as regular contact with consumer bodies, were all recommended. A review of Council's database of consumer contacts to ensure that it was sufficiently inclusive, particularly of minority groups, was suggested. These recommendations were agreed by the Third Council at its final meeting in March 1998.[72] Also during this period, discussions were taking place within the UKCC's professional directorates on the creation of a new Professional Officer post to help the Council develop its strategy for enhancing consumer involvement in the work of the Standards Promotion directorate. A Professional Officer for Consumer Affairs took up post in October 1998.[73] One year on from the end of the Third Council, in March 1999, Council agreed a new strategy in the area of consumer involvement, to be overseen by a consumer involvement steering group.[74]

Conclusion

For most of the twentieth century, involvement in the statutory self-regulation of professions has been fairly stable. It has been seen as the business of an elite within the professions, aided by a small number of others – the 'great and the good' – and has increasingly included specialists in education management and finance. In the case of the statutory bodies in nursing and midwifery, however, the other participant in all this was the Ministry of Health, whose interventions limited the claim to independent decision-making. The 1979 Act echoed earlier legislation in emphasising a balance of representation across all groups within the professions, and in its treatment of a small lay component. With its prospect of self-financing, and demands that there should be consultation with the profession on all key matters, there was scope for greater independence and for changes in thinking about who should be involved and how.

Change started to come with the Second Council and its more overt emphasis on serving the public interest. The creation of a standing conference of consumer organisations was a bold and unprecedented move in the statutory structures in the health field. The formation, at the start of its term, of the Standards and Ethics Committee began to enable Council to debate matters of more direct concern to both ordinary practitioners and service users. Legislative change in 1992 was disappointing in regard to questions of involvement. The review work had come too early to reflect new thinking, the terms of reference precluded direct engagement with the concept of self-regulation, and the recommendations that were put forward for more direct practitioner involvement, without the support of the UKCC, became a casualty of the legislative amendment process. Approaches to both consumer and practitioner involvement shifted into a new gear in the second half of the Third Council. This chapter has charted a whole series of ways in which both groups have become progressively more involved as participants in the work on standards of conduct, education and practice. Challenges of how to develop still further these more inclusive and open ways of working, how to create equality of opportunity to participate, how to combat charges of tokenism and how ensure that the full diversity of interests is heard, for example, certainly remain. Questions of what might be learned from the experience to date of bringing professionals and lay people together to make decisions about standards have barely even been posed. In a world where stakeholder organisations are increasingly the order of the day, perhaps there are lessons that can be learned from this remarkable series of developments in the life of the UKCC.

Notes

1 The Medical Act 1950 increased the total size of the Council to fifty, providing for forty-four medical members (eleven elected), five Crown nominees, twenty-eight university/royal college appointees, three dentists and three lay members.

2 Pyke-Lees, W., *Centenary of the GMC 1858–1958: The History and Present Work of the Council*, London, GMC, 1958, cited in M. Stacey, *Regulating British Medicine. The General Medical Council*, Chichester, John Wiley and Sons, 1992, p. 23. Stacey notes that George Bernard Shaw is said to have claimed credit for this change. The much quoted remark that 'all professions are conspiracies against the laity' came from Shaw's play *The Doctor's Dilemma*, 1911.

3 For a discussion of the elite character of GMC membership in the 1970s, see Stacey, *Regulating British Medicine*.

4 In addition to the four medical practitioners to be nominated by the Royal College of Surgeons, the Royal College of Physicians, the Society of Apothecaries and the Incorporated Midwives Institute, the Midwives Act 1902 provided for one nominee each from the Association of County Councils, the Queen Victoria Jubilee Institute for Nurses and the Royal British Nurses Association. There were also to be two others to be nominated by the Lord President of the Council – one of whom was to be a woman.

5 For the continuing prominence of the notion of public service in Edwardian and interwar Britain see Mandler, P. and S. Pedersen (eds), *After the Victorians. Private Conscience and Public Duty in Modern Britain*, London, Routledge, 1994.

6 Jean Donnison has remarked on the determination of the Ministry to exercise greater

control over midwifery. See Donnison, J., *Midwives and Medical Men. A History of Inter-professional Rivalries and Women's Rights*, London, Heinemann Educational, 1977, p. 188. For an account of the GNC's battles with the Ministry, see Davies, C., *Professional Power and Sociological Analysis – lessons from a comparative, historical study of nursing in Britain and the USA*, Ph.D thesis, University of Warwick, 1981. See also Rafferty, A. M., *The Politics of Nursing Knowledge*, London, Routledge, 1996.

7   Nurse Registration Act 1919, Schedule, section 2.

8   Nurses Act 1949, First Schedule.

9   By the early 1950s, there had been changes here too. Of the nineteen members of the CMB, six were appointed by the minister, of whom two had to be certified midwives and one a general practitioner. Places were reserved for nominees of the Royal College of Physicians, the Royal College of Surgeons, the Royal College of Obstetricians and Gynaecologists and the Society of Medical Officers of Health. There were still two nominees from the local authority sector, but there were also now four midwives nominated by the RCM. See Midwives (Constitution of CMB) Order, 1952.

10   *Report of the Committee of Inquiry into the Regulation of the Medical Profession* (Merrison Report) Cmnd 6018, London, HMSO, 1975.

11   Ibid., para. 383.

12   Ibid., para. 378.

13   Ibid., para. 403.

14   Stacey, *Regulating British Medicine*, p. 84.

15   Interestingly, while Merrison dismissed an all-lay body, there were alternative views. The Socialist Medical Association argued that control of the medical profession 'should be a service to the community as a whole not to the medical profession as such'. From that point of view the public should fund and control it. MIND, the mental health campaigning group, took a similar view: 'financing . . . should not depend on members' contributions, or it becomes impossible to avoid the suspicion of the body's being concerned with professional rather than public interest' (para. 426).

16   *Report of the Committee on Nursing* (Briggs Report), Cmnd 5115, London, HMSO, 1972, para. 616.

17   Ibid., para. 637d.

18   Nurses, Midwives and Health Visitors Act 1979, Section 1 (4).

19   Interestingly, the Briggs Committee had recommended that elections be held to the Central Council, since this was the body responsible for setting standards and maintaining discipline. Devolutionary pressures, however, had persuaded the government to legislate for elections to be held to the National Boards. See *Report on the Committee of Nursing*, paras 638–9, and Chapter 1 above.

20   See Chapter 2, note 9.

21   Quite a number of Council members held management posts in the NHS and might be said to bring a management perspective into the heart of the Council – not quite perhaps what Briggs had envisaged when he argued for a stronger separation and independence from service.

22   Boards also had appointed as well as elected members, but in the main they opted to send their elected members to Council. The NBNI was an exception here in choosing to send a Secretary of State educationalist nominee, Dr J. Bamber, to the UKCC.

23   Two of these, Tariq Hussain and Michael Jackson, were also qualified as RNMS and during the period of the First Council were managing services in the field at the time referred to as mental handicap.

24   As noted above in note 22, one of the NBNI's appointees to Council was also a 'lay' educationalist.

25   The position contrasted with that in medicine, where funding, for example, was available for locum cover for GPs. Resignations from Council were often for reasons of workload, though not necessarily due to clinical commitments.

26   In 1987, as many as eighteen Council members held posts as Directors of Nursing or

Midwifery Services, and a further fourteen had posts in nurse education, the majority at director level.

27 These were Mr P. Fletcher, a member of the Institute of Health Service Administrators, Mrs S. Webb, a member of the British Institute of Management, and Mr E. P. McNally from the Association of Health Service Treasurers.

28 Lindy Price was daughter of Lord Brecon, Minister of State for Welsh Affairs, who had been appointed to this post by Prime Minister Harold Macmillan in 1957. She had carried out a wide range of public duties in the education and nursery nursing fields. She had been a prison visitor and a member of the Parole Board for England and Wales. She had also served on the Police Complaints Board. She came to the UKCC from serving on the Maternity Services Liaison Committee and later went on to chair a health authority and NHS trust in Wales. In this career, she was the epitome of members of 'the great and the good' noted earlier. The Hon. Mrs Price died in 1999.

29 UKCC, *New Midwives Rules and Code of Practice: A Consultation Paper*, 1984.

30 Around 200 responses were received by the close of the consultation in September 1984. Also see Chapter 7, note 16.

31 MIN 62/84 (ii).

32 From the outset Council has divided its business into different agendas. For most of its lifetime it has operated a two-part agenda – closed and open – as a general rule. Members and officers attend the closed session which deals such issues as staffing and the appointment of members to committees or outside organisations. National Board chief executives, government health department observers, the press and the public join the meeting for the open session. The aim now is to take as much business as possible in open session, and the closed session is generally quite short. The President can invite outside persons to any session if it is appropriate, and may choose to call an extraordinary meeting of Council for members and officers only. Between 1987 and 1995 a three-part agenda (private, closed and open) was used. The private session was for members and officers only and was largely concerned with staffing issues and committee appointments. It was also used for certain policy matters on which Council had not reached a position that could be made known beyond its membership. The closed session contained material of a confidential nature, but which could be shared with National Board chief executives and government health department observers.

33 It was a small event with nine consumer representatives and five representatives of the UKCC. The Association of Community Health Councils for England and Wales, the Patients' Association, the Consumers Association, the College of Health, the Association for Improvements in Maternity Services, the National Association for the Welfare of Children in Hospital, MIND, the Marie Curie Foundation and Cancer Relief responded positively to the invitation to attend and sent representatives. Positive interest was also expressed by the Terrence Higgins Trust, MENCAP and Age Concern but these organisations were unable to send representatives.

34 CO/91/02.

35 CC/91/21; CC/91/74.

36 MIN 77/88 (a).

37 See agenda, minutes and papers of the Standards and Ethics Committee.

38 See the minutes of the Standards and Ethics Committee, 28 February 1990; SEC/90/12. See also the papers of the Registrar's Professional Group, eg RPG/90/50, RPG/90/44; RPG/91/03.

39 UKCC, *Standards for Records and Record Keeping*, London, UKCC, 1993.

40 Previous to establishment of the Joint Liaison Committee, liaison between the two Councils was arranged on an *ad hoc* basis, with meetings held to discuss a particular topic or a draft paper. The Joint Liaison Committee comprised a core membership of the President of the GMC, the Chairman of the UKCC, the Chairs of the bodies' ethical committees, both Registrars and supporting staff from both bodies. See Annexe to JLC/90/01. Biannual Joint Liaison Committee meetings continued into

UKCC's third term. In 1996, however, the Joint Liaison Committee was replaced by a less formal arrangement. Liaison is now maintained through routine communications and regular dinners.

41 See Joint UKCC/GMC Liaison Committee file for agendas, minutes and papers.

42 There was provision in the legislation to set up a practitioner panel, though Council preferred to wait to see whether, with its larger membership, the workload could be handled without this.

43 *Parliamentary Debates* [Commons], 201, 13 January 1992, cols 709–10.

44 Ibid., 205, 4 March 1992, col. 395.

45 These were Dr Eva Jacobs, a retired university lecturer and volunteer with the Patients' Association, and Mrs Rita Lewis, a former chair of the National Association of Community Health Councils – the nominating body in her case. A third 'consumer' member, Mr David Crowson, Divisional General Manager of Mencap in Wales was appointed in January 1997 following the resignation of one of the Secretary of State appointees.

46 Nurses, Midwives and Health Visitors Act 1992, Section 8(3). Council had determined, though, that it would not involve non-Council members in the work of the Health Committee. Consequently the Professional Conduct Rules (SI 1993 No. 893) were drafted to enable non-Council members to serve on the PPC and PCC but not on the panel of professional screeners and Health Committee.

47 Council agreed that the panel should comprise twenty members. Initially, though, only ten representatives were appointed. See CC/93/50.

48 Minute 22/96(3); CC/96/18.

49 The standing orders of the Education Committee initially specified the inclusion of two student members, but it was later agreed that three (one nursing student, one midwifery and one health visiting student) should be invited into membership. Nominations were sought from the RCN, RCM and HVA: EC/93/01; EC Minute 16/93(2); EC Minute 25/93(3). The inclusion of student members continued with the Joint Education Committee established following the organisational review of 1996. See EC/96/06; EC Minute 21/96(2).

50 These were Ms B. Lawrence Beech, Honorary Chair of the Association for Improvements in the Maternity Services and Mrs H. Lewison, Chairman of the National Childbirth Trust.

51 These consumer members included the two people appointed by the Secretary of State following nomination by consumer organisations, and also a third Secretary of State appointee – Jenny Hughes – who was the Chairman of Kensington, Chelsea and Westminster Health Authority.

52 Graham Pink was sacked from his job as a charge nurse in Stockport after 'blowing the whistle' on what he perceived to be dangerously low staffing levels and poor standards of care. His campaign for election to the UKCC drew heavily on this experience and his belief that the UKCC could do more to assist those in similar positions. Having won a seat on the Council, Pink continued to criticise the UKCC in the professional press, and in radio and television interviews. He was particularly critical of what he saw as its secretive approach to business. Having been given but declined an opportunity to discuss his grievances with fellow Council members, Pink resigned his seat in May 1994.

53 Turner, T., 'Tunnel vision', *Nursing Times*, 16 June, 89(24), 1993, p. 21.

54 Cassidy, J., 'The power of one', *Nursing Times*, 16 November, 90(46), 1994, p. 20; *Nursing Standard*, 9 November, 9(7), 1994, p. 3.

55 See Chapter 3, pages 61–2.

56 Uprichard, M., 'Foreword', *UKCC Organisation Review: Summary of the Steering Group Report*, 1996, p. 2.

57 The matter was discussed at the Oct 1995 meeting of the SEC at the request of Rita Lewis, one of the consumer members of Council. SEC Minute 32/95(5), October

1995. Support for the retention of the Committee was received from outside, from both nurses' and patients' representatives. Jean Robinson, the vice-president of the Patients' Association and herself a former co-opted member of the SEC, for example, questioned how the UKCC could fulfil its 'primary function' of 'the protection of the public . . . without such a key committee.' Beverley Lawrence, the honorary Chair-woman of the Association for Improvements in the Maternity Services, expressed similar concerns in a letter to the Chief Executive, noting that 'this bizarre and inexplicable action has decreased consumer confidence in the council.' See 'UKCC Ethics Committee plan rapped', *Nursing Times*, 4 October, 91(40), 1995, p. 9. See also a letter from Jean Robinson to the *Nursing Times*, 18 October, 91(42), 1995, p. 22.

58 Minute 23/96(2).
59 EAP Minute 20/97; EAP/97/08, 'Addressing Ethical Issues: future consideration and the working of the Ethics Advisory Panel', 1997, pp. 2–3.
60 UKCC, *Protecting the Public*, London, UKCC, 1997.
61 CC/99/36, para. 4.
62 The turnout for elections to the Third Council was 16.5 per cent across the UK as a whole. The figure for the Fourth Council was just 13 per cent.
63 During 1994 and 1995, for instance, the consumer members played an active role in encouraging Council to agree to the disclosure of cautions to employers and others seeking confirmation of a practitioner's registration, in the face of considerable opposition from professional associations and trades unions. See Minute 8/95(2); Minute 33/95(3); CC/94/76; CC/95/37.
64 It was hoped that the panel could be increased from ten to twenty members. Six people were appointed after nominations had been received from consumer organisations.
65 Minute 7/98(3); CC/98/09.
66 CC/99/39, para. 12.
67 Minute 26/98(3); CC/98/33; Registrar's Letter 33/98, 28 October 1998.
68 This is one of the strategic objectives agreed by Council in December 1998. See Minute 37/98(3.3).
69 Minute 8/99(3); CC/99/13.
70 CC/96/63.
71 CC/98/06, especially Annexe 1.
72 CC/98/06; Minute 5/98(6).
73 MG/98/15; MG/98/19.
74 CC/99/10; Minute 6/99(9); Minute 16/99.

9 Professional self-regulation in question

The work of this history came to an end with the final meeting of the Third Council, in March 1998. For anyone following events at the time, this was by no means a natural point to pause for review. It was a moment, indeed, when the professions were poised for the biggest change since the legislation that first set up the Council and National Boards. A government-initiated, fundamental review was under way. JM Consulting had already interviewed staff and members of the regulatory bodies and observed some of their proceedings. Under the title *The Future of Professional Regulation*, the UKCC had prepared a submission to the reviewers which set out – for the first time – what it saw as the key principles of regulation and the areas where it felt change was indicated. In January 1998, close to that last meeting of the Third Council, the consultants had issued an interim report. It was a hard-hitting document, containing one challenge after another to the complexities of the regulatory arrangements, the procedural rules that had been thrashed out and the advisory and guidance documents that had been issued. Twelve months on, it was to become apparent that government supported many, if not most, of JM Consulting's final recommendations. A new kind of regulatory machinery seemed set to be put in place – with a much transformed Central Council, with some significant new powers but without the National Boards. It is not possible to finish this account of the history of the UKCC without paying some attention to what JM Consulting said, why the proposals won acceptance and what, in the light of this history, might be said about them.

To embark on this, it is necessary to return once again to the position in 1979 as the present statutory structures were put in place, and to explore the stance of governments on the question of professional self-regulation (PSR). It is important to bring the other regulatory bodies in the health field into the picture, and to explore how their interests and concerns meshed or failed to mesh with government agendas. It was possible for governments of the 1970s – and, more surprisingly perhaps, it continued to be possible for governments of the 1980s – to assume that PSR could by and large be left alone. As this chapter will show, they assumed that as long as the different interests within professions were all adequately represented, the professions could be trusted to carry out regulatory affairs without interference. Merrison's equation – professional control of a register means protection of the public – held firm. The contemporary history of how this began to break down with a review by JM Consulting of the regulation of professions supplementary to medicine, how this presented problems for an incoming Labour government with a heavy legislative agenda of its own and how media criticism put that government under pressure is told in this chapter. It forms the context in which the JM Consulting report on nursing, midwifery and health visiting needs to be understood, and it is crucial to a critical appreciation of what happened next, as far-reaching powers (though not quite as far-reaching as the government initially proposed) were written into the Health Act of 1999. The chapter thus seeks to put the JM Consulting model of PSR in a wider context. It traces the ways in which questioning of the institution of PSR had started to build up by the late 1990s. It considers how the Labour government integrated these issues into its determination to 'modernise' and to raise the quality of public services and what position had been reached by the autumn of 1999, as this book went to press.

Reluctant engagements with PSR

It can often appear to those working inside the regulatory arena that change is very recent. It seems as if it is only since the mid- or even late 1990s, that the press has taken a keen interest in matters of professional conduct, and only perhaps since Labour took office in 1997 that regulation has really emerged onto the political agenda. A longer historical perspective, however, indicates that the question of PSR was being raised earlier. Consideration was limited to a small group of interested parties and, where debate did take place, it occurred, as did the discussions that preceded the 1992 Act, outside the glare of publicity. The debate on PSR has been – and in important ways still is – muted.

The 1980s – a government looking elsewhere

What was the incoming Conservative government's view of PSR at the time that the UKCC started its life?[1] Government views about the nature and value of the statutory self-regulation of professions in the 1979 Act were coloured by events in medicine. There had been new legislation the previous year, building on foundations laid by the Merrison enquiry.[2] This had strongly affirmed the importance of a body independent of government, composed mainly of members of the profession, free to make decisions about the direction of that profession. On this model, the key task for parliament was not to agree the directions for the profession, but to ensure that the profession was in a position to do so and that arrangements for consultation and representation of different internal groups were adequate. It was entirely consistent with this that emphasis in the 1979 Act was placed on 'due regard' to groups within the professions, and that the MP who wanted more substantial educational proposals in the legislation was told that this was a matter for the professions to decide.[3] It was equally consistent that the UKCC's plan for a largely internal enquiry into pre-registration education went unchallenged. Significantly, too, when it came to a government review of the work of the Council and Boards in 1989, the instruction was to examine questions of efficiency, but to take the principle of self-regulation as a given.

This did not, of course, mean that the 1980s' Conservative governments were content, as earlier governments had been, to defer to professions or to hold them in high regard. New Right philosophies, hostile towards the growth of the welfare state, distrusted the public sector professions for their drain on the public purse, and indeed were giving much attention to ways to control health care more closely. There were direct attempts to question the monopolistic character of professions, to bring them into the ambit of deregulation thinking, but these did not gain favour.[4] Instead, government eyes in the 1980s were focused on change at the point of care delivery. Attention first turned to new, industrial-style general managers whom, it was hoped, would question professional practice and introduce greater efficiency and value for money. The focus then shifted towards establishing an internal market, which it was hoped would create new incentives to change practice through consumer choice, and where performance criteria could be written into contracts. In the period building up to the NHS and Community Care Act 1990, and for some time after, PSR itself was all but ignored.

It was not being ignored altogether by the wider public, however. Individuals (fuelled by a government beginning to emphasise consumer choice in all spheres) were starting to question public services and expect more from them, and deference towards the professions was declining. Organised groups working on behalf of patients and service users were becoming more vociferous.[5] Media coverage of cases involving doctors whose actions appeared to put patients' lives and wellbeing at risk was starting to mount, and to call into question in particular the operation of the GMC. In the early 1980s, Nigel Spearing MP had attempted to get a legislative change to definitions of professional misconduct.[6] It is probably too strong to characterise the 1980s as the decade of the 'patients' revolt'[7] but certainly there was a noticeable increase in questioning of what might be expected from a professional. There was also questioning of whether the medical profession in particular had the will and the structures to give an effective response.

Piecemeal legislation

A number of issues relating to the regulation of health professions began to appear on the legislative agenda in the early years of the 1990s. There was little option, for example, but to find time for new legislation for the Council and National Boards, following the first review. As Chapter 5 has shown, however, the civil servants worked hard behind the scenes to keep the changes of the 1992 Act to the barest minimum, and certainly the government of the day was reluctant to include anything that might be regarded as controversial. There was also the matter, in an era of 'consumer choice', of the growing popularity of alternative or complementary medicine. Should there be more of a regulatory framework here? Time was found for legislation to create registers in the mid-1990s, for both osteopaths and chiropractors.[8] The question of poor performance of doctors was the subject of a Department of Health enquiry, and new procedures for dealing with poor performance in medicine were enshrined in legislation in 1995.[9] All this took valuable parliamentary time. When others started to press to be included in the list of professions regulated under the Council for Professions Supplementary to Medicine (CPSM) – in a context where many of those working in this sphere felt that legislation, first passed in 1960, now needed updating – the government called a halt.[10] In February 1995 it took the decision to commission a firm of management consultants to undertake an overall review of the regulatory machinery for the professions supplementary to medicine. JM Consulting won the contract. Twenty years on from the Merrison enquiry, in a very different climate, management consultants were about to offer an entirely new consideration of what PSR was and what it should entail.[11]

A new broom ...

JM Consulting were working in uncharted territory. It was near impossible to find their way between the myriad views about how regulation should be adapted and changed. The only answer seemed to be to start from first principles. In doing so, the consultants brought public protection to the fore as the single and central purpose of PSR. The public should be able to distinguish between a practitioner who was appropriately qualified and one who was not. Since opportunities for practice in a marketplace outside the NHS were increasing, the need for this was becoming more pressing. Anyone could offer services as a physiotherapist, for example. It was clear to the consultants that public protection required the legislation to be changed to give unambiguous protection of title.

The important thing to be guaranteed, JM Consulting argued, was a threshold level of safe practice. It was not necessarily the business of a regulatory body to set standards beyond the basic – professional associations might well be better employed dealing with matters of specialisms and more advanced practice. In maintaining safe practice, however, the regulatory body, they felt, had to get involved not only in removing practitioners who were not fit to practice but in administering lesser penalties to bring practitioners back into line. Professional associations, however, might be better placed to develop codes of conduct. Regulatory bodies should not set 'aspirational standards' nor should they get in the way of service development. They should intervene only when there is a threat to public protection. The individual occupational boards of the CPSM, the consultants felt, were both straying beyond the basic business of regulation and often 're-inventing the wheel'. The Council could and should take a stronger lead. Its work should be achieved and the boundaries of that work should be established by constantly asking 'is the public at risk?' To debate such a question effectively, the vision, potentially at least, was that employers and education commissioners should sit on a newly formed Council for Health Professions alongside members of the public and professionals, and be part of this dialogue. The consultants considered whether non-professionals should actually be in the majority on the new Council, believing that this 'could be a logical development of current trends in public policy on professional regulation'. This, however, was 'too radical a change at this stage'.[12]

Placed alongside the Merrison report, the contrast is a sharp one. Merrison's view of PSR had been one where the profession itself took on the responsibility of maintaining a register, policing standards of entry to and removal from it *in order to* protect the public. The JM Consulting team turned this on its head. A register was vital but they had an altogether less benign view of the disinterest of the professions. Public protection required a balancing of the interests of the profession with those of employers, service users, educationalists and others. What advanced the profession did not necessarily advance the public. And advancing the profession was the business of professional associations, not of the regulatory body.

The government gave broad endorsement to the report and seemed set to legislate for a new Council for Health Professions.[13] There was no wide public debate about this major change of thinking, however. Nor was there any clarity about where this change was going to leave the other health professions. Was the new thinking to be applied more generally? Was the idea that the inclusive-sounding Council of Health Professions at some later date was to bring in the UKCC and perhaps the GMC also? Nothing more emerged into the public arena before a change of government in May 1997.[14]

Labour – same or different?

Labour came to power after eighteen years in opposition. In a flurry of White Papers and consultative documents over its first eighteen months in office, it was clear that it wished to distance itself from the marketised forms of health and welfare service delivery of the previous governments, and to institute something new. Modernising government, social services and the NHS were all on the agenda. The aim was to implant a new kind of culture across the whole range of public services with a much stronger commitment to quality on the part of all those delivering and managing care. National service frameworks for clinical care delivery, mechanisms for strong clinical governance at local level and new kinds of inspection and monitoring of clinical performance were unveiled.

Where was PSR to stand in all this? To be sure, modification to PSR was not the top of the government's agenda, nor did this capture imaginations in the same way as primary care groups and trusts, or the work of the new National Institute for Clinical Excellence or the Commission on Health Improvement. But the message was nonetheless clear. In December 1997 the NHS White Paper envisaged that there would be developments to 'build on and strengthen the existing systems of professional self-regulation'.[15] The following summer a consultative document on quality, coming after considerable media attention to apparent failures in clinical care, particularly by doctors,[16] commented that public concerns about the effectiveness of regulation needed to be addressed. Rather more ominously it continued:

> The organisation of professional self-regulation still owes more to history than to the needs of patients in a modern NHS. The challenge now is for the Government and clinical professionals to work together to modernise that framework so that it is fit for the next century.[17]

As with its predecessor, it was the day-to-day health care delivery which was the central focus of government attention, but it was clear that PSR was not going to be allowed to act as a brake to the projected overall change.

By the time that these words on PSR were published, the government had to hand, though it had not yet made public, a review of the regulatory legislation for nursing, midwifery and health visiting.[18] JM Consulting had once again won the contract; the consultants began background work in July 1997 and in January 1998 they issued the interim report referred to at the outset of this chapter. Both in this and in the final report, they drew on their prior work on professions supplementary to medicine. Once again, there was the view that public safety required strong protection of title, and that regulation should be about threshold safety standards of practice. Much of the work regulatory bodies had been doing beyond initial registration – and this was particularly true of the UKCC – should shift, they felt, to professional associations. It is worth looking at the arguments in more detail.

The JM Consulting reports

JM Consulting's interim report in January 1998 was issued with a request for feedback from interested parties. The nursing press treated the event with some relish. The report was a 'grand plan to kick the bureaucratic stuffing out of nursing ruling bodies' proclaimed the *Nursing Times*. It went on to summarise the argument as urging that the UKCC should be 'less hidebound, less picky and less amateurish', and to quote Jim Port, the lead consultant, as saying that the Council meeting his team had attended 'seemed locked in a time warp'.[19] An editorial in the *Nursing Standard* underlined some of the management consultants' criticisms – 'who could argue . . . that there is a tendency to tribalism within the nursing profession? Who could but agree that our register is overly complex, or that the array of titles merging from postregistration education programmes is confusing?' While the editorial acknowledged that JM Consulting had praise for certain areas of work – on the scope of professional practice, for example – the overall charge that regulation protected its own rather than protecting the public was, the writer felt, not at all easy to counter.[20]

The consultants had been at work for just four months. Having already carried out the professions supplementary to medicine review, they had something of a head start. But they had to come to terms with the complex relationships between Council and Boards and with the detail of the functioning of the professional conduct and fitness to practice machinery, which was on an altogether different scale. They had listened, however, not only to those working inside the regulatory machinery, but to civil servants, employers, trade unions and professional associations. They concluded that the system had grown complex and cumbersome. It was losing sight of the fundamentals.

When it came to a final report, echoing their interim report and their previous study of professions supplementary to medicine, they argued that the legislation 'fails explicitly to put public protection as its paramount purpose' and that there was 'unhelpful complexity' that 'works against the principles of simplicity and transparency and reduces the flexibility to cope with future changes'.[21] While there was much good practice, what was needed was new legislation and a culture change to go with it. These should be based on a clearer understanding of the central purpose of regulation.

> The purpose of the statutory body is to protect the public through setting and monitoring standards of professional practice, education and conduct for nurses and midwives; and to influence the development of these professions in the public interest. The accountability of the Council in all these matters is to the public first, and secondly to the professions that establish and fund it.[22]

The consultants found a number of things to admire. Council deserved credit for the continuing professional development aspects of PREP, for example, and for the way it had acted to counter suspicions that the disciplinary machinery worked to defend practitioners. They accepted key parts of the Council's submission – the matter of placing a duty on employers to check registration status was a key example. They were sharply critical, however, of work on standards, arguing that it had been done piecemeal and was inaccessible to those not closely involved;[23] they wanted to see clear outcome standards in pre-registration education and better ways of ensuring they were achieved. They envisaged less prescriptiveness and more delegation in relation to post-registration education. They suggested guidelines on offences and sanctions, more collaboration with other regulatory bodies and new powers, including a power of mediation in matters of professional conduct. On the mattter of nursing and midwifery working together, the reviewers acknowledged the concerns of midwives that present arrangements were not facilitating 'genuine multi-professional working within the Council'[24] and stressed that any replacement body should bring 'full participation and parity of membership and esteem between the two professions'.[25] More particularly, they recommended the establishment of a Nursing and Midwifery Council, with equal numbers of nurses and midwives among its elected membership, and with rules of procedure to ensure that neither profession could be outvoted by the other on matters specific to their profession. For the first phase of the new Council's life, they felt there should also be professional Directors of Midwifery Regulation and of Nursing Regulation.[26] A streamlined register, with two live Parts – Registered Nurse and Registered Midwife – and no separate registration for health visitors was a further key recommendation.[27]

In proposing a new-style Council, the consultants envisaged a small body – of no more than twenty-seven members, and with lay members being at least one third. It should work strategically, and utilise consumer and practitioner panels for all parts of the work of fitness to practise. There should be Council offices in all four countries, probably with further regional offices in England to ensure close contact with employers, education providers and registrants.[28] The consultants wanted to see a streamlined register, a conduct manual giving registrants a single coherent document to guide their practice, greater protection of title and power to make rules for clinical supervision. Stronger financial and efficiency measures, imposed on Boards, should be extended to the new Council. The government should carry out a short review with the aim of establishing a practical scheme for regulation of health care assistants.

The report was substantial, and the list of proposals was long. The recommendations and the rationale underlying them amounted to a radical re-positioning of statutory regulation. In effect, though the consultants were too politically wise to put it in this way, the new model amounted to taking the 'self' out of self-regulation.

Working towards legislation

The JM Consulting review disappeared into the Department of Health in the summer of 1998.[29] The Queen's Speech in November, introducing the legislative programme for the next session, announced provision for a new Health Bill. Baroness Hayman, in the government's address in reply to the Queen's Speech, echoed the earlier White Paper in its promise of working with the professions and others 'to strengthen the existing systems of professional self-regulation by ensuring that they are open, responsive and publicly accountable'.[30] It was by now apparent that, faced with lack of parliamentary time, and a queue of health professions wanting legislative amendment, the government proposed to insert a clause in the Health Bill that would give it flexible powers to amend primary legislation by Order, that is without full-scale parliamentary debate.[31] Despite assurances that the government's intentions were 'benign', and were intended to ease 'the legislative logjam' in respect of professional regulation,[32] regulatory bodies in the health field were uneasy. Was the aim quietly to erode the fundamental principles of professional self-regulation? The statutory bodies worked closely together, taking joint action, sharing legal advice and information and co-ordinating action to lobby for limits to the scope of the legislation.[33]

When the Health Bill was introduced into the House of Lords at the end of January 1999, provision for Ministers to change primary legislation governing the regulation of the health professions by Order was included as expected. On 9 February, the JM Consulting report on the review of the Nurses, Midwives and Health Visitors Act was finally released, together with an announcement of the government's acceptance of its main recommendations. The report was described as 'sensible'; it was felt that since there had been widespread consultation during the course of its production, there was no need to consult further. There were just four topics on which the government wished to see further comment.[34] An amendment would be made to the Health Bill to make provision for the abolition of the existing statutory bodies and so open the way for the creation of a new

Council on the lines that JM Consulting had suggested. A brief review of the possible regulation of health care assistants was also announced, with a target report date of December 1999.

Intense activity between the statutory bodies on the need to limit the scope of the order-making power found a number of sympathetic ears in the House of Lords, and there were many proposed amendments during the Bill's passage through Parliament.[35] By the time the Bill became an Act, these amendments had made clear that the core functions of regulation would not be transferred between bodies or to any new body that was created, that a lay majority would not be imposed on the Council or any of the other regulatory bodies, and that the existing relationships that several of the bodies had with the Privy Council would remain unaltered.[36] A further set of lobbying activities was mounted by midwives concerned by the government's decision to give equal rights of membership on the new Council and its committees to nurses, midwives and also health visitors. It was a move that seriously compromised the JM Consulting model for parity between nursing and midwifery. The main aim of the lobbyists was to secure a Midwifery Board within the new Council, with statutory responsibility for determining conditions of admission to midwifery training, pre- and post-registration midwifery education, advice for midwives on professional conduct and Rules for midwifery practice.[37] Here, as in relation to the other amendments, government resistance was coupled with reassurances that detailed arrangements for any new regulatory bodies would be the subject of on-going consultation with interested bodies, and that there would be opportunities for members to scrutinise the resulting Orders when finally introduced.[38]

The Health Bill passed into law in June 1999. The previous month the five statutory bodies and the four health departments had met to discuss issues of implementation. A Change Management Group was set up to be chaired by John Wynn Owen,[39] and a Legislative Proposals Group established to work on drafting with the aid of a rather larger Reference Group. Overall, the professions had cause to be pleased. Government officials had worked hard to bring them on board; they had listened to concerns and reiterated that professional regulation, as the professions themselves acknowledged, needed to be modernised. However, for anyone with memories of the skeleton legislation of 1979, the work of the shadow bodies, the fundamental questions that needed to be addressed, and the sheer logistics of regulating so large and so diverse a group, it must have seemed like a rather uncomfortable action replay.

Could it be said, in the light of these events, that the question of self-regulation of professions had been fully aired? There had been more correspondence on this one matter of regulation than on the rest of the Health Bill put together, was the wry comment of one member of the House of Commons.[40] And yet, notwithstanding the volume of debate, a listener in the public gallery might have been hard-pressed to follow what had happened. Just what was the significance of questions about accountability to the Department of Health or the Privy Council,[41] or debates about negative or affirmative procedures?[42] If those taking part in the debate had been briefed by the regulatory bodies – as they certainly had

– what did this say on the matter of protection of the public? Was there another view on all this?

Indeed there was. The National Consumer Council (NCC) had been gathering information about regulatory bodies in health and asking just what kind of protection present mechanisms of PSR offered to users of services, and how these mechanisms linked – or failed to link – with voluntary registration and NHS regulatory procedures (clinical governance for example) at local level. In the summer of 1999, they were ready to report. The process of simply amassing and comparing information about the statutory bodies – how they were composed, what powers they had – and setting this alongside what might be other components of an overall system for public protection raised important questions. The NCC judged the position to be

> a patchwork of varying arrangements for different professions, differences in regulation between public and independent sectors and legislation governing many regulatory bodies which has not caught up with changes in public demand or with current health care practices.[43]

The NCC's concerns contrasted with the matters being so avidly debated between the professions and the government. They focused on the vulnerable public, and included problems of regulation in relation to team care, lack of regulation in the private sector, the continuation of unregulated groups, the grey areas where practitioners who should not do so nonetheless continued to practise and, not least, the sheer difficulty for consumers of finding their way around the system. The NCC recommended better links between different types of regulation, and consideration of a 'one-door' complaints system, more open business and more participation of lay members.[44]

The NCC set out a list of fourteen principles which, they felt, should underpin the regulation of health professionals (see Figure 9.1). For the long term, however, the NCC felt that a 'radical rethink' was needed. They questioned whether promoting professional work and regulating it did not represent a conflict of interests. They started thinking from what they saw as a consumer perspective and made clear that they were working further on the topic of regulation.[45] It was perhaps a sign of the times that a consumer lobby of this sort should have emerged. There was a distinct gap between the kinds of concern it was expressing and the matters being dealt with by legislative amendment. The place the NCC might play in future in the shaping of new regulatory arrangements remains to be seen.[46]

Conclusion

Governments of the 1980s and 1990s have been reforming governments as far as health services and the work of health services professionals are concerned. Yet they have not seen the long-established institutions of self-regulation as a matter that should be at the top of the political agenda. By the autumn of 1999, the events

- Clear and intelligible statements of principle and measurable standards – a Code that addresses consumer concerns, and identifies intended outcomes
- Good publicity, with maximum education and information directed at professionals and consumers
- Public accountability and transparency through reporting on the criteria for screening and handling complaints, the nature of, and resolution of complaints
- The ability to command public confidence
- Separation in operation and control from the institutions of the profession, with adequate resources, funded so the objectives are not jeopardised
- Regular review and updating in the light of changing circumstances and expectation
- The development of performance indicators to measure the scheme's effectiveness, with input at all stages from lay people and consumers
- Substantial representation (nationally and locally) of consumer, lay and other public interests on governing bodies or councils and committees, showing how various interests are balanced
- Clear criteria for appointment of lay and consumer representatives
- Strong external consultation and involvement with all relevant stakeholders in its design and operation
- Monitoring compliance through investigation of complaints and research
- Clear, accessible and well-publicised complaints procedures, and independence where resolving complaints
- Fairness to complainants and professionals, with appeal provisions for both and having regard to the wider public interest
- An adequate range of meaningful sanctions for non-observance of the standards, including interim measures to suspend registration or restrict practice while complaints are being considered, and reconsideration of the standard of proof required

Figure 9.1 The National Consumer Council Framework for Regulation.
Source: National Consumer Council 1999, pp. 30–2.

outlined in this chapter suggest, PSR seemed to be in process of being changed without being fundamentally challenged in public debate in parliament. The government repeatedly reassured the professions of its willingness to consult them on change, yet the public interest that the NCC made clear is at stake in the matter of setting and maintaining the standards of those who work as health professionals was not emerging in any clear way. Labour, like its predecessor, certainly wanted to change professional performance. It had introduced an array of new mechanisms in the Health Act to do so. It had laid down a series of strategic directions for nursing that had clear implications for the directions of regulatory decision-making. But the government was content to work behind the scenes with the professions on the question of their existing self-regulatory machinery, as though it were only a question of technical tidying. By muting the debate in the way that successive governments had done, the shadowy status of PSR, noted at the outset of this study, has been confirmed. There continues to be a distinct lack of public understanding and debate about how self-regulation works, how far it has or has not changed over the years and what the public really want and expect of the health care professions.

Notes (see Appendix 5)

1 For a more extended account of this, see Davies, C., 'The demise of professional self-regulation – a moment to mourn?', in Lewis, G., S. Gewirtz and J. Clarke (eds) *Rethinking Social Policy*, London, Sage, 2000.

2 *Report of the Committee of Enquiry into the Regulation of the Medical Profession* (Merrison Report) Cmnd 6018, London, HMSO, 1975.

3 Reading MP, Gerald Vaughan bemoaned the Bill's lack of detail on the educational reforms recommended by Briggs. *Parliamentary Debates* [Commons], 13 November 1978, 958, cols 37 and 55.

4 See the discussion by Margaret Stacey on this, citing government work on restrictive practices, fair trading and monopolies, Stacey, M., *Regulating British Medicine. The General Medical Council*, Chichester, John Wiley and Sons, 1992, p. 181. Right-wing analyses of professions, for example, Green, D., *Which Doctor? A critical analysis of the professional barriers to free competition in health care*, London, Institute of Economic Affairs, 1985, were not taken up.

5 In discussing how the GMC should be financed, Merrison noted that 'MIND (National Association for Mental Health) commented that the "financing of the regulatory body should not depend on members' contributions, or it becomes impossible to avoid the suspicion of the body's being concerned with professional rather than public interest." ' *Report of the Committee of Inquiry into the Regulation of the Medical Profession*, para. 426. The argument did not commend itself to Merrison, although it is one that continues to surface, most recently through the National Consumer Council (see note 43).

6 See Chapter 5, page 106. For more details see Allsop, J. and L. Mulcahy *Regulating Medical Work*, Buckingham, Open University Press, 1995, pp. 84–5. Stacey, *Regulating British Medicine*. pp. 182–5.

7 See Stacey, *Regulating British Medicine*, chapter 13.

8 A General Osteopathic Council was set up under legislation in 1993 and a General Chiropractic Council in 1994.

9 Department of Health, *Maintaining Medical Excellence: Review of Guidance on Doctors' Performance* (Chair: Sir Kenneth Calman), London, Department of Health, 1995; Medical (Poor Performance) Act, 1995.

10 In 1995 the CPSM covered chiropodists, dietitians, medical laboratory scientific officers, occupational therapists, orthoptists, physiotherapists and radiographers.

11 JM Consulting, *The Regulation of Health Professions: report of a review of the Professions Supplementary to Medicine Act (1960) with recommendations for new legislation*. Bristol, JM Consulting Ltd, 1996.

12 Ibid., para. 8.19a.
13 Government indicated its acceptance in July 1996 in an Executive Letter EL[96]67. Work was done in drafting a Council for Health Professions Bill but it was never publicly released.
14 Two further issues were important in this period. One had to do with the government's commitment to vocational qualifications and its hope that these would grow to encompass all levels of skill, including professional skill. The health professions, including the nursing, midwifery and health visiting professions, had not been enthusiastic and largely resisted government pressure on this (see Chapter 3). Social work, where there was no strictly comparable independent regulatory machinery, had gone along this route. See Weinstein, J., 'The use of National Occupational Standards in professional education', *Journal of Interprofessional Care*, 12(2), 1998, pp. 169–79. Also potentially important was new regulatory thinking in social work and social care where a 'joined-up' Labour government was to prove reluctant to read across. See Davies, C., 'Rethinking regulation in the health professions in the UK: institutions, ideals and identities' in Hellberg, I., M. Saks and C. Benoit (eds) *Professional Identities in Transition: Cross-Cultural Dimensions*. University of Gothenburg, 1999.
15 *The New NHS. Modern, Dependable*. Cm 3807, London, the Stationery Office, 1997, para. 6.15.
16 High-profile media criticism of the medical profession was particularly marked throughout 1998. A television programme in March (*Dispatches*, Channel 4) strongly questioned GMC disciplinary decisions, following which there was continued newspaper scrutiny. The lengthy GMC proceedings concerning paediatric heart surgery at Bristol Royal Infirmary, accompanied by protests and reports of parent anguish at babies' deaths attracted particular attention. The GMC's ruling in May was followed by a government decision to institute a public enquiry. The case was continuing to attract attention as this book went to press and was being widely regarded as the watershed event that strengthened government resolve to demand more in the way of information on and demonstrations of professional competence.
17 DoH, *A First Class Service: Quality in the new NHS*, London, DoH, 1998, para. 3.47.
18 Strictly speaking, the government was no longer able to review the UKCC since it had been de-designated as a non-departmental public body. This was clarified in a letter from J. Dorling, Department of Health to Sue Norman, Chief Executive and Registrar, dated 22 August 1996. It would have made no sense to review the National Boards alone, however. A review of the legislation enabled it to encompass the working of all five bodies.
19 Naish, J., 'Marching orders' *Nursing Times*, 14 January, 2(94), 1998, p. 18. The report also hit the national press, see Brindle, D., 'Tooth and claw', *Guardian*, 11 February 1998, p. 19 where views of the RCN and UNISON were sought.
20 Editorial, *Nursing Standard*, 14 January, 12(17), 1998, p. 1.
21 JM Consulting, *The Regulation of Nurses, Midwives and Health Visitors. Report on a Review of the Nurses, Midwives and Health Visitors Act 1997*, paras 12a, 12f. The report was released, as the text below indicates, in February 1999, together with NHS circular HSC 1999/030. Quotations here and in the following paragraphs are drawn from the thirty-page summary which preceded the main report, but was bound together with it.
22 Ibid., para. 17.
23 Ibid., para. 72.
24 Ibid., para. 12(d).
25 Ibid., para. 20.
26 Ibid., paras 22, 27(d), 35(b and c), 43, 48, 106.
27 Ibid., para. 62. See also paras 10–11. Health visitors were regarded as a 'specialist professional group within nursing'. Their 'exceptional treatment' under current legislation was deemed by JM Consulting as inappropriate.
28 Ibid., para. 108. It was acknowledged that the review had come at a time of renewed

attention to devolution and constitutional change. For this reason, if no other, there would need to be flexibility in any new legislation (para. 9).

29 One part of the government's dilemma was how to find time for it in the busy legislative programme. Another, as noted, was that devolution was once more on the agenda. Removing the National Boards at a time when devolved powers were actually being put in place in Scotland and Wales would be unlikely to be politically acceptable. It was widely assumed that devolution was the reason why publication of the report was delayed.

30 *Parliamentary Debates* [Lords], 595, 2 December 1998, col. 498. See also Secretary of State for Health, *The New NHS. Modern. Dependable,* para. 7.15.

31 This order-making power, known as the Henry VIII clause, enables the modification of primary legislation by secondary legislation. See Chapter 2, note 9.

32 CC/98/46, para. 10.

33 The GMC, the CPSM, the General Dental Council, the General Optical Council, the Royal Pharmaceutical Society of Great Britain and the UKCC all worked together closely during the passage of legislation.

34 Health Service Circular 99/030. The questions were: Should the Council's duty to collaborate with other stakeholders be reciprocal? Should the title 'nurse' be protected? Should there be a new sanction of reprimand, based on a lower level of proof? Should other interested parties be able to appeal misconduct or restoration decisions?

35 Baroness Hayman proved to be particularly sympathetic on this matter and was instrumental in introducing key amendments.

36 Legislation for nursing, midwifery and health visiting requires Secretary of State approval for key constitutional and financial matters, whereas formal responsibility in the case of medicine, for example, is to the Privy Council. The Privy Council, originally a body of advisors to the monarch does not play a major part in public affairs. Senior government and opposition members are appointed as Privy Councillors. They retain their title for life and the Privy Council meets only rarely to mark great occasions of state. In practice, if there are disputes, the health department is usually involved. Stacey regards the Privy Council as simply 'passing on messages from health ministers'. Stacey, *Regulation of British Medicine*, p. 218.

37 Two amendments concerning the position of midwifery under a future statutory structure were put forward during the committee stage in the House of Lords. In the House of Commons, four early-day motions, tabled on 15 April 1999, led to the introduction of an amendment providing for a Midwifery Board at the Standing Committee stage. See *Parliamentary Debates* [Lords], 597, 4 March 1999, cols 1844–7; *Parliamentary Debates* [Commons], Standing Committee A, 20 May 1999, cols 922–5, 928–30, 934.

38 It was not altogether clear whether the government would seek to draft separate orders for the CPSM and nursing and midwifery, though separate consultations were in train at the time of going to press.

39 Secretary of the Nuffield Trust.

40 *Parliamentary Debates* [Commons], Standing Committee A, 20 May 1999, col. 927.

41 See note 36 above.

42 For an explanation of negative and affirmative procedures in relation to statutory instruments, see Chapter 2, note 9. It was to the satisfaction of the statutory bodies that they won the right to the affirmative procedure.

43 National Consumer Council, *Self-Regulation of Professionals in Health Care*, London, NCC, 1999, p. 1.

44 The NCC report was debated at a meeting of Council on 8 September 1999. See Minute 27/99(9).

45 A further report on regulation covering both business and the professions was released by the NCC as this book went to press. See National Consumer Council, *Models of Self-Regulation,* London, NCC, 1999.

46 Since the NCC lobbied for and won the right to be consulted about any changes that might take place under the new powers of the 1999 Health Act, it is possible that it could become a more powerful player in future. It was critical of the way that government had assured the professions that it would not impose a lay majority on them.

10 Conclusion

The UKCC has travelled a considerable distance in the years since it was first established together with the four National Boards under the 1979 Act. New thinking about issues of professional conduct and ideas about giving more meaning to the concept of an active register began to take shape even before the appointed day when the shadow body handed over functions. Procedures for dealing with those who were unfit to practice on grounds of ill-health were put in place for the first time. Efforts were made to draw lessons from the cases that came forward and to open up proceedings to the public gaze much more than had occurred in earlier years. Project 2000's 'new preparation for practice' set out a framework for substantial change in an experience of education for nurses that had long been seen as deeply unsatisfactory. The work involved much lobbying and compromise given the the entanglements of education and service and the cost to the NHS of training for the professions. A decade on from the initial report, moves were once again made to carry out a major review, adjusting educational programmes with a view to responding to tensions and fitting them more closely to current health needs and to the requirements of the professions of nursing and midwifery. Establishing a post-registration framework in the face of a patchwork of provision across the UK and of employer suspicion about the potential inflexibilities and the costs of any new scheme proved elusive; yet the systems the UKCC has put in place on requirements for continuing professional development linked with periodic re-registration are recognised as highly significant, and lessons from this are being picked up in developments in medicine, dentistry and elsewhere. A name on the register today means more than it did in 1979.

This book shows how much development and change there has been over the lifetime of the first three Councils. With skeleton legislation, and unease between the constituent groups within the professions, there was much to do to put systems in place and to establish working relationships. Just how difficult that was in the context of five statutory bodies was evidenced in the protracted process of agreeing an initial strategic plan. The central focus at that time was on delivering the long-awaited report on pre-registration education and on gathering sufficient support for its proposals to enable these to go forward to Ministers. The educational agenda to an important extent overshadowed the pioneering work on devising a code of conduct and on creating an active register for more than half a million registrants. It deflected attention from reflection on the challenges of handling a more diverse and growing volume of professional conduct work and the questions this was beginning to raise about how nurses were being deployed and the role and remit of the UKCC in relation to matters of practice.

By the time of the Second Council, sitting from 1988 to 1993, new thinking was under way on internal organisation and on communication, and the government's first review of the statutory bodies was about to take place. But while in many ways the Second Council was a time of organisational upheaval, it was by no means only that. The ambitious agenda of post-registration education and practice began to be mapped out and consultations with the professions began to reveal the complexity of the issues at stake. This was the moment in which the notion of regulation *in the public interest* came more firmly to the fore, and when a start was made in refocusing the Council to be more responsive both to the professions and to the public more generally. The house style changed and important first steps were taken towards a dialogue with consumers on the work of the professions. By the end of the second term, the UKCC was altogether more outward-looking than it had been previously. It was also set, under the 1992 legislation, to become a directly elected body and to take on more responsibilities in relation to professional conduct.

The Third Council, larger and more diverse than ever before, involved people in immediate clinical practice and people with strong trade union backgrounds as well as educationalists and managers. They came into office as dissatisfaction among the professions with the new NHS was mounting, and at a time when there was more public questioning of the shortcomings of health care service provision and more criticism generally of the services that the professions were offering. Members faced a turbulent time, with hostile press and public commentary both about the style of Council's decision-making and about the nature of a number of decisions – particularly in relation to a number of restorations to the register. This Council, however, brought a more vocal and questioning stance concerning its own remit than had emerged at any point before. Significant organisational change was piloted through in 1995, and action was taken to revise professional conduct procedures in relation to restoration. This was also the Council that brought the theme of the balance between protection of the public and support for the professions to overt attention and built on previous practice to involve consumers in ways that would have been unimaginable in 1983. It was also during the time of the Third Council that the concept of standards began to be considered in a more overt way. Figure 10.1 offers a summary of the key changes of approach that have been discussed in earlier parts of this book.

A list such as this focuses on *what* the UKCC has done rather than *who* has done it and *how*. The work of PSR has been carried out with a Council membership that rose from 33 on the Shadow Council ultimately to 60 following the changes of the 1992 Act. The Shadow Council was an all appointed body, drawing from a recognised leadership in the profession. By the time of the Third Council, elections brought in more of a rank and file perspective and there was also a rising amount of lay participation.

- from a focus mainly on education . . . to a focus also on practice
- from addressing the professions . . . to a clearer focus on the public
- from expert discussions and authoritative publications . . . to greater consultation, networking and open debate
- from dealing with individual episodes of misconduct . . . to also defining issues and acting positively to promote standards
- from establishing a predefined and limited practice . . . to encouraging extended autonomy and scope
- from responding to consultation documents . . . to being more proactive in setting aspects of the health policy agenda
- from avoiding 'political' positions . . . to at times challenging health policy where it can be seen adversely to affect practice.

Figure 10.1 Transitions across three Councils

Who is available to do the work of PSR inevitably shapes the vision of what PSR is and what it can and should achieve. Self-regulation has relied on the good-will of employers to release people, and on the willing contributions of those who are retired. It is this that – at least until recent years – resulted in a membership weighted towards the most senior ranks of the professions, those who combined their own sense of public duty with their employers' acceptance that their contribution to UK-wide debates would bring the benefits of a broadened vision locally. Younger professionals, those in clinical posts, those who work part-time, or have family commitments outside work, who are in independent practice, or work for small employers, are unlikely to be directly represented on a council of the sort that has existed since 1979. Charges that the UKCC is out of touch or elitist can be traced to this. Direct financial recompense and other support may be needed in future if regulatory bodies are to get the diversity of members they require.[1] Modes of inviting potential participants through recommendation or advertisement, as well as adjustment to the roles and responsibilities they are offered also need to be examined. Whoever Council members have been, and wherever they have come from, the load that they have taken on has been substantial. Involvement in PSR has meant giving up many evenings and week-ends to prepare for meetings and for examination of professional conduct cases. Some of the current recommendations about the need for a more strategic focus to the work of Council and more use of panels[2] could serve to open up the work and to redress the unfair and unrealistic demands that regulatory work has made.

It is also important to acknowledge that what the UKCC has done it has had to do on a massive scale. Day-to-day work has been carried forward by a staff of around 100, no more than a dozen of whom at any one time are registered practitioners. Consultation and communication on policy are formidable under-takings – if ambiguity or error creep in they do so very publicly and on a massive scale. Handling comments and responses can be challenging. Managing entry to, changes in and removal from the register and operating the confirmations service for employers, involves literally thousands of queries on every working day. The update of the overseas registrations system in early 1996 marked the start of a series of changes to integrate and improve computer systems, and an automated telephone switchboard came on line later that year and allowed for a significant increase in call handling. For the majority of those working in nursing, midwifery and health visiting, such matters are vital. The UKCC's speed and efficiency in answering queries and handling registration can have a direct effect on their employment. Registrants are more likely to judge the regulatory bodies by their efficiency in relation to these matters rather than by the position Council might take on standards for education or criteria for removal and restoration.

Yet the debate that the Council has had and continues to have about the standards to be met for admisson to the register, for maintaining a position on it, removal from and restoration to it – together with the extent to which it can control or at least influence employment and deployment decisions – are crucial to the quality of care services and to public satisfaction with nursing and midwifery. On these matters, the JM Consulting report, known popularly in regulatory circles as the 'fundamental review', in some respects was perhaps not fundamental enough, or not perceived as fundamentally as its authors intended. Four issues exemplify this.[3]

Concerning the *protection of title*, the starting point for JM Consulting had been an examination of therapy professions in a context where private practice was growing and small health care businesses were getting under way either independently or in contracts with the NHS. The public, they argued, needed to be assured that any therapist they encountered had undergone the necessary training and was competent to practise. Regulatory legislation therefore had to give strong protection of the title and sanctions against anyone using the occupational title unless they were on the register.[4] Midwifery, they now noted, had this clear protection of title; should it not be extended to nursing? It was one of the matters on which the government decided to consult and the outcome to date is unknown.

On the one hand this looks a retrograde step. The question has arisen at a time when employers and a number of practitioners too are looking for greater flexibility to practise across traditional boundaries and to provide team care. The UKCC has eschewed close definition of tasks and acknowledged and supported flexibility in providing a framework whereby individual practitioners can extend the scope of their practice while remaining safe. This has been widely seen as a move in the right direction. On the other hand, it could be argued that the absence of this 'fundamental' of self-regulation legislation has had a negative effect. It has allowed employers to use students as labour, to substitute untrained for trained nurses, and has left the position unclear to the public just how much input from a registered nurse they are receiving. Would protection of title give a necessary area of power to the profession and greater transparency and protection to the public – or would it mean rigidity and loss of employer freedom? The way to *re-balance powers* between the employer, the public and the profession is by no means clear.

Nor are matters entirely clear on the *establishment of standards*. Just what standards are at the point of registration and beyond, and the form in which they are to be expressed in a changed and still changing context, requires more debate. The consultants were strongly critical of a 'piecemeal' approach and of confusing terminology. They wanted to see a clear threshold standard of safe practice at the point of registration. They wanted codification of the variety of guidance documents about standards in practice, and argued that standards beyond this point were not a question of safety in the same way and need not necessarily be the business of a regulatory body at all.[5] Over the lifetime of the UKCC, however, both its own understanding of the term 'standards' and that in the wider environment have undergone a number of changes.

In the 1990s, for example, there has been a rapprochement between the professions and the vocational qualifications movement, and a greater acceptance on the part of a number of professions in the health field and elsewhere that pre-registration education and training needs not only to specify learning outcomes but to be more clearly competence-based. Yet with such education now firmly in the higher education sector, how is this to be achieved and what adjustments to quality assurance systems are needed? To take one example, full registration at the point of qualification – something that made sense under a hospital-based nurse training – may need to change. The now acknowledged period of mentoring and supervised practice perhaps demands a form of provisional/probationary registration as in medicine. Then there is the matter of standards beyond registration. The UKCC has taken an immense step in setting its continuing professional development standard for maintaining eligibility to practice. It would be the first to acknowledge that this is not a direct guarantee of continuing practice competence, of the form, for example, that has been recently mooted for medicine. Whether direct and continued competency testing is or should be acceptable to professionals, whether it is logistically possible to apply it given the numbers involved, are important and at present unanswered questions. An alternative route may well be to ensure that the conditions are in place in employment settings, through clinical supervision or other means, to enable practitioners to review and develop their practice. We have perhaps reached a time when more active management, through clinical governance, can and should fulfil a role that in the past has been left to the individual professional alone. The point here is not to make alternative recommendations to those of JM Consulting, but to indicate the issues of principle, not only for nursing and midwifery but for the regulation of professions more broadly, that their recommendations have highlighted but not necessarily explored in full.

Similar points may be made in relation to recommendations on *the machinery of professional conduct* and its mechanisms and procedures. Chapter 5 gave an indication of the complexity of the processes, the reasoning that lay behind reluctance to define misconduct narrowly, the continuing efforts to review the implications of cases and the way in which particular cases generated widespread disquiet and calls for life bans for some offenders. JM Consulting made a wide range of recommendations here, some procedural but some more far-reaching.

They suggested restructuring the Code so that offences could be linked to specific clauses. They took on an issue the UKCC had encouraged them to grapple with in recommending procedures for poor performance as well as misconduct. They called for a mediation approach for certain cases 'where no serious threat to the public is involved'. Several of these suggestions, however, blur the line between matters of employer discipline and matters of professional discipline which the UKCC has repeatedly sought to draw. Does it make sense to use the very costly professional conduct machinery unless there is a real issue of public safety where the practitioner's very right to practice is at stake?[6] There is an underlying and unanswered question here about the extent to which, and the ways in which, contemporary professional practice needs to be monitored by the individual professional, by peers, managers and employers in the workplace and by a statutory body. Some might want to argue that less rather than more should come forward to be processed through the machinery of professional conduct.

Finally, there is the matter of *sharing regulation* – between professional and lay people and between adjacent occupations and groups within occupations. The professions' unease about the potential extent of lay representation is reflected in their successful lobbying to ensure that any future regulatory councils should not have a lay majority. This is notwithstanding the UKCC's record on developing and increasing lay involvement in the different areas of its business (see Chapter 8), and the recognition of the value that lay perspectives can bring to decisions about matters of professional conduct, for example. The question of what constitutes a branch within a profession and what constitutes a different profession and how both gain a voice in regulation also continues to dog the debate. JM Consulting took a strong line on a role at the centre and integration and sharing in their review of the professions supplementary to medicine legislation, but a different one in relation to midwifery and nursing. The question is how to devise a structure in which real difference can not only be aired but at times fostered and developed – while at the same time making the most of the commonalities that exist and avoiding duplication in establishing and maintaining standards. Unifying and simplifying organisational arrangements is vital for a public confused by the array of regulatory structures and divisions between professions, several of which contribute to the quality of their care, as the NCC has pointed out. It is also important for the education providers and for practitioners themselves, faced at present with multiple, overlapping and sometimes conflicting requirements for monitoring and review. Establishing organisational forms that can nourish stakeholder dialogue and work strategically enough to give professionals what they feel is the right mix of freedom and control is the key challenge for the decades to come.

Behind the changes in the UKCC and the calls for reform from different quarters is an even more fundamental and still unanswered question of what it means to be a professional as the twenty-first century opens, what level of autonomy and clinical feedom professionals should be granted and what role they should play in the wider professional arena. The 'postwar settlement' that put professionals (or more accurately in the health case, doctors) at the heart of the policy process and granted them autonomy and deferred to their expertise both in the consulting room and at the policy table has been overtaken by events.[7] Merrison's argument that the medical profession should maintain the register and police its members because it is the only group that has the knowledge and skills and because it can be trusted to do so – looks increasingly outmoded and unacceptable. Yet it is not at all clear what is being or what should be put in its place. Is it a contradiction to ask a profession both to improve its practice and at the same time to regulate its members in order to protect the public? Interestingly, sociological commentators, ready in the 1970s to challenge professional power and to accuse professions of using PSR to protect their own interests, are now beginning to be concerned that the pendulum has swung too far against the professions in trying to respond to questions such as this.[8] What is needed is a new contract between the state, the professions and the public, one in which the rights and obligations of all parties are rethought. It is clear that the current mix of regulatory powers in medicine by no means offers a model that others should emulate.

The situation is further complicated by the fact that nursing, midwifery and the professions called 'supplementary to medicine' won the form but not the substance of PSR that doctors achieved. The medical profession has always been in a more powerful position *vis-à-vis* government and employers. The history of nursing and to some extent midwifery, too, is of efforts to use the regulatory machinery in order to win something of the control over education and practice that the doctors have always enjoyed. They have by no means always been successful. The Briggs Committee recognised this in their argument that nursing education in particular needed to be freed from service and the nursing and midwifery professions and institutional structures needed to be more united if they were ever to exercise a proper degree of professional leadership and be able to exert an influence on policy.[9]

Following the 1999 Health Act, we are poised to see some very different regulatory institutions in relation to nursing and midwifery and the professions supplementary to medicine, and perhaps in relation to medicine too. These new institutions are likely to be ones that are consciously designed to bring stake-holders further into the standards debate and to create a stakeholder dialogue at the very heart of professional regulation. Those who take part in such institutions in the future, however, deserve to be provided with a better understanding of the regulatory task that they are asked to undertake, and of the balances it needs to hold between public protection and practitioner support, than is currently available or is likely to be clarified by the use of the Order-making powers of the new legislation. Nearly a decade ago, Margaret Stacey concluded her study of the regulation of medicine with a call for a new committee of enquiry into regulation – a new Merrison, she implied – for the health field as a whole.[10] Such an enquiry would need to bring together a diversity of representatives of public and profes-sions, employer and trade union interests. It would need to be prepared to create a dialogue between interests, to disseminate its ideas widely among practitioners and public and to adapt and develop in the light of that dissemination. It would need to consider developments in related fields and have power to examine other forms of regulation that professionals at present experience. It would be a route to a new exploration of principles of professional regulation fit for the twenty-first century. There can be no greater tribute to the work of the statutory bodies in nursing, midwifery and health visiting than that others attend to and reflect on the lessons to be learned from their struggles to uphold standards of health and health care.

Notes

1 The NCC makes this point in relation specifically to lay and consumer involvement, but it applies to members of the professions regulated also. See *Self-Regulation of Professionals in Health Care*, London, NCC, 1999, p. 42.
2 See JM Consulting, *The Regulation of Nurses, Midwives and Health Visitors. Report on a review of the Nurses Midwives and Health Visitors Act 1997*, Bristol, JM Consulting, 1999, esp. para. 4.91.
3 Left out of account in this discussion is the question of devolution and the nature of the regulatory presence in the four countries. It is widely believed that this delayed publication of JM Consulting's report. The reviewers did not engage closely with the proposals put forward and the matter remains to be settled (see Chapter 3, note 110).
4 JM Consulting, *The Regulation of Health Professions: Report of a Review of the Professions Supplementary to Medicine Act (1960) with recommendations for new legislation*. Bristol, JM Consulting, 1996, paras 431–7 and 5.40–5.49. The issue remained masked while the majority of employment was in the NHS since NHS employers are required to employ only those on the register.
5 For press coverage of the tensions that were generated between the RCN and UNISON at the idea that the former might take on this work, see Brindle, D., 'Tooth and Claw', *Guardian*, 11 February, 1998, p. 19.
6 Despite the acknowledged complexities in attributing costs, it was clear that costs have risen and are now very substantial. Estimates suggest a rise from around £4000 per case early in the 1990s to over £10,000 per case in 1998. See Minutes and Papers of Finance Committee, FC/91/26, FC/98/27.
7 See Clarke, J. and J. Newman, *The Managerial State*, London, Sage, 1997.
8 Stacey, analysing the medical profession in 1992, was pessimistic about the extent to which that profession was prepared to engage in regulatory reform. Writing at the heart of the competition era in the NHS, however, she took the view that professions can be a bulwark against an overly powerful state and that a strong and united profession can 'oppose government proposals . . . in the interests of the health of the people'. Stacey, M., *Regulating British Medicine. The General Medical Council*, Chichester, John Wiley and Sons, 1992, p. 258. The arguments in the final part of her book, including her argument for an independent enquiry, bear re-reading and are highly pertinent to the present day. For another prominent sociologist who has changed position on professions, see Freidson, E., *Professionalism Reborn*, Oxford/Cambridge, Polity Press/Blackwell, 1994.
9 *Report of the Committee on Nursing (Briggs Report)*, Cmnd 5115, London, HMSO 1972, para. 618.
10 Stacey, M., *Regulating British Medicine*, part 5.

Appendix 1
Chairmen, Presidents and senior officers[1]

Chairmen and Presidents of the United Kingdom Central Council, 1980 onwards[2]

1980–3 Dame Catherine Hall DBE OStJ HonDLitt SRN SCM FRCN
1983–5 Dame Catherine Hall DBE OStJ HonDLitt SRN SCM FRCN
1985–8 Dame Audrey Emerton DBE DL DStJ DCL RGN RM RNT
1988–93 Dame Audrey Emerton DBE DL DStJ DCL RGN RM RNT
1993–8 Dame Mary Uprichard DBE RSCN RGN RM MTD
1998– Ms Alison Norman CBE HonDSc RGN RM RHV

Chairmen of Council Committees

First Council 1983–8

- Educational Policy Advisory Committee
  1983–8 Miss Margaret Green OBE MA(Ed) BA(Hons) RGN RNT FRCN
- Midwifery Committee
  1983–8 Miss Mary Uprichard OBE RGN RSCN RM MTD
- District Nursing Joint Committee
  1983–8 Mrs Margaret Damant RGN CMB(Pt 1) RHV QN HVT DNT Soc Stud Cert
- Health Visiting Joint Committee
  1983–6 Miss Sheila Jack BA RGN RM QIDNS RHV HVT RNT
  1986–8 Miss Susan Mowat RGN RM RHV FWT
- Health Committee
  1983–5 Dame Catherine Hall DBE OStJ HonDLitt SRN SCM FRCN
  1985–8 Dame Audrey Emerton DBE RGN RM RNT
- Finance Committee
  1983–8 Mr Roger Holland MA CEng MIEE
- Committee on Research
  1983–6 Dr James Bamber MA Med PhD ABPsS APsSI

Second Council 1988–93

- Educational Policy Advisory Committee
  1988–93 Professor Margaret Green OBE MA(Ed) BA(Hons) RGN RNT FRCN
- Midwifery Committee
  1988–93 Miss Sarah Roch RGN RM MTD FPA Cert
- District Nursing Joint Committee
  1988–90 Miss Kathleen Munro RGN RM NDN RNT PWT DNT
  1990–3 Mrs Mollie Antrobus RGN DNCert PWT DN(Lond)
- Health Visiting Joint Committee
  1988–91 Ms Jean Orr MSc BA RGN RHV HVT CertEd
  1992–3 Miss Margaret McIntyre BA RGN RM RHV HVT QN
- Health Committee
  1988–93 Dame Audrey Emerton DBE DL DStJ DCL RGN RM RNT
- Finance Committee
  1988–93 Mr Roger Holland MA CEng MIEE
- Standards and Ethics Committee
  1988–93 Dame Audrey Emerton DBE DL DStJ DCL RGN RM RNT

Third Council 1993–8 [3]

- Education Committee 1993–6
  1993–6 Mrs Eileen Walker BEd(Hons) MA RGN RM RNT
- Joint Education Committee 1996–8
  1996–8 Professor Ann Lowis DipN(Lond) RGN OHNC PgCertTLT
- Midwifery Committee
  1993–6 Miss Sarah Roch RM RGN MTD FPACert
  1996–8 Miss Alison Scouller RGN RM DAM PGC(FE)
- Nursing and Community Health Care Nursing Committee
  1993–6 Professor Jean Orr BA MSc RGN RHV HVT
  1996–8 Mrs Mary Hanratty MSc BA RGN RMN RCI RNT
- Finance Committee
  1993–8 Mr Chris Grimes IPFA FCCA
- Standards and Ethics Committee 1993–6
  1993–6 Mrs Audrey Males OBE RGN ONC RCNT DipN(Lond) MIPD MIMgt BA

Registrars and Chief Executive Officers of the UKCC, 1980–98

1981–7 Miss Maude Storey RGN RM RNT FBIM
1987–94 Mr Colin Ralph MPhil RN DN(Lond)
1994–5 Miss Catherine McLoughlin (Acting) CBE RGN RMN
1995– Ms Sue Norman RGN DNCert RNT BEd(Hons)

Notes

1   Titles and honours are given for the end point of an individual's service on or employment with the UK Central Council.
2   The title of Chairman was changed to President under the 1992 Act, but the method of selection – appointment by the Council from among its members, did not alter.
3   A new structure for Council committees was established at the start of the Third Council term. This was reviewed during the internal organisation review of 1995 and a new structure was introduced in 1996.

Appendix 2
The work of registration

The UKCC's registration processes enable names to be entered on one or more parts of the register on completion of approved courses of education and training. They allow but do not require that certain additional specialised training can be recorded against the name of a practitioner. The registration department provides a confirmations service to enable employers to check the registration status of current and prospective employees, and will also on request verify registration for relevant bodies overseas.

Following the Nurses Midwives and Health Visitors Act 1979, eleven parts of the register were established (SI 1983. No. 667). Project 2000 preparation was associated with the opening of further entry routes. There are currently fifteen parts of the register into which individuals can be admitted. These cover first and second level nurses in the general, mental and learning disabilities fields, first level nurses associated with nursing sick children, midwives and health visitors. Courses of training for enrolled nurses are no longer available, but enrolled nurses can maintain their registration on the relevant parts of the register or take conversion courses to attain first level status.

In the early years of the UKCC there were around forty other qualifications which could be recorded against the name of a registrant. The number of recordable qualifications rose as the National Boards established post-qualifying courses.

Admission to the Register

The legislation recognises three types of registration process: that arising out of training in the UK, that arising out of training covered by EU Directives and that arising out of training outside the UK and in what is now termed the European Economic Area (EEA).

In regard to registration from within the UK, the formal process is that all training is approved by one of the four National Boards. On completion of training, details of the course undertaken and personal details about the applicant are transferred electronically to the UKCC. The UKCC then collates the training information with an application completed by the applicant, a declaration of good character in support of the applicant from the educational institution and a fee. When all the information is received, registration takes place. On first registration, applicants are issued with a card stating their name, professional identification number (PIN) and the date on which their registration expires. In 1988, the National Boards began to withdraw from the shared registration database. Enquirers concerned about the status of their applications for registration then found that queries could not be handled until the UKCC received confirmation of completion of training. This continues to have a negative effect on perceptions of the UKCC.

Applicants who hold a general nursing or midwifery qualification from countries covered by the European Directives are simple to handle. Sectoral directives for nurses responsible for general care (77/452/EEC, 77/453/EEC, and 89/595/EEC) and for midwives (80/154/EEC, 80/155/EEC and 89/594/EEC) set out agreed equivalents, and essentially registration occurs when it is confirmed that the applicant holds a qualification deemed by the Directive to be equivalent. Since 1989, applicants from these countries, who are not recognised in the category of midwife or general nurse, may be covered by General System directives (89/48/EEC and 92/51/EEC). The first provides for the mutual recognition by member countries of higher education diplomas awarded on completion of professional training of at least three years' duration. It came into force on 1 January 1991. The second relates to programmes of less than three years' duration or part-time equivalent. This Directive came into force on 1 January 1994. Applications from EEA countries that do not meet these requirements, and those from other countries, are more complex to deal with. Here, the UKCC's officers undertake an individual review of the applicant's pre- and post-registration education and training and determine either that the applicant is suitable for registration, or that the applicant needs to undertake some additional education or clinical practice. Guidance on the latter is available.

Renewal of registration

While a system of annual notification of intention to practise for registered midwives was inherited from former bodies for midwives, periodic renewal of registration for the professions as a whole was implemented in 1987. The initial statutory instrument under which this took place was replaced in 1995 when the UKCC introduced its requirements for continuing education as part of renewal. To remain on the live register, it is now necessary to renew registration every three years. This involves completing a Notification of Practice form, which includes a declaration that PREP requirements for continuing professional development have been met, and providing a fee. From April 2001, the UKCC aims to have in place a procedure to audit compliance with the continuing professional development standard.

The development of policy

The Registration Committee was established in 1983 as a Committee of Council which convened when necessary to consider policy matters and non-routine applications for registration. It comprised all members of Council. The Committee met frequently in early years as policies and guidelines were established on matters such as procedures for handling overseas applications and for temporary registration while applicants gained the necessary instruction and experience to meet registration requirements. Individual cases, especially ones where a Head of Institution had refused to sign the declaration of character, were part of its business. Establishing a statute to allow periodic renewal of registration proved challenging. SI 1986, No. 1345, envisaging removal for non-payment, was deemed *ultra vires* by the Lord Chancellor's Department and a replacement was only signed the day before periodic fees came into effect. Two particular controversies occurred in 1989. One was when an application was made for a judicial review in respect of Council's powers to impose periodic fees (see Chapter 3 note 29); the other was when Council successfully defended an industrial tribunal case brought under the Race Relations Act.

Towards the end of the Second Council, it was recommended that the Committee be established on a more formal basis to consider cases where a precedent had not been established, to handle appeals against officer decisions and to provide a regular review and analysis for Council of registration statistics. Its work was subsequently subsumed into that of the Education Committee. Information and procedures for overseas applicants were reviewed and substantially revised; work was under way in establishing the option of an automatic electronic confirmations service for employers, which is in operation today, and attention began to focus on the trends in registration statistics. After 1995, new arrangements needed to be in place to deal with notification of practice and steps were taken to develop new computer systems to speed up renewal processes. By 1998, large users of the confirmations service could dial in direct to the register, and internet access and other information technology developments were in hand.

Registration statistics

The work of the registration department was at its height in the early years as records were amalgamated and updated (see Chapters 2 and 3). It continues to handle a considerable volume of activity, and periodic re-registration has significantly added to this. There are currently over 20,000 admissions to the register annually; this includes a significant proportion of registrants completing subsequent registration courses and adding their names to more than one part of the register. There are also around 10,000 applications to record further qualifications. In 1997–8 the department processed almost 6,000 decisions on overseas registrations and issued 3,400 verification documents. The registration department also undertakes approximately 150,000 confirmations of registration each year.

A number of patterns and trends can be gleaned from the statistical data compiled by the UKCC. The total number of persons on the effective register in March 1998 was 637,449, and the names of approximately one-third of these appear on more than one part of the register. The number and proportion of registrants in the four countries of the UK are shown annually, and details of overseas applicants for registration are given (see *Statistical Analysis of the UKCC's Professional Register*, various dates).

Table A2.1 shows total numbers on the effective register from 1989 to 1998 and the numbers of initial registrants each year. It demonstrates a slow overall increase until 1994, followed by fluctuations and a noticeable drop in 1998. Initial registrations declined over the whole period, most dramatically in 1997 and 1998. The number of nurses, midwives and health visitors on the register at any one time is a function of overall NHS policy and decisions by NHS and other employers, together with decisions of individuals not in employment to keep or not to keep effective registration. Figures for numbers of students in pre-registration programmes are the result of local negotiations between NHS authorities and educational institutions over which the UKCC has no authority. As a result of a shortage of nurses in some areas of the UK, the number of applications from overseas handled by the registration department rose from 4,177 in 1993/4 to 5,946 in 1997/8. Preliminary statistics for 1998/99 suggested this increase had continued.

The UKCC's registration statistics enable a number of features of the overall nursing midwifery and health visiting labour force to be highlighted. Less than 10 per cent of those on the effective register, for example, are men. Less than 15 per cent are under 30 years of age and this proportion has been steadily decreasing. From 1995, with the implementation of PREP, it has started to become possible to show the field of practice of registrants. While some information can be found in the annual *Statistical Analysis of the Council's Register*, the complexity of capturing fields of practice is considerable and new ways of recording this information are planned for the year 2000.

Table A2.1 Changes in the effective register 1989–98

Year ending 31 March	Total on the register		Initial registrations	
	Number	Per cent change per annum	Number	Per cent change per annum
1989	584,447	–	–	–
1990	607,103	+4	22,350	–
1991	622,001	+2	22,164	−1
1992	633,119	+2	21,159	−5
1993	641,749	+1	20,755	−2
1994	638,361	− 0.5	20,072	−3
1995	642,951	+1	19,863	−1
1996	645,011	+0.3	19,632	−1
1997	648,240	+0.5	17,984	−8
1998	637,449	− 2	16,382	−9

Appendix 3
Professional conduct: procedures, cases and statistics

This appendix is in three parts. Section one describes the procedures used to process and consider allegations of misconduct and reports of potential unfitness to practise on health grounds. Section two provides brief case summaries (in order of mention in Chapter 5), and section three provides statistical tables. The major part of section one describes arrangements in the period immediately following the 1979 Act. Much of this still pertains, and to indicate this parts of the account are written in the present tense. Leaflets describing key features of the contemporary procedure, designed for employers and others considering bringing a complaint, are available from the UKCC. Further information can be found in R. Pyne, *Professional Discipline in Nursing Midwifery and Health Visiting*, Oxford, Blackwell, 1998 (third edition).

Section one: Procedures

The 1979 Act created a two-tier structure for professional conduct, with initial investigations undertaken by the National Boards and hearings by the Central Council. Amending legislation in 1992 brought the whole process under the remit of the Central Council.

On receipt of a complaint (either through the criminal courts upon the conviction of a registered nurse, midwife or health visitor, or as reported by colleagues, managers, patients, relatives or members of the public) the National Boards assembled the available evidence and obtained a written response to the allegations from the practitioner concerned. The matter was then passed to an Investigating Committee to decide whether the case should be referred to the PCC of the Council. Membership of an Investigating Committee was drawn from among those members of the National Board who were not also members of the Central Council, and was to include at least one member from the professional field of the practitioner under investigation.

The Investigating Committee had three possible courses of action.

- If sufficient evidence to substantiate the allegations was presented, and if the matter was sufficiently grave to warrant removal from the register, the committee could decide to refer the case on to the PCC of the Council.

- If there was insufficient evidence, or if the facts of the case (even if proved) would not warrant removal of the practitioner's name from the register, the committee could decide to take no further action.
- If evidence of ill-health was perceived to be pertinent, the committee could direct the case to the Health Committee of the Council.

Details of the conduct of the proceedings of the PCC are laid down by the Council following consultation, and are enshrined in rules in secondary legislation. Hearings are conducted in public, in recognition of the fact that professional regulation is concerned with the protection of the public from unsafe practitioners. A quorum of three members is required for each committee, though in practice, Council has chosen to constitute committees with a minimum of five members. The committee is empowered to subpoena witnesses and must ensure that a legal assessor (a barrister or a solicitor with at least ten years' experience) is present at each hearing. A practitioner who is to be the respondent in a PCC hearing is formally notified of the inquiry in writing and informed of an entitlement to be represented at the hearing by a friend, by counsel or a solicitor or by an officer of a professional organisation or trades union. A copy of the rules is sent to the respondent. In cases other than a 'true conviction' (i.e. where the person having been found guilty by a court was given a conditional or unconditional discharge) the respondent will already have received copies of the statements of the witnesses who are called to give evidence, so as to be fully aware of the case to be defended.

Hearings begin with a formal reading of the charges and a plea in response and then proceed through four stages.

- It first needs to be established whether the allegations can be proved. The rules of evidence are similar to those of the criminal court, and it is the role of the legal assessor to ensure that the rules concerning admissibility of evidence are observed. The required standard of proof is similarly high.
- It must be determined whether any of the established facts constitute professional misconduct. Before this is decided, the respondent or their representative is given further opportunity to address the committee and to call additional evidence. In making their decision, the members of the Committee consider the episode or events in the context of their occurrence, in the light of the advice given to practitioners in the UKCC's Code of Professional Conduct and with regard to the definition of misconduct given in the Professional Conduct Rules – that is 'conduct unworthy of a nurse, midwife or health visitor'.
- If misconduct is proved in respect of any of the charges, the Committee is informed of the previous history of the respondent and any evidence presented in mitigation.
- Following deliberation in camera, the judgement of the PCC is given by the chairman.

The Professional Conduct Rules framed under the 1979 Act provided for three possible judgements: removal from the register, with immediate effect; misconduct proved but removal from the register not deemed to be an appropriate sanction or postponement of judgement for a stated period. The chairman of the PCC may pass comment on the respondent's actions and also, where appropriate, on the setting or context in which the incident occurred. The chairman may also refer the respondent to an appropriate part of the Council's Code of Conduct, but the 1979 Act gave no power to issue a formal caution or reprimand.

A respondent has a statutory right to appeal to the High Court in England, Wales or Northern Ireland, and to the Court of Session in Scotland, against a decision to remove from the register up to three months after the hearing. The decisions of the UKCC professional conduct committee may also be examined through judicial review. This latter provides a mechanism by which individuals or groups other than the respondent in a case can challenge a decision. Council is informed of decisions of the PCC and can consider the pattern of cases that has emerged. It cannot, however, discuss or revisit specific decisions, something that has given rise to both confusion and frustration in controversial cases.

The PCC of the UKCC is also empowered to hear applications for restoration to the register. Those seeking restoration must confirm that they are not the subject of any recent or pending convictions and must provide two character references. If at any point during their proceedings, the PCC, or indeed, the Investigating Committee of the National Board, form the view that the fitness to practise of the person whose case is being considered is impaired by illness, they are able to refer the case to the Health Committee.

Under the 1979 Act, the Health Committee had two different sets of procedures: one for those cases of alleged unfitness to practise due to illness directly referred to the Council by professional colleagues, managers, patients or their relatives; and one for cases referred to the Health Committee by an Investigating Committee of the National Board or by the PCC of the Council. In both situations a panel of professional screeners, drawn from the Council's membership, is assembled, and the practitioner is asked to undergo medical examination by two of the Council's specifically appointed medical examiners. Detailed medical reports are then submitted to the relevant UKCC staff and copies sent to the practitioner concerned. At this stage, the practitioner may choose, either with the support of a professional organisation, trade union or other adviser, or as a personal decision, to commission further reports from their general practitioner or another medical specialist. All relevant material, including documents seen by the referring committee, is then assembled and presented to the Health Committee for its consideration. In cases referred by an investigating committee or by the PCC, the panel of professional screeners simply selects the categories of medical examiner required. In direct referral cases, the panel has a wider role. Their first task is to consider whether there is any evidence of illness of a significant nature. Then, if significant ill-health is apparent, the panel goes on to consider the reports of the Council's medical examiners (if the practitioner has agreed to undergo examination) and any additional medical evidence submitted. It decides whether or not there is sufficient evidence to indicate that the practitioner's fitness to practise is impaired. If this is the case, there is reference to the Health Committee; if not, the case is closed.

Twenty-five members formed the pool from which a Health Committee could be convened. A quorum was set at three, though five became standard. The field of work of the practitioner is taken into consideration when a Health Committee is constituted, and one of the medical examiners who reported on the case must be present. The proceedings of the Health Committee are conducted in private. The practitioner is encouraged to attend the hearing. He or she may be accompanied, can require that both medical examiners attend and may bring additional medical advisers. In the majority of cases, the hearing is based on the assembled documents rather than on evidence from witnesses. The rules established under the Act allowed for four decisions:

- Adjournment of the case in order obtain further medical reports or evidence
- Postponement of judgement to a later date
- Decision that a practitioner's fitness to practise is seriously impaired by illness, in which case it must remove the practitioner from the register
- Decision that fitness to practise is not seriously affected by illness. In direct referral cases, the case will then be closed, but in cases referred by either the investigating committee or the Professional Conduct Committee, the health committee may refer the case back so that the 'misconduct' issue can continue to be addressed.

The practitioner has the right to appeal to the High Court against a decision by the Health Committee, and may also seek restoration to the register at a later date. Restoration is subject to a further medical examination by UKCC-appointed medical examiners.

Practitioners involved in the professional conduct and health committee process have access to the Nurses Welfare Service, an independent charitable body established under the auspices of the GNC for England and Wales in 1972. Staffed by qualified professional social workers, the Nurses Welfare Service provides a casework and counselling service, providing the PCC or Health Committee with objective social background reports and helping those involved in disciplinary or fitness to practise cases to understand the procedures and the powers of the Committees. It also helps those preparing for a restoration hearing to work through their plans for the future.

Section 14 of the 1979 Act gave powers to act in cases of persons who falsely represented themselves to possess qualifications in nursing, midwifery or health visiting or to be on the Council's register. Initially the penalty was a fine of £500, but this has subsequently been raised to £2,500. Annual reports show action regularly being taken against a small number of people under this clause and police forces being given help with their enquiries.

The Nurses, Midwives and Health Visitors Act 1992 placed the responsibility for investigations at Council level and gave new powers of caution and suspension. A discussion of the rationale for this and the negotiations preceding the new legislation can be found in Chapter 5. The new Act also removed the restriction on including non-Council members on committees dealing with removal and restoration to the register (so long as a majority of those present were members of Council).

Investigation is now handled through a PPC. Until March 1998, membership of the closed PPC remained restricted to Council members. A quorum of three is required and membership is drawn with 'due regard' to the professional field of the practitioner concerned. The Committee makes its judgement on the basis of written reports and evidence. The PPC, in exceptional circumstances, may decide to impose an interim suspension of a practitioner's registration, pending further investigation and/or early referral to the PCC or Health Committee. In these cases, the practitioner concerned has a right of audience and representation before the PPC.

Both the PPC and the PCC may now caution respondents where the facts alleged have been proved to the required standard and are deemed to constitute misconduct. A caution remains on the practitioner's registration entry for five years. Since January 1995, it has also been Council policy to disclose a caution to any person seeking confirmation of a practitioner's registration status.

Section two: Cases coming before PCC

The following are brief accounts of the facts in the cases discussed in Chapter 5. They have been drawn, with the agreement of the UKCC, from files and transcripts. Transcripts of professional conduct cases can be purchased from the UKCC. Where cases are not proven, where the committee takes no action or where the respondent's case is upheld at appeal, however, the transcript is destroyed.

Ms J. Rosser

This case was brought by a local supervisor of midwives against an independent midwife and came to a hearing in September 1988. Ms Rosser faced seven charges, four of which were found proved and judged as constituting misconduct. Ms Rosser was struck off the register. The committee, having heard the evidence of expert witnesses and being uneasy about this, on the advice of its legal assessor, had called for rebuttal evidence. An appeal was heard in February 1989, during the course of which the UKCC, judging that the appeal decision was likely to focus on criticism of the use of rebuttal evidence, reversed the decision, and Ms Rosser was reinstated on the register.

Mr P. Donnelly

The respondent, a Director of Nursing Services at a children's hospital, had been convicted in October 1988 of indecent assault on two thirteen-year-old boys. He had been sentenced to two years imprisonment and served a reduced period of this sentence. A hearing in December 1989 was postponed for seven months to obtain medical reports and to give the respondent a chance to prove that he could work satisfactorily. He was in employment from May 1989 to April 1990, at which point he was dismissed because he had been found alone in the kitchen area with a fourteen-year-old boy employed to do washing up. This was felt to be inappropriate in the light of his previous conviction. The respondent maintained that he was checking breakfast trays. No incident was alleged. A resumed hearing in August 1990 proved misconduct but allowed the respondent to remain on the register.

Mr J-P. Jhugroo

The respondent, a former SEN, had been fined and disqualified from driving for having excess alcohol in his blood on three separate occasions in 1987, 1988 and 1989. On the third occasion he was imprisoned for three months. There was no evidence that he had ever been on duty under the influence of alcohol and he stated that he did not have a health problem. In giving a judgement of removal from the register at a hearing in August 1989, the chairman referred to 'persistent and irresponsible' behaviour that brought the profession into disrepute, and suggested that the respondent should supply an employer report and a psychiatric report should he wish to apply for restoration. The respondent appealed on the grounds that the case ought to have been referred to the Health Committee; that it was wrong to find misconduct and that the rules were *ultra vires*. In dismissing the first two grounds of the appeal at a hearing in December 1991, it was argued that the health issue was clearly in the minds of the committee, that it was not obliged to make a referral and that misconduct (defined in rules as 'conduct unworthy of a nurse') is not limited to the discharge of duties. An interpretation of the legislation was given indicating that the committee had power under the legislation to remove for a specified period even though it was not explicitly written into the rules and that the UKCC did not regard itself as having this power. The court referred the matter back for the original committee to have the opportunity of considering whether removal for a specified period was a more appropriate penalty. The committee duly considered the matter and decided not to take this course.

Mrs F. Leeming

This case came before the PCC in May 1993 for a decision in respect of restoration to the register. In 1990, Mrs Leeming had given an account of the death of a patient to the police as a result of which she was convicted of conspiracy to pervert the course of justice. The inquest had returned a verdict of unlawful killing due to gross neglect, the pathologist having concluded that the cause of death was asphyxia due to compression with bedding and the toxicologist giving evidence that the amount of drugs administered had been greater than that prescribed. In 1992, Mrs Leeming had appeared before the PCC, charged with failure to disclose her conviction on a job application. There was no assumption that she had caused the death of the patient, but her name had been removed from the register. The 1993 hearing resulted in restoration. There was some public questioning of this, and the shadow Minister of Health, David Blunkett, took up the matter. The son of the patient who had died took the case to a judicial review in May 1994. The grounds were: that relevant facts (the inquest findings) had not been put, that Mrs Leeming's account of the death had not been sought and that the decision was perverse and unreasonable. The judge concluded 'regretfully' that the appellant's interest in the matter was remote, that the committee was right to confine itself to the facts in the case and that delays in the hearing, only some of which were due to the complainant, had caused hardship to Mrs Leeming who had been thus deprived of her livelihood. The case was dismissed. No order for costs was made. The sister of the patient who died wrote in strong protest copying her letter to the Prime Minister and other parties.

Mr S. Bhundun

In February 1991, Mr Bundhun was convicted of rape and sentenced to five years imprisonment. At the time he was working as a charge nurse with responsibility for elderly and continuing care wards and supplementing his income by working as a bank nurse at night. He was the qualified nurse in charge of the night shift at a private nursing home and the victim was a confused, frail elderly patient at the home. At a PCC hearing in July 1992, he was removed from the register. At the restoration hearing in June 1995, the respondent supplied references from professional colleagues and family friends as well as supportive reports from his probation officer and a psychiatrist who had treated him in 1990 after the offence. These latter both linked alcohol dependence with the offence. The respondent stated that he had stopped drinking while in prison and had studied a range of alternative subjects but failed to get a job. He was restored to the register.

Mr D. Thorpe-Price

The respondent was convicted in 1991 of smuggling £1,000 worth of heroin into the country. He was sentenced to a total of four years' imprisonment for his offences. He was further convicted in 1993 of three thefts of National Savings Certificates worth nearly £60,000 from an Alzheimer's Disease patient whom he had befriended. He was sentenced to one year's imprisonment for these offences which, though taking place earlier, had only come to light after the drugs conviction. The PCC considered his case in June 1995 and decided to adjourn to allow him to obtain medical reports in relation to his former drug dependence and evidence from his employer. The hearing resumed in September 1995 at which time the respondent produced the evidence the committee had requested. He was given a caution.

Mr O. Winn

In April 1990, the respondent had been convicted of manslaughter and sentenced to five years' imprisonment. Three sets of intruders had broken into his home and tried to use his swimming pool. He had persuaded the first group to leave, and had taken an unloaded shotgun with him to remonstrate with the second group who had been throwing stones and shouting abuse. On the third occasion the gun was loaded and one of the intruders lost his life. In September 1991, the respondent was removed from the register. At a restoration hearing in June 1995, the respondent provided references attesting to his rehabilitation and evidence of studying for a degree. He spoke at length of his ambitions for a career in nurse education. He was restored to the register.

Mr Y. Choy

Mr Choy had first appeared before a disciplinary hearing in 1972 following a conviction, on two counts of theft and of administering drugs to obtain sexual intercourse, that had resulted in two years' probation. A GNC hearing arising from this conviction postponed judgement for one year. Following this, in November 1973, the case was closed. In June 1984, the respondent had been convicted of rape. The victim had been a patient of below normal intelligence and the respondent had gained access to her home by falsely holding himself out to be a doctor or community nurse. He was given a two-year prison sentence, twelve months of which was suspended. In December 1986, at a hearing following this conviction, the committee was also informed about his previous conviction. They determined on his removal from the register. In June 1995, the PCC heard and rejected an application for restoration to the register. In March 1996, a further hearing was scheduled. This was supported by four references. The committee was aware of both previous convictions and of failure to disclose the first conviction to a subsequent employer. It was in this employment that the rape was committed. The committee determined on restoration. This decision generated strongly adverse coverage in the national as well as the nursing press, and a quantity of critical correspondence from individual nurses. The RCN applied for judicial review of the decision. It then emerged that Mr Choy had made no reference to his convictions on an application form for a post in 1995. It also became clear that his referees for the restoration hearing had not been fully informed of his history and, in the light of their greater knowledge, they withdrew their references. In the context of these new facts, the UKCC came to an agreement with the RCN that the decision to restore should be overturned. There was no further hearing. The decision was formally quashed in January 1997.

Mr S. Wallymahmed

The respondent, working as an agency nurse, had applied for a post as a staff nurse in a forensic unit in an adult mental health service in the NHS without indicating that he had previously had criminal convictions. The prospective employer had been alerted to this and had made a complaint which resulted in a disciplinary hearing in November 1996. The respondent had been convicted in 1990 of two of offences of buggery and one of indecent assault. The victims were his nephews aged eight and five. He had served a sentence of five years' imprisonment. The case had been the subject of a professional conduct hearing in 1991 where misconduct was proved, but the case was referred to the Health Committee. Following health reports and evidence of the respondent's involvement in long-term psychotherapy, the Health Committee had closed the case, concluding that fitness to practise was not seriously impaired. The second PCC hearing found that failure to disclose (the cause of the second complaint) was misconduct and issued a caution.

Section three: Statistics

The following information is included to give some idea of the workload and range of decisions. Tables have been compiled from the annual *Statistical Analysis of the UKCC's Professional Register*, Annual Reports, and with the help of staff in the Professional Conduct Department. The more recent annual statistical analyses contain further information, including a very detailed table on the type of alleged offence. The years in the tables run from 1 April to 31 March.

The workload of members

Professional conduct work has consumed a large amount of member time since the beginning of the UKCC, and overall workload and the logistical problems of scheduling cases remain considerable. Currently, members average between ten and eighteen days of professional conduct work each year. Some, however, do much more than this. One group of members sits on the PCC and the Health Committee, the other on the PPC and the panel of screeners.

Table A3.1 Meetings of committees and panel by year

Year	PCC (full days)[a]	Health Committee (full days)[b]	Panel of professional screeners meetings	PPC (full days)[c]
1983/4	31	–	–	–
1984/5	81	4	–	–
1985/6	78	16	8	–
1986/7	92	13	9	–
1987/8	102	15	9	–
1988/9	97	11	9	–
1989/90	108	14	13	–
1990/1	148	16	10	–
1991/2	137	14	13	–
1992/3	143	21	12	–

Table A3.1 (continued)

1993/4	109	12	17	10
1994/5	96	17	27	17
1995/6	167	25	19	15
1996/7	134	29	22	20
1997/8	140	29	23	23

Notes
a   The first meeting was in July 1983, so the statistics are not for a full year.
b   First meeting September 1984.
c   Prior to 1993, investigation work was carried out by the National Boards.

The preliminary investigation stage

Following legislation in 1992, the UKCC gained powers to carry out the preliminary investigations in relation to all allegations of misconduct. In almost every full year since 1993, the PPC has handled over 900 cases. Table A3.2 indicates that very high proportions of these are closed at the preliminary stage and that the proportion reaching the PCC has remained below 20 per cent. The UKCC has always argued that it received many inappropriate referrals, and the decision to involve lay members in this work, taken at the end of the Third Council in March 1998 (see Chapter 8) is thus a particularly important one.

Table A3.2 Decisions of the Preliminary Proceedings Committee[a]

Year	Total cases considered	Investigation completed	Closed	Referred to screeners[b]	Cautioned	Referred to PCC	Proportion referred (%)[c]
1993/4	475	389	334	26	8	21	5
1994/5	964	772	569	64	24	115	15
1995/6	871	728	556	48	25	99	14
1996/7	941	767	591	71	22	83	11
1997/8	997	785	571	49	23	142	18

Notes
a   A number of cases are required to be considered twice by the PPC and these are included in the figures in the 'total cases' column but excluded from the other columns as the investigation has not been completed. Such cases will be included in the remaining six columns when investigation is complete, which may be the next year.
b   Reference would be made on health grounds.
c   This represents the percentage of completed cases where the decision is to refer to PCC.

The numbers of hearings

Between 200 and 250 persons come before either the PCC or the Health Committee each year. The figures show the number of persons even where there is a joint hearing. They also include cases resumed from a previous year and, in the case of the Health Committee, those appearing at the end of a period of postponed judgement. Chapter 5 concentrated on the work of the PCC; the figures here show that the work of the Health Committee is also substantial and the number of cases dealt with in recent years has exceeded that for the PCC. While figures of this magnitude, taken together, represent a considerable workload for members and for the professional conduct department, they remain a tiny fraction of the 650,000 on the register.

Table A3.3 Number of persons appearing before the Professional Conduct Committee and the Health Committee by year

Year	Total[a]	PCC	Restorations (PCC)	HC[b]	Restorations (HC)[c,d]
1983/4	129	102	27	–	–
1984/5	251	208	36	7	–
1985/6	254	158	39	57	–
1986/7	304	200	37	67	–
1987/8	282	170	38	73	1
1988/9	268	187	22	59	0
1989/0	271	154	36	77	4
1990/1	315	218	19	76	2
1991/2	312	207	29	73	3
1992/3	316	137	22	153	4
1993/4	228	136	18	70	4
1994/5	195	83	14	98	0
1995/6	272	132	24	110	6
1996/7	263	118	0	141	4
1997/8	260	109	18	121	12

Notes
a   A small number of cases at the PCC may not be concluded in the year in which they start and so the figures in the first column may not tally with figures elsewhere.
b   The number of respondents appearing before the Health Committee will include respondents appearing for the first time and those appearing at the end of a period of postponed judgement.
c   From 1993 the Health Committee had the power to suspend registration as well as remove, and the figures include respondents applying to have their registration restored following removal and those applying to have the suspension of their registration terminated.
d   A rule changed in 1988 enabled the Health Committee to deal with restorations.

The judgements reached concerning professional conduct and fitness to practise

The question of how strict or lenient the UKCC has been in cases of alleged misconduct has been raised at a number of point and figures have been quoted from time to time about the percentage of cases removed (see Chapter 5, note 87). No convention has yet been established for compiling such a figure, however. The information in the following tables should be examined with care and ways of calculating a removals statistic other than that shown should be considered.

Table A3.4 Judgements reached by the Professional Conduct Committee[a]

Year	Total cases concluded	Misconduct proved			Not proved	Removals as percentage of cases proved
		Removed	Cautioned	No action		
1983/4	65	32	–	18	15	64
1984/5	146	75	–	59	12	60
1985/6	100	41	–	52	7	44
1986/7	148	71	–	68	9	49
1987/8	150	72	–	67	11	52
1988/9	159	71	–	68	20	51
1989/0	122	53	–	55	14	49
1990/1	194	92	–	60	21	61
1991/2	180	90	–	55	8	62
1992/3	131	52	–	44	24	54
1993/4	118	58	38	10	12	55
1994/5	77	45	22	5	5	63
1995/6	125	73	32	9	11	64
1996/7	115	96	15	0	4	86
1997/8	107	84	18	3	2	80

Note

a   The total cases concluded excludes cases that are part heard in the year and those where judgement is postponed for a specified period. The judgement in the cases that are part heard or where judgement is postponed will be reflected in the year in which the final judgement is made. A small number of cases referred to the Health Committee are also excluded.

Table A3.5 Judgements reached by the Health Committee (concluded cases)[a]

Year	Total cases concluded	Fitness not impaired – case closed	Fitness impaired – – removed or suspended[b]	Removed or suspended (%)
1983/4	–	–	–	–
1984/5	4	4	0	0
1985/6	37	23	14	38
1986/7	43	27	16	37
1987/8	52	33	19	64
1988/9	37	25	12	68
1989/0	83	68	15	82
1990/1	58	45	13	78
1991/2	53	30	23	57
1992/3	115	90	25	78
1993/4	37	22	15	60
1994/5	65	28	37	43
1995/6	91	45	46	50
1996/7	101	31	70	31
1997/8	86	30	56	35

Notes

a   The total number of cases concluded includes new cases (those being considered by the committee for the first time) and those that are resumed after a period of postponed judgement. Once again postponed cases are shown in the year in which they are concluded.

b   From 1993/94 the Health Committee has been able to suspend a person's registration as an alternative to removing their name from the register. As the process is the same, no distinction has been made between removal and suspension in the fourth column.

Appendix 4
UKCC publications

The UKCC distributes a wide range of documents, including circulars, Registrar's letters, consultation documents, press releases, explanatory leaflets, research reports, guidelines, standards and position statements. It also sends copies of *Register*, a quarterly information bulletin, to all registrants. There is no comprehensive list of documents issued by the UKCC over the lifetime of its three Council terms. The Annual Report of 1983/84 carried a list of new UKCC publications, a practice that recommenced in 1995/96. The list compiled here includes documents that have been available on application to the Publications Department, or sent, as in the case of the Code, to all registrants. The items listed are often the culmination of a consultation process, details of which are not included. The listing extends to the summer of 1999, shortly into the period of the Fourth Council. Items marked with an asterisk were no longer current at that date.

Key publications

- July 1983 *Handbook of Midwives Rules**
- July 1983 *Code of Professional Conduct for Nurses, Midwives and Health Visitors (based on ethical concepts)* (first edn)*
- July 1983 *Notices concerning a midwife's code of practice for midwives practising in England and Wales**
- November 1984 *Code of Professional Conduct for the Nurse, Midwife and Health Visitor* (second edn)* (Third and current edn June 1992)
- March 1985 *Advertising by Registered Nurses, Midwives and Health Visitors**
- May 1986 *Project 2000 - a New Preparation for Practice**
- May 1986 *A Midwife's Code of Practice for Midwives Practising in the UK* (first edn)* (Second edn March 1989; reprint March 1991; third edn May 1994)*
- April 1986 *Administration of Medicines**
- April 1987 *Confidentiality: an elaboration of clause 9 of the second edition of the UKCC's Code of Professional Conduct for the Nurse, Midwife and Health Visitor**
- March 1989 *Exercising Accountability**
- November 1990 *'With a view to removal from the register'?**
- June 1992 *The Scope of Professional Practice*

- October 1992 *Standards for the Administration of Medicines*
- April 1993 *Standards for Records and Record Keeping**
- August 1993 *Complaints about Professional Conduct* (first edn)* (Second and current edn March 1998)
- March 1994 *The Future of Professional Practice - the Council's standards for education and practice following registration: position statement on policy and implementation**
- June 1994 *Professional Conduct – occasional report on standards of nursing in nursing homes**
- March 1995 *PREP and You factsheets**
- September 1995 *The Council's Proposed Standards for Incorporation into Contracts for Hospital and Community Health Care Services*
- April 1996 *Position statement on Clinical Supervision for Nursing and Health Visiting*
- June 1996 *Guidelines for Professional Practice*
- August 1996 *Reporting Misconduct – Information for Employers and Managers*
- August 1996 *Reporting Unfitness to Practise – Information for Employers and Managers*
- November 1996 *Issues Arising from Professional Conduct Complaints*
- February 1997 *Scope in Practice*
- October 1997 *PREP and You*
- October 1997 *Midwives' Refresher Courses and PREP*
- October 1997 *Enrolled Nursing – an Agenda for Action*
- November 1997 *The Nursing and Health Visiting Contribution to the Continuing Care of Older People*
- December 1997 *The Future of Professional Regulation*
- April 1998 *Guidelines for Mental Health and Learning Disabilities Nursing*
- April 1998 *Standards for Specialist Education and Practice*
- April 1998 *Welsh Language Scheme for Wales*
- June 1998 *Making a Complaint*
- October 1998 *Guidelines for Higher Education Institutions on Registration for Newly-Qualified Nurses and Midwives*
- October 1998 *Guidelines for Records and Record Keeping*
- December 1998 *Midwives Rules and Code of Practice*
- April 1999 *A Higher Level of Practice*
- July 1999 *The Continuing Professional Development Standard*
- September 1999 *Fitness for Practise. Summary. The UKCC Commission for Nursing and Midwifery Education*

Information documents on the work of the UKCC

- August 1992 *A Guide for Students of Nursing and Midwifery** (revised edition July 1998)
- January 1997 *This is the UKCC*
- July 1997 *Protecting the Public*

- April 1998 *The UKCC in Wales*
- February 1999 *A Guide to the UKCC's Professional Advice Service*
- March 1999 *Protecting the Public – an Employer's Guide to the UKCC Registration Confirmation Service for Nurses, Midwives and Health Visitors*
- April 1999 *How the UKCC Works for You*
- May 1999 *UKCC Handbook 1999–2000*

Appendix 5
Notes on sources

The records of the United Kingdom Central Council for Nursing, Midwifery and Health Visiting are not yet archived and remain at the offices of the UKCC in London. Papers of the UKCC that are worthy of permanent preservation will be sent to the Public Record Office in due course. Access was afforded for this project to all non-confidential files in the UKCC and to both open and closed session papers of Council. No closed session papers for the more recent period have been cited. This is not as restrictive as it might appear, since matters initially discussed in closed session have usually later found their way into open session.

Readers may be helped by a brief explanation of the referencing conventions used for citing the primary source material of the UKCC. In the main, we have followed the conventions used by the UKCC itself, changing where these change. Council records the minutes of its open and closed sessions numerically through years. Before March 1992, minutes were given the prefix 'MIN' or 'C MIN'. After this date, the house style changed to 'Minute' and 'C Minute'. For clarity, we have also included the date of the Council meeting for each minute reference. Council papers are also identified through a numerical and chronological reference, for example, CC/90/07 (for a paper considered in open session) or CC/90/C07 (for a paper considered in closed session). The full titles of the papers are not given in the chapter notes. Similar conventions have been adopted for the minutes and papers of Council's committees. Some of the primary material cited in the text has come from UKCC topic files, for example those compiled for Project 2000 or PREPP. Where possible we have included the original Council or Committee paper reference. However, some material, for example the drafts of task or working groups, do not fit within these conventions. In these cases, we have given as much information as possible to aid identification. Other Council sources, such as press statements, circulars and Registrar's letters are identified as far as possible by reference number, title and date. For ease of reference, a list of major Council publications is also included as Appendix 4.

Unpublished sources

United Kingdom Central Council for Nursing, Midwifery and
Health Visiting

- Minutes and papers of the Shadow Central Council 1980–3
- Minutes and papers of Central Council 1983–98
- Minutes and papers of Midwifery Committee 1983–98
- Minutes and papers of Health Visiting Joint Committee 1983–93
- Minutes and papers of District Nursing Joint Committee 1983–93
- Minutes and papers of Nursing and Community Health Care Nursing Committee 1993–8
- Minutes and paper of Educational Policy Advisory Committee 1983–8
- Minutes and papers of Education Committee 1993–6
- Minutes and papers of Joint Education Committee 1996–8
- Minutes and papers of Standards and Ethics Committee 1989–95
- Meeting papers of Standards Group 1988
- Meeting papers of Registrar's Professional Group 1989–95
- Meeting papers of Registrar's Management Group 1987–95
- Meeting papers of Management Group 1995–98
- Meeting papers of Professional Conduct Committee and Health Committee Review Group 1989–91
- Meeting papers of Ethics Advisory Panel 1996–98
- Meeting papers of Working Group on Community Care 1989–90
- Meeting papers of Working Group on the NHS and Community Care Bill 1990
- Meeting papers of Informal Group on Research 1981–2
- Meeting papers of UKCC Annual Standing Conference with Consumer Organisations 1991–97
- Elec1.1   Papers of Working Group 1 – UKCC first election scheme, 1980–3
- L2.1.1   Papers of Working Group 2 – Single professional register, 1981–2
- K3.1   Papers of Working Group 3 – Education and training, 1981–2
- M2.1.1   Papers of Working Group 4 – Professional conduct, 1981–2
- COM1.1   Papers of Working Group 5 – Standing and joint committees, 1981–2
- R1.1   Papers of Working Group 6 – The handover of functions, 1981–2
- PROP1.1   Papers of Working Group 7 – Properties of former nursing, midwifery and health visiting bodies, 1981–4
- 1/1   UKCC Inaugural Reception, 1983
- 1/8/1/2   Nurses, Midwives and Health Visitors Bill/Act, 1991/1992
- 1/8/2   Papers of the UKCC Legislative Review Group, 1988–9
- 1/8/3   Review of the Council and National Boards by Peat Marwick McLintock, 1988–9
- 1/8/3/1   Papers and correspondence relating to the Nurses, Midwives and Health Visitors Bill, 1991/2

- 1/9   Programme of work, 1980–3
- 1/9/2   Strategy Document – Into the 1990s and beyond, 1984.
- 3/10/1   Review of Professional Committee, 1983.
- 55/11   A Strategy for the Statutory Bodies, 1984–5.
- K3.2   Project 2000
- K3.2   Project 2000 implementation
- K3.3   Nurse selection project
- K4.4   Post-Registration Education and Practice Project
- L2.1.3   Securing viability 1981–4
- Current files: B1.4 – B1.8; B4.10; B 4.10 – B4.15; B5.1 – B5.6; B6.1 – B6.7, K5.1; K6.1– K6.7, M2; M3; M4.
- UKCC Annual Reports, 1983–98
- UKCC circulars and Registrar's letters
- Statistical Analysis of the UKCC's Professional Register (various dates)

Public Record Office, London (PRO)

- MH 156/131–4
- MH 165/77–136; 146–212

Official publications and parliamentary papers

- *Parliamentary Debates* [Commons]
- *Parliamentary Debates* [Lords]
- Department of Health, *Working for Patients*, Cm 555, London, HMSO, 1989
- Department of Health, *Education and Training. Working Paper 10*, London, HMSO, 1989
- Department of Health, *Maintaining Medical Excellence. Review of Guidance on Doctors' Performance* (Calman Report), London, Department of Health, 1995
- Department of Health, *Choice and Opportunity. Primary Health Care: the Future*, London, HMSO, 1996
- Department of Health, *The New NHS. Modern – Dependable*, Cm 3807, London, The Stationery Office, 1997
- Department of Health, *Making a Difference. Strengthening the Nursing, Midwifery and Health Visiting Contribution to Health and Healthcare*, London, Department of Health, 1999
- DHSS, *Neighbourhood Nursing. A Focus for Care. Report of the Community Nursing Review* (Cumberlege Report), London, HMSO, 1986
- DHSS Northern Ireland Office, *Fit for the Future: A new Approach. The Government's Proposals for the Future of the Health and Personal Social Services in Northern Ireland*, Belfast, DHSS, 1998
- Ministry of Health and SHHD, *Report of the Committee on Senior Nursing Staff Structure*, (Salmon Committee), London, HMSO, 1966

- National Audit Office, *Nursing Education: Implementation of Project 2000 in England.* Report by the Comptroller and Auditor General, London, HMSO, 1992
- National Board for Prices and Incomes, *Pay of Nurses and Midwives in the National Health Service (Report No. 60)*, Cmnd 3585, London, HMSO, 1968
- NHS Management Executive Task Force, *New World, New Opportunities. Nursing in Primary Health Care*, London, NHSME, 1993
- NHS Wales, Welsh Office, *Putting Patients First*, London, The Stationery Office, 1998
- Office of Population Censuses and Surveys, *Nurses Working in the Community. A survey carried out on behalf of the DHSS in England and Wales in 1980*, London, HMSO, 1982
- *Report of the Committee on Nursing*, (Briggs Report) Cmnd 5115, London, HMSO,1972
- *Report of the Committee of Inquiry into the Regulation of the Medical Profession* (Merrison Report), Cmnd 6018, London, HMSO, 1975
- *Report of the Committee of Inquiry into Mental Handicap Nursing and Care* (Jay Report), Cmnd. 7468, London, HMSO, 1979
- Scottish Office, Department of Health, *Designed to Care: Renewing the NHS in Scotland*, Cm 3811, Edinburgh, The Stationery Office, 1997
- National Assembly for Wales, *Realising the Potential. A Strategic Framework for Nursing, Midwifery and Health Visiting in Wales into the 21st Century*, Cardiff, National Assembly for Wales, 1999

Other reports

- Annual Reports of GNC for England and Wales; GNC Scotland; CMB for England and Wales; CMB Scotland; NICNM; UKCC; ENB; NBS; WNB; NBNI
- CETHV, *An Investigation into the Principles of Health Visiting*, London, CETHV, 1977
- CETHV, *The Investigation Debate*, London, CETHV, 1980
- HVA, *Weights and Measures. Outcomes and Evaluation in Health Visiting*, London, HVA, 1995
- JM Consulting, *The Regulation of Health Professions. Report of a Review of the Professions Supplementary to Medicine Act (1960) with recommendations for new legislation*, Bristol, JM Consulting Ltd., 1996
- JM Consulting, *The Regulation of Nurses, Midwives and Health Visitors. Invitation to Comment on Issues Raised by a Review of the Nurses, Midwives and Health Visitors Act 1997*, Bristol, JM Consulting Ltd., 1998
- JM Consulting, *The Regulation of Nurses, Midwives and Health Visitors. Report of a Review of the Nurses, Midwives and Health Visitors Act 1997*, Bristol, JM Consulting Ltd., 1999
- National Consumer Council, *Self-regulation of Professionals in Health Care*, London, NCC, 1999

- RCM, *Midwifery Legislation. The Issues and the Options. Position Paper 14*, London, RCM, 1996
- RCN, *Administering the Hospital Nursing Service*, London, RCN, 1964
- RCN, *A Reform of Nursing Education* (Platt Report), London, RCN, 1964
- RCN Commission on Nursing Education, *The Education of Nurses: a New Dispensation*, London, RCN, 1985
- Peat Marwick McLintock, *A Review of the UKCC and the Four National Boards for Nursing, Midwifery and Health Visiting*, London, Department of Health, 1989

Journals and newspapers

- *British Journal of Nursing*
- *British Medical Journal*
- *COHSE Journal*
- *Health Service Journal*
- *Health Visitor*
- *Journal of District Nursing* (continued as *Journal of Community Nursing*)
- *Midwife and Health Visitor* (continued as *Midwife, Health Visitor and Community Nurse*)
- *Midwifery*
- *Midwifery Matters*
- *Midwives' Chronicle and Nursing Notes*
- *Nursing Mirror*
- *Nursing Standard*
- *Nursing Times*
- *Senior Nurse*

Selected secondary sources

Books

Allsop, J. and L. Mulcahy, *Regulating Medical Work. Formal and Informal Controls*, Buckingham, Open University Press, 1996.

Bendall, E. and E. Raybould, *A History of the General Nursing Council for England and Wales 1919–1969*, London, H. K. Lewis and Co. Ltd., 1969.

Crossman, R. H. S., *The Crossman Diaries. Vol. 3*, London, Hamish Hamilton/ Jonathan Cape, 1977.

Clarke, J. and J. Newman, *The Managerial State*, London, Sage, 1997.

Davies, C., *Gender and the Professional Predicament in Nursing*, Buckingham, Open University Press, 1995.

Dingwall, R., *The Social Organisation of Health Visitor Training*, London, Croom Helm, 1977.

Dingwall, R., A. M. Rafferty and C. Webster, *An Introduction to the Social History of Nursing*, London, Routledge, 1988.

Donnison, J., *Midwives and Medical Men. A History of Inter-professional Rivalries and Women's Rights*, London, Heinemann Educational, 1977.

Green, D., *Which Doctor? A Critical Analysis of the Professional Barriers to Free Competition in Health Care*, London, IEA, 1985.

Freidson, E., *Professionalism Reborn*, Oxford/Cambridge, Blackwell/Polity Press, 1994.

Heywood Jones, I. (ed.), *The UKCC Code of Conduct: A Critical Guide*, London, NT Books, 1999.

Kirkham, M. (ed.), *Supervision of Midwives*, Hale, Books for Midwives, 1996.

Klein, R., *The New Politics of the NHS*, (third edn), London, Longman, 1995.

Lathlean, J., *Policy Making in Nurse Education*, Oxford, Ashdale Press, 1989.

Pyne, R., *Professional Discipline in Nursing, Midwifery and Health Visiting* (third edn), Oxford, Blackwell Science, 1998.

Rafferty, A. M., *The Politics of Nursing Knowledge*, London, Routledge, 1996.

Stacey, M., *Regulating British Medicine. The General Medical Council*, Chichester, John Wiley and Sons, 1992.

Wallace, M., *Lifelong Learning. PREP in Action*, Edinburgh, Churchill Livingstone, 1999.

Webster, C., *The Health Services since the War. Vol. 2. Government and Health Care. The National Health Service 1958–1979*, London, HMSO, 1996.

Webster, C., *The National Health Service. A Political History*, Oxford, Oxford University Press, 1998.

Wilkie, E., *A Singular Anomaly. A Case Study of the CETHV, 1962–1974*, London, RCN, 1984.

Chapters and Articles

Davies, C., 'Policy in nursing education: plus ça change? . . .' in *The Politics of Progress. Proceedings of 19th Annual Study Day of the Nursing Studies Association,* Edinburgh, University of Edinburgh, 1985.

Davies, C., 'The demise of professional self-regulation – a moment to mourn?', in Lewis, G., S. Gewirtz and J. Clarke (eds), *Rethinking Social Policy*, London, Sage, 2000.

Davies, C., 'Rethinking Regulation in the Health Professions in the UK: Institutions, Ideals and Identities' in Hellberg, I., M. Saks and C. Benoit (eds), *Professional Identities in Transition. Cross-cultural Dimensions*, Gothenburg, University of Gothenburg, 1999.

Humphreys, J., 'English nurse education and the reform of the National Health Service, *Journal of Education Policy*, 11, 6, 1996.

Le Var, R., 'Project 2000: a new preparation for practice – has policy been realised? Part 2', *Nurse Education Today*, 17, 1997.

Meerabeau, L., 'Project 2000 and the nature of nursing knowledge', in Abbott, P. and L. Meerabeau (eds), *The Sociology of the Caring Professions* (second edn), London, UCL Press, 1998.

Stacey, M., 'Collective Therapeutic Responsibility. Lessons from the GMC' in Budd, S. and U. Sharma (eds), *The Healing Bond*, London, Routledge, 1994.

Stanwick, S., 'The market for education: supply and demand', in Humphreys, J. and F. M. McQuinn (eds), *Health Care Education: The Challenge of the Market*, London, Chapman & Hall, 1994.

Index

Donnelly, P. 107, 223–4
Dorling, J. 201n.18

EDS 38n.32
education and training: admission to
register 215, 216; Briggs Committee
3–4, 5–7, 9–10; First Council 43–4,
45, 204–5; Nurses, Midwives and
Health Visitors' Act (1979) 25, 26;
reform 33–5; register 30; Second
Council 48, 49, 50; Third Council 58,
62; *see also* post-registration education
and practice; post-registration
education and practice project; pre-
registration education and training;
Project 2000
Educational Policy Advisory Committee
(EPAC) 28–9, 144: district nursing
153; First Council 43, 76; lay people
173; professional practice 121;
specialties 157; time pressures 41
Education Commission 63, 91
Education Committee 56, 144: lay people
179; registration process 217
elderly people, position statement on 65
elections 26–8, 172: legacies 168–72;
Third Council 55–6; turnouts 182
Electoral Reform Society 26, 27
Emerton, Dame Audrey 48, 54, 84, 88,
93, 95, 96, 124, 138, 212, 213:
PREPP 124; pre-registration education
84, 88; Second Council 48, 54, 55
England: Briggs Committee 8, 9, 13–14,
15; midwives 162n.9
enhanced practitioners 130
Ennals, David 15–16
enrolled nurses (ENs) (second level
nurses): Briggs Committee 6; First
Council 45; pre-registration education
77, 79, 80, 83, 85–6, 88–9;
professional conduct 98–9; reform
34–5; Second Council 50; Third
Council 63–4; *see also* State Enrolled
Nurses
Enrolled Nursing – an agenda for action
63–4
Ethics Advisory Panel 70n.83, 181
European Directives: admission to register
216; General Care Nurse 38n.38, 87;
specialist nursing 158–9
European Economic Community/Union:
Advisory Committee on the Training
of Midwives 47; Advisory Committee
on Training in Nursing 47; Briggs

Committee 8; First Council 47; Third
Council 59
Eustace, Winifred 19n.17
Euston Road premises 36n.7
expenses 67n.1
extraordinary meetings 40–1

false representation of qualifications 222
Faull, David 100
fees: periodic *see* periodic fees; registration
46, 68n.30
Finance Committee: development 28;
First Council 41, 43; lay people 173
finance officer 41
finances: Central Midwives Board 145;
First Council 46; periodic fees *see*
periodic fees; PREPP 126–7, 129;
pre-registration education 82–3, 88;
professional conduct 99–100, 211n.6;
recompense 67n.1, 206; registration
fees 46, 68n.30; Second Council 48,
55; shadow period 35–6; Third
Council 62
First Council (1983–8) 40–7, 204–5, 212:
pre-registration education 75–8;
professional conduct 42, 43, 45,
97–102
first level nurses 34: First Council 45;
Third Council 63, 64
Fletcher, P. 186n.27
flexibility issues: Briggs Committee 6, 7,
10; JM Consulting Review 202n.28;
midwives 146
foreign-trained professionals 216, 218
Fourth Council (1998–) 91–2, 133, 182
Friend, Phyllis 15
Frost, Winifred 8
fundholding GPs 155
Furlong, Jackie 63
Future of Professional Practice, The 130
Future of Professional Regulation, The 189

gender factors 12, 218
General Chiropractice Council 200n.8
General Medical Council (GMC):
appointments 168–9; disciplinary
system 106, 117n.61; history xv;
questioning of 191, 201n.16; Second
Council 54; and UKCC, contact
between 177
General Nursing Councils (GNC) 18n.3:
appointments 169; Briggs Committee
9, 12, 13, 15; computer technology 30;
dissolution 25; Educational Policy

General Nursing Councils (GNC) (*cont.*)
  Advisory Committee 37n.24;
  education and training 5; enrolment
  and registration 6; professional
  conduct 98; retention fees 170
General Osteopathic Council 200n.8
governance 61
governments *see* Conservative
  governments; Labour governments
GP contracting 155
Great Portland Street *see* Portland Place
  premises
Green, Margaret 76, 212, 213: PREPP
  121, 136n.14, 138n.43
Griffiths Report 46
Grimes, Chris 213
*Guidelines for Mental Health and Learning
  Disability Nursing* 134, 160
Guidelines for Professional Practice 64, 134,
  181

Hall, Dame Catherine 24, 41, 172, 212:
  Code of Professional Conduct 33; *Into
  the 90s* 67n.14; professional conduct
  116n.32
Hancock, Christine 137n.19
Handbook of Midwives Rules 45
Hanratty, Mary 213
Hanson, Mike 24, 41, 69n.47
Hayman, Baroness 196, 202n.35
Heal, Sylvia 158–9
Health Act (1999) 151, 190, 196–7,
  203n.46, 210
Health and Personal Social Services Order
  (Northern Ireland) (1972) 20n.34
health care assistants: JM Consulting
  Review 197; pre-registration education
  85, 89; professional conduct 113;
  Second Council 50; second level nurses
  employed as 63, 64; Third Council 57
Health Committee (HC): establishment
  31; First Council 98, 99; judgements
  230; lay people 182; numbers of
  hearings 228–9; procedures 220,
  221–2; Third Council 108, 109, 111;
  workload 227–8
Health Visiting Joint Committee (HVJC)
  152–5, 161n.3, 173
health visitors 151–7: Briggs Committee
  5, 7–8, 10, 12, 16; election scheme 27;
  JM Consulting Review 195; Nurses,
  Midwives and Health Visitors Act
  (1979) 17, 143; registration statistics
  218

Health Visitors' Association (HVA) 12,
  75, 155
hearings: numbers 228–9; procedures
  220–1
Holder, Stan 68n.27
Holland, Roger 68n.37, 173, 212, 213
Hughes, Jenny 187n.51
Hussain, Tariq 99, 109, 110, 160,
  185n.23

identity: national 8, 9, 12; professional 12,
  16
illness, unfitness to practise due to 31,
  221–2
Institute of Employment Studies 63
international dimension 51
*Into the 90s – A Plan for Action for the
  UKCC* 41–4, 48, 99
Investigating Committee 219–20, 221,
  222
Irvine, Donald 45–6
*Issues Arising from Professional Conduct
  Complaints* 112

Jack, Sheila 212
Jackson, Michael 185n.23
Jacobs, Eva 70n.62, 187n.45
Jay Committee 20n.36, 166n.88
Jhugroo, J.-P. 107, 118n.81, 224
JM Consulting Review 113, 189–90,
  192–7, 207–9: health visitors 157,
  195; midwives 11, 152, 195
Joint Board of Clinical Nursing Studies
  (JBCNS) 18n.3, 25, 46, 157
Joint Committee for Health Visiting 25
Joint Education Committee 62, 90–1,
  162n.7
Joint Liaison Committee 177
Joint Nurses and Midwives Council
  (Northern Ireland) Act (1922) 162n.9
Joint Staff Consultative Committee 35
Joseph, Sir Keith 11
Judge, Harry 77
judgements concerning professional
  conduct 229–30
judicial reviews: periodic fees 46, 217;
  professional conduct 109, 117n.56,
  221

Keen, Ann 167n.95

Labour governments: Briggs Committee
  11–12; health visiting and community
  health care nursing 157, 164n.52;